# HOW TO BUILD YOUR BRIGHT FUTURE TODAY

# How to Build Your Bright Future Today

A Comprehensive Guide to Prepare Physicians
for the Current Health Care Era

## Rashed Hasan, MD, FAAP

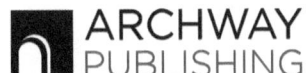

ARCHWAY
PUBLISHING

Archway Publishing books may be ordered through booksellers or by contacting:

Archway Publishing
1663 Liberty Drive
Bloomington, IN 47403
www.archwaypublishing.com
1-(888)-242-5904

Because of the dynamic nature of the Internet, any web addresses or links contained in this book may have changed since publication and may no longer be valid. The views expressed in this work are solely those of the author and do not necessarily reflect the views of the publisher, and the publisher hereby disclaims any responsibility for them.

Any people depicted in stock imagery provided by Thinkstock are models, and such images are being used for illustrative purposes only.
Certain stock imagery © Thinkstock.

ISBN: 978-1-4808-0767-9 (sc)
ISBN: 978-1-4808-0769-3 (hc)
ISBN: 978-1-4808-0768-6 (e)

Library of Congress Control Number: 2014909670

Printed in the United States of America

Archway Publishing rev. date: 05/23/2015

# *Preface*

If you are a Medical student, a budding physician or a seasoned physician who has made it through the grueling process of getting into a medical school, the residency and fellowship training *you are* the cream of the crop. We say this because getting into a medical school, in North America in particular, but anywhere else for that matter is not a picnic. You deserve to have a bright future in all aspects of your life. Therefore, it is critical that you are well informed through every step into your future so that, hopefully, you make the most appropriate decisions that are most suitable for your career, your family life, the financial and emotional aspects of your life and any other issues that are relevant to you. This book has something for current and future physicians at different stages of their education and career. For instance if you are a full-fledged physician and you are already in practice, you may skip the initial portions of the book that deals with residency and fellowship training and read the portions of the book that discuss the financial aspects of your life and how to protect your assets that you have worked very hard for. If you are a physician who is approaching retirement you may focus on the latter portions of the book which emphasizes this area of the life of a physician or a health care provider. We made an attempt to provide you with guidance from choosing your field in medicine and selecting a residency training program, to deciding on where to work after residency, what type of practice setting would be a better fit for you, how to negotiate a contract, how to organize your finances, and how to build a sound future that is conducive to a successful career, a stable personal life, and sound financial future. In addition we have provided you information on securing your medical licenses state by state. For physicians in the middle of their career, the financial sections and the sections on taxes and retirement should provide you with guidance that may be conducive to a retirement, that we hope, will be most appropriate for you. We wish you the best in your education and career.

# Contents

# Becoming a physician, Is it (did you make) the right choice?

Physician shortage is already here and will continue into the distant future in the USA and perhaps in Canada. In the US, 22 states and 15 medical specialties reported shortage of physicians in the US in June 2010. In the US, physician shortage is expected to balloon to approximately 63,000 physicians in the next five years (as of 2010 data) and 91,000 by 2020, according to the projections by the Association of American Medical Colleges. This projected shortage of physicians is up by more than 50% from previous estimates.

The Department of Health and Human Services of the US, estimates that the physician supply will increase by just 7% in the next 10 years and there will be a decrease in the number of physicians in the specialties of urology and thoracic surgery. During the same period, one-third of practicing physicians are expected to retire and the number of Americans 65 and older is projected to grow by 36%, according to figures released in September 2010 by the Association of American Medical Colleges (AAMC) Center for Workforce Studies. Thus, there is widening of the gap between supply and demand in favor of higher demand. Officials at the Association of American Medical Colleges attributed the widening gap between supply and demand to increased demands from the aging population of the USA coupled with increased demand for health care professionals and expansion of coverage by 2019 to 32 million uninsured Americans under the new health system reform law introduced in 2010 by the federal government. According to a report published by the American Medical Association (AMA) in 2013 on the subject of supply and demand, more than 50% of physicians received up to three employment solicitations per week around that time. Another survey conducted by the recruiter firm, Medicus, released in June 2013, showed that more than half of practicing physicians receive at least three employment solicitations per week, and almost 29 and 23 percent, respectively, receive three to five and six to 10 notices per week. The Medicus Firm's survey also reported that nearly 28 percent of physician in training received three to five solicitations per week and 9 percent received 21 to 50 notices weekly.

These findings were interpreted to mean that although the physician shortage was one reason for increased recruitment of physicians, with a shortage of 46,000 primary care physicians and about 45,000 specialists estimated by 2020, another factor is the change in the pattern of practice of physicians. An ongoing trend has been that more physicians are working for health care systems and hospitals (read the section on W2 vs. 1099 later in the book) and therefore, physician turnover was predicted to be higher. As of 2013, AMA and Medical Group Management Association-American College of Medical Practice Executives, project that only 36 percent of physicians will own stakes in practice by the end of 2013, down from 57 percent in 2000. In 2012, 63 percent of recruiting assignments were hospital employment of physicians, an increase from 11 percent in 2004, according to Merritt Hawkins & Associates a well-recognized physician recruitment firm. Merritt Hawkins & associates also explains that improving economy (as of the middle of 2013) may be a contributing factor towards increased demand for physicians at this time.

One way to deal with this shortage is to increase the number of residency training programs positions (which is funded primarily by the Center for Medicare and Medicaid) for new graduates from medical schools. Indeed the American Association of Medical Colleges has urged the federal government to lift limits on Medicare funding for residency positions, which have been capped at 100,000 slots since 1997. However, the heated debate that is ongoing in the US congress (as of 2013) over increasing the debt ceiling for the US or cutting spending is likely to delay any bill that is associated with increasing spending by the federal government. Therefore, the equation is likely to continue against increasing supply of physicians in the US.

During the past decade, new medical schools have opened and existing schools have expanded class sizes, but there has not been a parallel increase in the number of residency positions across the US. One piece of good news is that in September 2010,The Department of Health and Human Services stated that it has allocated approximately $ 320 million dollar towards expansion of primary care medicine and that it was releasing $167 million in grants to create an additional 889 primary care residency positions by 2015. Though this funding will help, it is only a fraction of the thousands of new positions needed to counter future physician shortages. For example if the number of residency training program positions was increased by 15%, it would produce an additional 4,000 physicians annually. Because it takes a long time (roughly 11-12 years) to produce full-fledged physicians it is not easy to keep up with increasing demand.

In addition to training more physicians, there needs to be a focus on finding ways to use the existing physician work force more effectively by collaborating with other health care professionals so that our society can do better with the physician supply we have to meet the needs of our population.

Following completion of the residency training program (during which physician train on one broad specialty of medicine) some physicians go on to complete additional training in a specific field called "subspecialty fellowship training". This requires additional 2-3 years of training, which would mean the need for additional funding for these physicians. Financial barriers to subspecialty fellowships training will also need to be minimized in order to produce more subspecialists. One of the barriers for some physicians to complete a fellowship is the large amounts of debt that they have accumulated and that they will have to deal with while they are completing additional years of training. A new issue that was introduced in 2010 is the affordable health care act (The media outlets have also called it Obamacare), a new law that will mandate that the approximately 38 million Americans who currently do not carry a health care insurance will be required by law to carry health insurance. Some argue that blaming future shortage only on the affordable health care act of 2010 (introduced by the administration of President Obama) is not really accurate because these uninsured individuals have always had needs for health care, which means that demand for physicians has always been there in the first place.

The table below shows the supply, demand, and the projected shortage of physicians for the next 15 years (as of 2010) as reported by the American Association of Medical Colleges (AAMC) center for Workforce studies.

|  | **Supply** | **Demand** | **Shortage** |
|---|---|---|---|
| **2010** | 709,000 | 723,000 | 14,000 |
| **2015** | 735,000 | 798,000 | 63,000 |
| **2020** | 759,000 | 851,000 | 92,000 |
| **2025** | 785,000 | 916,000 | 131,000 |

*Source: Modified from AAMC Center for Workforce Studies, June Analysis (figures approximated to nearest 1000)*

A survey conducted by the American Association of Medical Colleges in 2009 found that 41 states provide Graduate Medical Education (GME) Medicaid funding, seven less than in the previous survey in 2005. Nine of the 41 states were considering cutting GME Medicaid funding. While this funding is at risk, the new funding (by the Department of Health and Human Services) to create an additional 889 primary care residency positions nationwide is an important step toward meeting the growing demand for health care professionals as stated by experts in the field and this change comes following several years of calls by physicians organizations and other concerned parties for more funding for residency training programs. This new funding is just a portion of what's needed in the long-term, *it is a good start and good news for individuals planning on choosing medicine as a career.*

Eighty-two residency training programs nationwide will benefit from the $167 million funding from the Department of Health and Human service, which will go towards expansion of primary care residency training programs over five years. This funding is also expected to create new residency positions in pediatrics, internal medicine and family medicine, and were part of the $320 million in awards the Department of Health and Human Services plans, announced on September 27, 2010 and is aimed at boosting the primary care physician work force.

According to data published in the September, 2010 issue of the American Medical Association Journal (JAMA), there are about 110,000 residency training positions nationwide. This includes 40,000 primary care positions. Expanding the primary care work force is a priority for the Department of Health and Human Services. In addition to increasing residency training programs slots, the grants support community-based training programs viewed as strong motivators for young physicians to choose a primary care career. The Department of Health and Human Services issued a call on November 29, 2010 for applicants for another $230 million that will go toward increasing training opportunities for primary care residents and dentists in community-based ambulatory care centers.

At its Annual Meeting in June 2010, the American Medical Association House of Delegates adopted policies calling for more GME funding from a variety of sources and promotion of community-based training programs to encourage more trainees to become primary care physicians.

The Patient Protection and Affordable Care Act calls for the redistribution in July 2011 of residency positions that have gone unfilled for at least three years to train primary care and general surgery physicians. That is expected to amount to about 1,000 positions that will be redistributed largely to hospitals in medically under-served communities. The bottom line for you if you are considering a career in medicine as a physician is that we are facing physician shortage and any efforts at increasing the number of physician training spots is a step forward for the nation and an encouraging news for you.

## Cutting the USA federal deficit: GME funding is a target! Relevant to medical students and current physicians!!

### What are the potential impacts of a possible reduction in funding for the graduate medical education (GME) by the federal government?

As a result of the decisions made in the middle of 2011 to reduce the federal deficit of the USA, a Joint Select Committee on Deficit Reduction, which was named the "Super Committee" was formed to recommend to the Congress of the US by December 2011 reductions in federal spending to be accomplished over the next 10 years. One of the "entitlement programs" being examined by this Super Committee where "there is an opportunity for deficit reduction", is Medicare reimbursement for Graduate Medical Education (GME), the primary source of GME funding in the USA.

The Medicare Payment Advisory Commission (MedPAC) has in-dicated that approximately 50% of the Indirect GME Reimbursement is not "empirically justified" on the basis of current costs of teaching hospitals intended to be covered by that reimbursement. Furthermore, the Simpson Bowles Commission (another Committee on deficit re-duction) recommended a reduction in total GME funding in excess of 50% ($60 billion over 10 years) as a component of a comprehensive strategy to reduce federal deficit spending.

Because these discussions are occurring during a time period when there are projected physician shortage in the US and when the number of medical school seats are being increased across the nation, the Accreditation Council for Graduate Medical Education (ACGME) attempted to estimate the impact of reductions in GME funding of the magnitude under discussion in our nation's capital on the educational pipeline for physicians.

In order to assess the impact of the funding cuts for the GME, the ACGME conducted a survey of the current programs about their response in such an event. The total response rate was representative of 68% of all the residency positions in the USA. 60-75% of responders stated that if the funding remains the same, they would keep the same numbers of positions in their residency and/or fellowship programs. However, if the funding to the GME was reduced by 1/3, then 60-70% of the programs stated that they would decrease the number of positions in their programs and 4% would close their training program.

If the federal funding is decreased by 50%, 70-80% of programs stated that they would decrease the number of positions in their programs (some by a significant number) and 14% stated that they would close their program. According to the ACGME data, these figures represent 538 programs (193 core and 345 subspecialties) and 6600 positions (5000 core and 1600 subspecialty positions). Apparently the medical specialties and fellowship programs would be most affected with slightly over 3000 positions at stake.

The potential impact per state:

The number of positions lost will vary from state to state, however, at least 12 states would lose 500 positions or more. Furthermore, taking the above figures into consideration, with significant cuts (50% or more) in the GME budget, the following states are projected to lose > 5000 residency positions:

Massachusetts, New York, Pennsylvania, Michigan, New Jersey, Ohio, Virginia, Georgia, Illinois, Texas, Minnesota, Arizona and California.

The ACGME report stated that extrapolating from the 69% sample to the entire population of sponsors, it estimates the following reductions in programs and positions:

Among all ACGME accredited programs, it estimates that if there is 1/3 reduction in funding, about 1600 programs would close (representing 18 % of all residency/fellowship programs) and close to 20,000 positions will be lost. If the funding cuts reaches the 50% mark, then close to 33,000 positions would be lost representing approximately 2500 programs (30% of all GME positions).

The Association of American Medical Colleges projects that in the academic year 2020–2021, approximately 20,000 students will enroll into the first year class across all Liaison Committee on Medical Education accredited medical schools in the USA. If indeed a 50% reduction in GME funding does take place, and the 68% sample in the ACGME survey is representative of the entire GME effort in the US, we would have 19,711 positions available for that class when they graduate. This impact is magnified when one considers that there are over 2,500 graduates of osteopathic medical schools, and over 7,000 International Medical Graduates (approximately 3,500 of those are US citizens) currently enrolled in ACGME accredited entry level pipeline positions.

What are possible solutions?

The majority of responders to the ACGME survey stated that they would seek private funding (45%) followed by community or other hospital support (37%) and faculty practice plan support (36%) to replace or augment reduced federal support for GME. These are positive suggestions if you are planning on becoming a physician.

### *Becoming a physician: The process*

If you are a medical student or a new graduate of a medical school, you probably know some of what we will discuss in the next few pages, but if you are neither, then here is the process of making a physician in North America.

The making of a physician in the US and Canada is a lengthy process and involves Undergraduate education, Medical school completion, and Graduate Medical Education (GME). The latter involves training in a residency program which ranges from 3-5 years, and may be followed by further training in a fellowship program in one of the subspecialty fields of medicine, which take another 2-3 years. A brief detail of these processes is discussed below:

**Undergraduate education:** involves 4 years of education at a university or a college to earn a bachelor degree. The degree usually has a strong emphasis on basic science in the fields of chemistry, biology, physics and mathematics. Some students may be able enter a medical school with other areas of emphasis.

Others have additional education such as a master degree in a particular field such as a master degree in public health, yet others have a PhD in a field that may or may not be related to medicine. For most Medical Schools having one of these additional degrees (a Master or a PhD) will give the candidate additional bonus points in the competitive process to enter a medical school. So, if you have one of these additional degrees you should consider it a strength towards your application.

Over the years, we have seen individuals with a PhD in Mathematics, informatics, Marine biology, and even individuals with a degree in Law who subsequently applied to a Medical School, became accepted, successfully completed a medical school curriculum and became physicians.

Some Medical schools in the US or Canada have combined MD/ PhD programs that span anywhere from 6 – 8 years. Most candidates who join these programs, complete the program in 6 years. If you are already a medical student and you are reading this book, it is probably too late for you to join an MD/PhD program, however, if you are still conducting your "undergraduate education", then it is still a good time to consider this pathway. This pathway may be more appropriate for physicians who plan to pursue a fellowship program following completion of their residency training program (GME, see below) and then plan to work in the very "pure academic centers", which have strong emphasis on basic science research.

**Medical School:** often referred to as "undergraduate medical education". It involves 4 years of education at one the US medical schools accredited, by the Liaison Committee on Medical Education (LCME), or the Canadian medical school association. Following completion of medical school, students in north America earn their doctor of medicine degree (MD), however they must complete additional training (at least 1-2 years in most states in the US and/or Canadian provinces (graduate medical education) before they can be granted a license to practice as independent physicians. A technical term that is applied to this pathway to becoming a physician is "Doctor of Allopathic Medicine" as opposed to the "Osteopathic Medicine" discussed next.

Some physicians in the US earn a doctor of Osteopathic Medicine (DO) degree from a college of osteopathic medicine as opposed to "allopathic Medicine" discussed above. These doctors also will have to complete additional training in a "Graduate Medical Education" program before they are able to practice medicine on their own. The rules are slightly different for a DO in some states. For instance in some states a graduate of DO program may have to complete one year of internship at an osteopathic residency program before he/she can join an allopathic (MD program) residency program, otherwise she/he may have difficulty getting licensed in that particular state. So, clarify these issues with your osteopathic medical school and your state licensing board about the specific rules and restrictions before you embark on an allopathic residency program if you are a graduate of DO Medical school. International graduates who wish to train in the US and possibly practice medicine in the US must a medical degree that is equivalent to the Medical Doctor degree. Many countries have different names for medical degrees. Examples include, Bachelor of Medicine and Bachelor of Surgery (MBBS), which is usually a 7-8 program of basic science and Medicine. Countries that follow the British system of Medical education usually grant their medical graduates this degree. Regardless of the type of the medical degree, all graduates must pass the United States Medical Licensure Examination (USMLE) before they are eligible to participate in a residency training program.

**Residency Training program:** referred to as "Graduate Medical Education". A new graduate of a medical school enters into a training program referred to as "Residency program" that is 3- 7 years of professional training under the supervision of physician educators in a residency program accredited by the Accreditation Council in Graduate Medical Education (ACGME). With rare exceptions, in order for your training to be valid you must complete your residency training in an ACGME accredited program. These programs are listed at the American Medical Association (AMA) website (http://www.ama-assnorg) and are also published annually in the so called "Green Book", which is also published by the AMA.

The length of residency program varies from one field to another. Medical fields such as Family Medicine, Pediatrics, Internal Medicine, and some emergency Medicine programs require 3 years of training. General surgery and Orthopedic surgery require at least 5 years of training. Fields such as Otolaryngology, Ophthalmology require one year of general surgery followed by 3-4 years of residency.

**Fellowship training programs:** Following completion of a residency program, a physician can practice Medicine independently if he/she can secure a full and unrestricted license to practice in medicine in a particular state. Most states grant a license to practice medicine without specifying the specialty, which suggest that you can practice in any field provided that you have the expertise and the knowledge to practice in a particular field.

Physicians who would like to become highly specialized in a particular field in medicine e.g. Adult cardiology, adult pulmonology, pediatric intensive care, neonatal intensive care or pediatric gastro-enterology, will have to complete 3 additional years of training in that particular subspecialty. This part of training is called "Fellowship". It involves clinical training as well as training in research, leadership, management and scholastic activities.

### *Should I apply for a Fellowship following completion of your residency?*

We will discuss this issue later in the book. The decision involves many factors including time, lifestyle, and of course money! In the next several pages we will discuss the process of applying for and securing a position in a residency program in the US.

### Are you currently a Medical Student or a new Medical School graduate?

We assume that you are either a medical student or you have graduated from a medical school (if you have Congratulations!! Well done) and waiting to enroll in a residency program. With rare exceptions you will have to complete a residency training program before you can practice medicine as an independent physician.

Today in the US, applications for a residency program are processed online through the Electronic Residency Application Services (ERAS) and the National Resident Matching Program (NRMP). You will have to register with both of these organizations, pay the fees and receive an identification numbers (or tokens as it is called at ERAS) before you can apply to any residency programs. Their websites are: www.nrmp.org and www.aamc.org. The registration process usually starts in late summer, early fall. We will discuss these processes in details later.

ERAS: If you a medical student in one of the medical schools in the US, your Dean's office will help you with starting the process of applying for ERAS as follows:

- The Dean's office will issue you what is called "an electronic token", which you will use to access the ERAS website and register.
- After completing the registration at "My ERAS" you will have to complete an application (on line), select programs and assign supporting documents. There are guidelines at the ERAS website to help you complete your application under the title: "My EARS user guide". The ERAS registration process opens July 31 and remains open until May 31 of the following year. The deadlines for submitting applications are set by the individual Residency programs, therefore you need to contact each program to inquire about the deadline for applications. Often this is posted at the specific residency website.
- Following completion of an application, your designated Dean's office will receive notification that you have completed your ERAS application and begin scanning and transmitting your supporting documents to ERAS.
- The examining boards such the United States Medical Licensure Examination (USMLE) will receive a request and will process the request for score reports to be sent to your designated residency programs
- At this point Residency programs may access their account at ERAS regularly to download applicants' materials.
- If you are a graduate of an Osteopathic Medical School, you may apply to an Osteopathic Residency Program following the same steps.

–   If you are a graduate of a Medical School that is not located in the US, then your designated Dean's office is the Educational Commission of Foreign Medical Graduates (ECFMG). You may access their website at: www. ECFMG.org. You will also be able to register with ERAS from a link at the ECFMG website.

ERAS has simplified the process of application to residency programs. Twenty years ago, you had to contact residency programs, request a paper application, fill out the paper application, add the supporting documents and then you had to mail it into each and every single program. This obviously was more labor intensive, time consuming, and involved extra money for copying and mailing the applications. Technology has indeed simplified our lives.

You can also apply to NRMP online. We will discuss this later in the book. At this stage we would like to provide you with ideas about different residencies and what strategies you should take in order to increase your odds of securing a position in your desired residency program.

The United States has the largest number of structured residency programs in the world. There are approximately 8500 residencies in various specialties in the US. They range from surgical to medical programs and from pediatrics to adult programs.

You can and you should start early in your medical school career on exploration of specialty options and career pathway. We suggest that you do some of the ground work for choosing your specialty during your preclinical years in order to become more informed about your specialty choice options. You may want to consider volunteering at a hospital or a clinic in the specialties in medicine that you believe you are attracted to. Try to narrow the number of fields that you might be interested in as much as possible. Consider rotating in fields you are less likely to have an opportunity to rotate through during your clinical rotations. That is true! You may not rotate through certain fields such as Otolaryngology (also known as Ear, Nose and Throat [ENT]), Ophthalmology, Orthopedic surgery, Physical Medicine and Rehabilitation, etc. Most of the core rotations during the clinical years in medical schools will be in: general surgery, Internal Medicine, Pediatrics, Psychiatry, and Obstetrics and Gynecology.

If you do this initial ground work during your preclinical years, then when you start your actual clinical rotations, you can actively gather more information about the fields that you have not excluded and that you believe you may be interested in. One of the major decisions that we suggest you make towards the end of your third year in medical school is whether you feel that you are more surgically inclined or you are more medically inclined.

Fields such as general surgery, cardiac surgery, colorectal surgery, and plastic surgery are obviously surgically inclined. However, fields such as Otolaryngology and ophthalmology are also surgically inclined and most of them require at least one year of residency training in general surgery before the candidate can start training in that particular field. On the other hands Family Medicine, Internal Medicine, Pediatrics, and physical Medicine and Rehabilitation are not surgically inclined. Obstetrics and Gynecology involves a combination of Medical and surgical issues.

To be a surgeon you have to be good with your hands and have a very good hand-eye coordination especially in the current era of robotic surgery. If you don't think you will like cutting into a person's body or skull at 7 am, or you don't enjoy the site of blood or seeing a person with a severe fracture where the bones are sticking through the skin of a limb, then surgery is probably not a good choice for you.

Be honest with yourself when you go through different clinical rotations as a medical student (or even as a volunteer on different hospital wards if you are still doing your undergraduate education). If you are already a medical student, the 4- 6 week rotation in one field is not a real test of what a particular field is like, when you have to practice it day in and day out for many years to come, but it should give you a good feeling about that field. If you have an inclination towards certain field, do additional electives to get a better feel for what that specialty is like. However, the way the residency application process is structured is that you begin your application in the fall of your 4th year in medical school, when you have not yet completed any elective rotations and you do not have a good idea about what a particular field of medicine is like!

Some physicians begin in a certain path, but change along the way. For instance, some physicians have changed their field from family medicine to emergency medicine, or pediatrics to ophthalmology, and so on and so forth. Another reason for optimism is that Medicine is one of the most flexible professions. Having a medical degree will open the door for you to practice medicine in various clinical fields and in different settings (Hospital based or Clinic based), but it will also allow you to change your path into other areas such as a biomedical research, public health, policy making fields, or administration of a hospital or a health care system. So, with your medical degree the sky is the limit as long as you have the energy and the motivation to reinvent yourself and change along the way, you will always have the opportunity to change your career later.

In choosing your career, we suggest you consider the following questions:

- What were your goals for entering a medical school and are these goals still valid?
- The type of life style you envision for yourself (and later for your family)?
- Your geographic preferences?
- What aspects of Medicine are appealing to you: Medical, Surgical?
- What areas of medical practice make you uncomfortable or you find difficulty in handling (Adults vs. Children, Hospitals or clinics, Men, Women)?

— What are your skills that you value and do these skills match the residency training you contemplate to embark on?

Choosing a field in medicine is sometimes difficult and setting your mind on one field happens over time, however you know yourself better than anyone else, be honest with yourself and set realistic aspirations for your future. The decision you make today will be with you for many years to come, but as we said earlier having a degree in medicine gives you the flexibility to work in various settings and that is a good piece of news.

Here are some suggestions on how to choose a specialty:

The first step is to judge yourself whether you like surgery or non-surgery.

Did you like dissection during your science classes in high school or in college?

Do you mind the site of blood?

Do you like long hours of standing on your feet and performing a procedure?

Are you good with your hands? Are you mechanically inclined? With the advent of non-invasive surgery (mostly done through endoscopes) and robotic surgery you have to be good with your hands and have a very good hand-eye coordination?

Do you like to wake up very early in the morning to be in the operating room and start surgery at 7 a.m.? and make rounds on your post-operative patients at 9 p.m.?

If you answer *yes* to all these questions you are probably surgically inclined?

> Do you believe you would want to do what you like today 25 years later when you have a family, children, and perhaps grandchildren? OR
>
> You prefer to see patients in the ambulatory clinic, take a good history, perform a good physical examination and then go through the mental work of differential diagnosis, reach a diagnosis, then prescribe a plan for the patient, which may include prescription of a medication? If the latter is what you like then you are probably more medically inclined. Always think about these questions as you conduct your clinical rotations.

Once, you have made the decision that you are more medically or surgically oriented, then it is time to narrow it down further to adult medicine or pediatric medicine. There is a big difference between adult medicine and pediatric medicine, this leads us to the next step.

Overall children are healthier than adults, they are more fun to be with, and there is a mystique about them: You never know what the child you are treating today is going to be 20 years from now. He or she may be a famous artist, an actor or actress, an economist, an engineer, a physician or even a president.

Children grow up very fast both physically and mentally. If you are a pediatrician you see the baby immediately after birth in the hospital and then at two weeks (if not sooner) of age, then at 1, 2,4,6, 9,12,15,18, and 24 months of age for well child examination, assuming the child remains perfectly healthy. During these visits you will also see and interact with the parents and perhaps other family members. As you can imagine the parents of this baby probably see you (the pediatrician) more than they see many of their own family members in the first two years of their child's life. You become a part of their lives!!

It is a great deal of fun and enjoyment to see the child grow from a helpless baby to an older child who may talk to you and addresses you by your name. In some pediatric practices, parents grow up and become parents themselves and then bring their children to the same pediatrician. As a pediatrician you may see more than one generation of patients throughout the entire length of your career in your practice.

Pediatric medicine is more emotionally laden than adult medicine. You will have to deal not only with the patient (the baby or the child), but also the parents, the grand-parents, the uncles, etc., especially when the child is sick and is in the hospital.

In pediatrics you have to deal with more social issues and the legal ramifications are more complicated than adults. For example, an adult patient can refuse a medical treatment you are recommending and if she/he is mentally competent, signs consent against medical advice, then that is the end of the story. On the other hand, a parent cannot simply refuse a treatment for her/his child if the physician believes that it is in the best interest of the child to have that particular treatment or procedure. In case of refusal the physician will have to first make every attempt to convince the parent to give permission for the procedure or the treatment. However, if the parent(s) still continue to refuse physician's recommendations, then the physician may have to secure a court order for that treatment or procedure. You can imagine all the extra energy, time, and emotions that will be invested in this process. In the hospital setting, you often get help from others, however, in the clinic setting, you have to do it on your own.

Another medico-legal ramification of pediatric medicine is that the stature of limitation for filing a medical lawsuit is up to 18 years of age for the child, which means that parents will have up to that age to file a malpractice lawsuit against you as a physician. On the hand, in most states, the stature of limitation for adults is only two years.

Adult medicine on the other hand is about "grown up human beings", who don't change physically and emotionally as fast as children. Unlike children who are innocent, adults sometimes have diseases that are self-inflicted such as smoking and its consequences of chronic bronchitis and emphysema, overweight and obesity which are the result of overeating combined with a sedentary life. Obesity leads to diabetes, hypertension, sleep apnea etc. Some adults do not take good care of their diseases such as controlling their blood pressure or diabetes by being non-compliant with their medications or treatment plans.

Some physicians have a difficult time dealing with these self-inflicted issues. Children on the other hand are innocent and at least in the earlier years of their lives are cared for by their parents or guardians. If they get a disease it is usually not out of their fault. There are individuals who are incapable of dealing with children in general and particularly when they are stricken with diseases. They will tell you that "it is heart-breaking to see a child sick and suffer from diseases or trauma." The point to emphasize again is: dealing with children is more emotionally laden.

*So what are your thoughts so far?* Do you like adult medicine or Pediatric Medicine? We are giving you some ideas about each field and what they are like.

-Once you have made these two major decisions (Medicine or Surgery, Adult or Pediatrics), then you can develop strategies to successfully get into a particular residency of your choice. Unfortunately, it is not easy to make these decisions in a matter of months during your third year in a Medical School. By the time you enter your fourth year you really will have to make decisions fast.

-If you think you are interested in a particular field e.g. surgery, but you will not be doing your surgery rotation until the end of your third year, try to spend some time with one of your classmates who is doing that particular rotation. You may have to go to the hospital on weekends or holidays to accomplish this. By spending time with your classmate on a surgical floor and even going to the operating rooms, you will have a good idea of what the field of surgery is like and this may facilitate your decision-making process. You may take a similar approach for other specialties by joining a classmate on hospital floors or certain clinics.

## What is your strategy?

**Useful strategies that you may use to get into a particular residency:**

Some residencies are harder to get into than others. Fields like Neurosurgery, Ophthalmology, Otolaryngology, Orthopedic surgery, and dermatology are more competitive and difficult to get into for one major reason: Supply vs. Demand. The number of residency positions offered are very limited in these fields and there is more demand than supply. Most of these programs have 1, 2 or 3 positions each year and therefore competition is fierce. On the other hand Internal Medicine, Family Medicine, and pediatrics are easier to get into simply because the number of positions available in each program is large. For instance it is not uncommon for a large program in Internal Medicine in a major academic center to have 50 positions for PGY 1 (Post-graduate year 1) and so as you can imagine it would be easier to get into internal medicine with 50 positions than Ophthalmology with one only one position in the program.

Secondly from an economic standpoint, physicians in some of these more competitive fields have the potential to generate higher incomes compared to other "less competitive fields" after graduation. In addition fields such as Dermatology and Ophthalmology are primarily outpatient practices with little or no night calls, which is conducive to a better lifestyle.

Here is a list of the approximate physician income by specialty for 2010 according to data published by the American Medical Group Association and SK& A, A Cegedim Company in 2011:

| Specialty | Median Income | Starting Income |
|---|---|---|
| Allergy/Immunology | 249,000 | 186,000 |
| Cardiac and Thoracic surgery | 516,000 | 356,000 |
| Colorectal surgery | 379,000 | n/a |
| Critical Care Medicine (Adult) | 277,000 | 232,000 |
| Dermatology | 375,000 | 254,000 |
| Gastroenterology (Adult) | 405,000 | 286,000 |
| Geriatrics | 218,000 | 163,000 |
| Obstetrics/Gynecology | 295,000 | 226,000 |
| Hematology/Oncology | 320,000 | 234,000 |
| Hospitalist | 215,000 | 168,000 |
| Nephrology | 259,000 | 189,000 |
| Neonatology | 274,000 | 180,000 |
| Orthopedic surgery (spine) | 675,000 | n/a |
| Orthopedic surgery (Hand) | 489,000 | n/a |
| Orthopedic surgery (pediatrics) | 446,000 | n/a |
| Radiation Oncology | 427,000 | 356,000 |
| Diagnostic Radiology | 300,000 | 327,000 |
| General Surgery | 357,000 | 273,000 |
| Urology | 413,000 | 319,000 |
| Anesthesia | 370,000 | 329,000 |
| Neurosurgery | 566,000 | 465,000 |
| Plastic surgery | 402,000 | 310,000 |
| Ophthalmology | 325,000 | 277,000 |
| Otolaryngology | 368,000 | 302,000 |
| Emergency Medicine | 268,000 | 200,000 |
| Neurology | 236,000 | 188,000 |
| Pathology | 354,000 | 246,000 |
| Internal Medicine | 214,000 | 152,000 |
| Family Medicine | 208,000 | 153,000 |

| Specialty | Median Income | Starting Income |
|---|---|---|
| Psychiatry | 214,000 | 168,000 |
| General Pediatrics | 209,000 | 139,000 |
| Pediatric cardiology | 253,000 | n/a |
| Pediatric endocrinology | 192,000 | n/a |
| Pediatric gastroenterology | 213,000 | n/a |
| Pediatric Hematology/oncology | 213,000 | n/a |
| Pediatric Intensive Care | 275,000 | n/a |
| Physical Medicine | 244,000 | 181,000 |
| Sports Medicine | 221,000 | 165,000 |
| Transplant surgery/kidney | 360,000 | n/a |
| Transplant surgery/Liver | 448,000 | |
| Trauma surgery | 481,000 | |
| Urgent Care | 222,000 | 165,000 |
| Vascular surgery | 417,000 | 293,000 |

However, these figures changes on an annual basis and vary from region to region in the US. For example a hand surgeon (Orthopedic surgery/hand) has a median income of $ 728,000.00 in the west, $ 483,000 in the south, and $ 488,000 in the north. The Medical Management Group Association (MGMA) publishes compensations for physicians across the US on an annual basis. You may access their website at: www.mgma.com. However, you will have to pay a fee to receive detailed information on physicians' compensations.

## What is a hospitalist?

A trend that has become popular over the past 5-10 years is to have physicians who are primarily hospital-based and care for patients who are hospitalized. These physicians are appropriately named "hospitalists" and a new field has evolved which is called hospitalist medicine.

These are physicians who has completed a residency in Internal Medicine and who choose to work primarily in the hospitals caring for hospitalized patients. Most of these physicians are employed by the respective hospitals, although there are some groups who operate independently and sign contracts with hospitals. Physicians who have office practices and do not wish to take care of hospitalized patients may turn the care of their patients to hospitalist.

Hospitalist medicine is also expanding to include pediatricians who care for hospitalized children and surgeons who care for hospitalized surgical patients. If you do not enjoy office practice and you like to care for sick patients who need hospitalization this is another option for you. The median compensation for hospitalists in the US was $ 171,000.00 for 2006, but increased to $ 215,000.00 for 2010.

The following the range of compensation for hospitalists (Adult Medicine) for various regions of the US for 2010 based on 2009 data:

- Northeastern states: $ $ 162,000 - 179,000
- Mid-Atlantic states: $ 205,000.00
- Midwestern states $165,000- 211,000
- South and Southeastern states: $ $ 180,000 – 235,000
- Western and Northwestern states: $165,00 – 213,000.00

A word of caution about any physician compensation including the ones listed here, is that they are based on surveys, which are voluntary and are not audited by any entity and therefore, you should understand some of the limitations of these figures. However, according to practice management guidelines, these are the best data available with regard to physician compensation. You may also consider inquiring from friends and colleagues about individual physician's compensations and benefits in different fields.

**So, what is your strategy?**

In order to secure a position in one the competitive residency programs, you must have a strategy. Here are some strategies to help increase your chances of getting into one of the competitive programs:

- Get a high score on USMLE (United States Medical Licensure Examination); high 90s would be great, but definitely above 90. Over the years the contents of qualifying examinations have changed and with advent of the internet it has become easier to find knowledge. If you were a medical student in early eighties, the best source was a good textbook or review articles in certain journals, both of which were in hard copies only. Today any information on any topic in Medicine is in the palm of your hands or few clicks away on a computer. You can surf the internet for written topics, radiographic images, videos and other relevant images 24 hours a day, seven days a week. You can even find medical knowledge on *Youtube.com*! As a result it is easier to acquire knowledge.

  The contents of qualifying examinations have become more practical and it our impression that it is easier today to get a higher score. In the days of the National Board of Medical Examiners (NBME) and the Federation Licensure Examination (FLEX), the two examinations that preceded the USMLE, a score in the 90s was uncommon. Today, the scores on USMLE are often high, sometimes surprisingly high, and scores in the high 90s are much more common nowadays compared to 25 years ago. So your odds of getting a high score on the USMLE are higher today especially if you study hard, attend all the medical school classes in the basic sciences and the laboratory sessions, attend all of your clinical rotations and get involved in direct patient care, and perhaps take short courses offered by various organizations on USMLE. One example of an organization that offers these courses is *The Kaplan education Centers* available throughout the US. You may visit their web site at: www.kaplan.com.

- Plan on doing an elective rotation during the third or fourth years of medical school in few programs that you like and that you believe you will be considered a competitive applicant.

*How do you know if you are a competitive applicant for that program?*

Well, be realistic. If you are not a graduate of an Ivy league Medical school, you probably will not be able to be competitive in an Ivy league residency program which has a limited number of positions. For example, your chances are low to get into a residency at Brigham and Women's Neurosurgery residency program unless you are a graduate of Harvard or Yale or similar schools. Applying to these programs and keeping your expectations very high is unrealistic and may end up in disappointments on the Match Day.

While you should be realistic, you should also have a methodical approach to securing a residency position. Personal communications is very important in everything we do in life. It has been said that "it is who you know, and not what you know". People want to see you in action. They want to know you at the personal and professional levels. What is your personality like? How do you work with people? How is your interaction with peers and patients and their families. If you get an opportunity to do an elective rotation in your field of interest in a program that you think you have a realistic chance of getting accepted, make every effort to know the leaders in that program including the program director. In every program, there are a handful of people who make the major decisions about ranking of the applicants on the NRMP match list. If you work with these people during an elective rotation and they get to know you first hand it is a big plus because now you are no longer another candidate on another application.

Residency training programs receive thousands of applications every year, and the time available to sort through these thousands of applications are very limited. Programs start receiving applications in September. They have only few weeks to sort out through these applications because the interview process starts in November and goes through February. With a number of holidays spanning from September through January, programs have very limited time to work with thousands of applications.

So, as you can imagine if no one knows you, your application may not go past the administrative assistance. Furthermore, Programs have the ability to filter applications using various parameters: USMLE score (of say) 85% or less, LCME medical school, specific medical schools in specific regions, etc. If you have a USMLE score of 84 and the program uses a filter to exclude any candidate with a score of less than 85%, then surely your application will not go past the administrative assistance (or Secretaries as they used to be called). These secretaries or administrative assistance (usually female) have some power and therefore you should be nice to them whenever you interact with them over the phone, by email or in person. For instance if you ask her nicely, she may,*and she can*, pull your application and hand it over to the program director for review and put in a good word for you. Such as "this is the candidate who did an elective with you last month and he is really good!". If you have already worked with the leaders in the program (such as the program director) and you have done well during your elective rotation, this may open the door for you for a good letter of recommendation from an authority in that field which in turn may land you an interview.

- Letters of recommendation: The Dean's letter goes only so far. If your goal is to get into one of the competitive residencies you will need recommendation letters from individuals who are well-known in that field either because they are known in the community they serve, or they are recognized nationally for their clinical and scholastic contributions. When you ask for a letter of recommendation for a specific competitive program we suggest that you ask the person who will be writing a letter in your support to address the letter to the program director with their specific names and title(s). I know this would involve extra work and resources, but it will make the letter more personal. If the letter is addressed "To whom it may concern" it may be construed that you did not do your homework or you did not care enough. So, make a real effort to get the name of the program director, their academic credentials, and their title on top of the letter. In this way you will make the letter of recommendation more personal. We do recognize that the ERAS application process does NOT allow for the letter to be personal, but you should make an effort to make it as personal as possible in whatever way you can.

- Your personal statement: Make it concise and informative. Do not sound that you are begging or desperate in your cover letter. Do not exaggerate facts because if you do eventually people will find out the truth. It is better to stick with facts and figures to state your accomplishments. You can effectively communicate your brilliance by stating what you have accomplished and what you can offer to the program and the field you are applying for. Pay attention to details in your personal statement: double-check your spelling, grammar, dates, etc.

- Geographic location of the program. This is important from a number of aspects. First, it may be important for you to live in an interesting city while you are conducting your residency. Other people care more about being close to family and friends rather than moving away to live in an interesting city. For most people, cities like San Francisco, Los Angeles, New York, Boston, Miami, and Chicago are very interesting places and they may want to live in one of these cities during their residency training. In general, programs in these cities are more competitive compared to smaller cities, therefore if you are applying for one of the competitive fields take this factor into this consideration.

## Is the specific residency programs I am applying to competitive?

Historically, one measure of the competitiveness of a specialty or a program within a specialty is the percentage of the positions that is filled by US allopathic graduates (USMDs).

According to 2010 data from the National Resident Matching program (NRMP) 25,520 positions were offered in 2010. There were 30,543 registered applicants for these positions. 24,378 positions were filled. So as you can see there were over 1000 positions in various residencies that were unfilled. The number of positions in Family Medicine filled by US allopathic graduates (MDs) increased from 43.2% to 44.8%. For Internal Medicine the number of positions filled by US allopathic graduates increased from 53.5% to 54.5%. 78.5% of positions offered in anesthesiology were filled by US allopathic MDs.

Here is a list of some of the other specialties and the % filled by USMDs:

Urology 100%

Internal Medicine/Dermatology 100%

Radiation Oncology 93%

Otolaryngology 92%

Orthopedic Surgery 91%

Neurosurgery 90%

Plastic Surgery (Integrated) 88%

Internal Medicine-emergency Medicine (a combined 5 year program) 87%

Diagnostic Radiology 85%

Transitional Year 84% (this is a good back-up option for you if you are applying for a very competitive residency program and you are not sure if you are going to match with one of your first choice programs. It will also count towards a PGY-1 year requirements for programs such as Diagnostic Radiology)

Internal Medicine-Pediatrics (a combined 4-year program) 83%: This is a good and broad residency if you like both adult and pediatric medicine and you plan to practice medicine in a general practice setting the future.

General Surgery (categorical) 83%

Emergency Medicine 76%

Pediatrics 70%

Pathology 65%

Psychiatry 61%

As you can see half of the positions in Family Medicine and Internal Medicine remained unfilled by US graduates, whereas 100% of positions in Urology were filled by US graduates. The unfilled positions are usually filled by International Medical graduates (IMG) or as they used to be called in the past "Foreign Medical graduates (FMGs)".

By the way even if you are US citizen by birth, but you received your medical degree from outside the US you are categorized as IMG. e.g. If you are a US citizen who has graduated from the American University of the Caribbean, you will be categorized as an IMG.

In the same manner you can assess how competitive a specialty is, by evaluating the percentage of US graduates who fill positions in these specialties. Obviously, that makes Family Medicine and Internal Medicine less competitive than Urology and Dermatology which are usually filled by US MDs 100% of the time. Ophthalmology data are not available through the NRMP, but 95% of positions are filled by USMDs.

It is important to recognize that these data provide a summary of categorical residency programs available for US senior medical students. The data pertain to the overall match result, but they do not necessarily provide a comprehensive review of all the potential training positions available in each specialty in the US. Also, the competitiveness of certain residency programs may change over time. For instance more recently (as of 2012), there are anecdotal observations that the field of Radiology may be coming less competitive than it used to be in the past 10-15 years and there are early indications that it may be not as difficult to secure a position in Radiology compared to 15 years ago. Also keep in mind that if the GME budget cuts continue and the number of residency position are slashed over the next 10 years, it may become even more difficult to secure a position in any residency or a fellowship training program.

## Do All residency programs participate in the match?

The NRMP is the single largest matching program in the US. It matches applicants to programs according their preferences. However, there are separate matching programs for residency training in Ophthalmology (The San Francisco Match), Child Neurology, and Urology. These matching programs notify program directors and applicants for the matching results in January (instead of March) of each academic year. So, if you plan to apply to one of these specialties, it is important that you contact the respective programs earlier so that you do not miss important deadlines.

## Do all residency positions start in July?

In general yes, however you may be able to start your residency at some other time especially if the program has unfilled positions (positions that were not filled through the match when that NRMP match results were announced in March). The NRMP publishes a list of unfilled position in all the programs across the US every year after the match results are released in March. If you were a participant in the NRMP for that year, you may have access to these data without paying additional fees. If you were not a participant in the NRMP, you can still contact the NRMP and purchase a copy of the unfilled positions for a fee.

## Can we apply and match to the same program or institution as a couple?

**Yes you can.** Some residency programs have special arrangements where couples can apply to the same institution or program. The institution/program will make an attempt to synchronize your interview process and assist couples with matching to the same program (if they qualify) so that couples can conduct their residency in the same institution and in the same city.

**Decision time!:**

Your time and resources are limited. Unless you have access to unlimited resources and time, you can practically apply only to a limited number of programs through the NRMP. Usually the first 10 programs are included in the initial fee that you pay towards registering with ERAS and/or NRMP. If you want to add more programs to your ranking list you will have to pay extra fees.

If you do apply for more programs, and you are invited for an interview, the travel involved requires time and money and as a medical student or a new graduate who is not a doctor yet your resources are limited. Therefore, you will have to narrow down your choices as much as possible if your resources are limited. Here is what you will have to do to narrow the choices down:

- First decide whether you like surgery or Medicine

- If you like Surgery, do you want to be a general surgeon or a surgeon in one of the sub-specialties such as Urology, Neurosurgery, plastic surgery, etc.

- Urology Residency Programs require 1 or 2 years of general surgery before you can start the Urology residency, but most programs will help you match with a preliminary surgery residency within their institution if they believe that you are a competitive applicant. The same is true for Orthopedic surgery in most programs. Plastic surgery is a bit more complicated. There are programs that are integrated and would allow you to do so many years of general surgery then transition to plastic surgery; others would want you to complete a 5-year general surgery and then join a plastic surgery program. Cardiothoracic surgery, colorectal surgery, trauma surgery, bariatric surgery and hand surgery are the same.

- Once you have decided on what field of Medicine you like, the next step is to answer the following question:

    *Is the field I am applying to is very competitive?* If you are applying for Dermatology, Urology, Ophthalmology, Otolaryngology, Orthopedic Surgery, Radiation oncology, Neurosurgery, diagnostic radiology, or Emergency medicine, then you are applying to one of the competitive residencies.

- Select about 5-10 programs that you believe you have a realistic chance of being a competitive applicant based on your USMLE scores, your medical school ranking nationally, your Medical School GPA, your research experience and publications.    Let us use an example: you are a graduate of an average Medical School, your GPA is 3.5, but you have no research experience, and have no publications in reputable journals, but you would like to apply for a neurosurgery residency. It is highly improbable that the Brigham and Women's Hospital program (Affiliated with Harvard Medical School) will invite you for an interview. Look for programs in your region. By now you should have done an elective in some of these programs and have established some relationships with the leadership in these programs. If you have not, your chances are low

- Once you have selected these 5-10 programs in the competitive field that you would like to join, add these programs to your list on ERAS (Electronic Residency Application Services). You should apply for ERAS in late summer, early fall, pay the fees and get an ERAS number. That is how programs identify you and your application.

- However, Always remember that when you are applying to very competitive residency programs there is always the possibility that you may not be invited for an interview or if you are invited you may not be ranked high enough on the program match list in order to match to a program of your choice. *So you need a back-up plan! What is your back-up plan?*

- The back-up plan would be to apply to programs in other fields that you are almost sure you will be matched to comes the match day and you have a position, which means you have a job next year! The options are as follows: a Transitional year, Internal Medicine, Family Medicine, Pediatrics, etc.

- The transitional years residency program (as the name implies) is for candidates who would like to start a residency in a field which requires one year of post-graduate training before joining the program such as radiology.

- If you don't match with your preferred program the first time, you do one year in one of the other fields and apply again to your favorite field next year.

- An alternative is to find an investigator in your preferred competitive field such as Neurosurgery, Orthopedic surgery, or Otolaryngology and spend a year doing research while waiting to get into a residency in that specialty. In this way physicians in that field will get to know you, your personality and your abilities. Then they can recommend you to other programs or better offer you a position in their own program. We suggest that you discuss these issues with the program director in an honest and realistic way as far in advance as possible.

During the meeting with program director you could say something like " I am really interested in Otolaryngology and this is the only field I would like to train in and have it as my career... I am willing to do whatever it takes to get into this field. If I have to spend a year or two doing research in the field while waiting for a position then I am willing to invest the time. Realistically do you think I will be able to secure a position next year or the year after?". OR "I really like your program, but I am willing to relocate if you think my chances are better in another program next year". Program Directors are often well connected and they should be able to give you a realistic answer.

Several years ago a physician who was very interested in completing a fellowship in Pediatric Surgery (which is a very competitive field and there are limited positions available in the US). He was board certified in General Surgery and was a physician and had a Law degree. He did one year of Surgical Critical Fellowship and during that year he planned to apply for a Pediatric Surgery Fellowship. He was told clearly that his chances are not good getting into Pediatric Surgery, but he thought he could get in. Two years later he was still doing Surgical Critical Fellowship and was not able to secure a position in a Fellowship program in Pediatric Surgery.

The lesson here is that if the program tells you that your chances are not good to get into that particular field *move on.* There was another surgeon who went to Canada to get into a fellowship in pediatric surgery fellowship because he could not get into a residency in pediatric surgery fellowship in the US. So, the Canadian residency programs are another option.

On the other hand, there was a physician who was a graduate of a Medical School in France and who was very interested in Neurosurgery, but he was not able to get into a residency in Neurosurgery in USA. He spent few years doing research in that field with physicians who were considered pioneers in the field and he finally succeeded in getting into the same Neurosurgery residency program where he conducted his research..

- Like we alluded to above, another option for you is to apply for a residency program across the northern border. Sometimes certain Canadian programs accept Medical students from the US to enter certain Residency or Fellowship programs. However, I suggest (if you have the resources) you make a trip to large programs such the University of Toronto programs and discuss these issues with the specific program directors before you rely on getting into one of the Canadian programs based only on your application.

So far we have discussed strategies to help you get into the very competitive residency programs. But, what about programs that are less competitive such as Internal Medicine, Family Medicine, Pathology, or if you like dealing with children and families, Pediatrics?

## Applying for a Residency program in Internal Medicine, Family Medicine, Pathology, Psychiatry or Pediatrics

- These programs are usually larger in size, which means that there are more PGY- I positions available and as a result your chances are higher to get into one of these programs

- This does not mean that these fields are less important. In reality most patients receive their medical care through a physician in one of these fields whether in clinics or in a hospital. A survey conducted by Merritt Hawkins, which is a nationally recognized physician recruitment firm, from April 1, 2009, to March 31, 2010 showed that Family Medicine and Internal Medicine are the most requested specialties.

• If you are interested in one of these fields then your chances are very good that you will match into one of the programs that you rank on your list. So how do you decide which programs you should apply to and spend the time and money to go for an interview?

• The answer to the question is: it depends on what you would like to do after you complete your residency.

    Would you like to work in an academic center, where research is a major component of your daily work? Where you have to do bench research, apply for and secure multi-million dollar, multi-year grants and also be active in publishing scientific work in journals with a high-impact factor? If these are your goals, then you need to apply for and secure a position in a residency program in a high-quality academic center preferably a program that is affiliated with an Ivy League school. Examples of these schools according to descending ranking in 2010 are:

Harvard Medical School

Johns Hopkins

Washington University in St Louis

University of California San Francisco

Duke University

Stanford University

University of Washington

Yale

Columbia University.

These programs *are* very competitive, however because these programs are very large your chances of getting into one them is good especially if you apply to a program which has up to 50 PGY-1 positions. For example the Massachusetts General Hospital program in Internal Medicine has 66 PGY-I positions and University of California San Francisco program in Internal Medicine has about 60 PGY-I positions in Internal Medicine (based on 2010 data). As you can imagine with so many positions chances are that you will get a position, provided your GPA is reasonable, you have good letters of recommendations and *especially* if you have done an elective with them as a medical student prior to your interview.

These programs have a good number of physicians who are multi-million dollar, multi-years National Institute of Health (NIH) grant recipients and they have conducted quality research and have published in high quality Medical journals. If you join one of these residencies the probabilities of working with one these outstanding investigators are good provided you work hard at it. In the process you learn about research, grant writing, and scientific writing. If you are lucky to have one of these investigators agree to be your mentor, then you are on the right track to become a world renowned investigator yourself.

- If you are not interested in working in pure academic medical centers because you are not into basic science research, which may involve dealing with rodents and other animals and you don't want to deal with the pressure of securing grants, then you may be interested in what we call "quasi-academic settings". These are institutions which have residency programs and often medical students from the medical school that they are affiliated with. Part of your responsibilities will be teaching of residents and medical students in addition to taking care of patients in hospitals or in clinics. If you are interested in working in this type of environment, then you can still apply and join one of the above programs, but you don't necessarily have to. You can instead match with and join one of the thousands of other programs across the US, which are located in hospitals which have residency programs in various specialties and often have medical students. If you join one of these programs as resident you will still receive high-quality training in your field and you will learn the art of teaching.

After you graduate from one of these residencies if you decide to work in one these hospitals you will have the opportunity to teach residents and medical students and your contract usually states that part of your duties would be teaching of residents and medical students. However, there isn't the intense pressure to secure grants and publish in high-impact journals. You can still do clinical research and in some select institutions some bench research, but not with the same intensity as in the "pure academic centers". In these centers part of the revenues for the hospital comes from the federal funding for the residency programs. Other sources of funding could come from teaching medical students.

- The final option is for those of you who would like to work in private practice in an office setting or in a hospital setting. These settings usually don't involve teaching residents or medical students and the only focus is on patient care and the revenue generation in these setting is only from patient care.

- One last factor to consider is the geographic location you would like to be in during residency training. We will discuss this issue further in the book

## What are the probabilities of not matching with your first choice?

In 2010 only 52% of US MDs matched to *their first choice program*, down from 57% in earlier year. However, 93% of US MDs matched to a program. So the lesson to learn before we proceed further is that your chances of matching to your first choice is only about 50%, and the chances of you matching into a program is 93% not 100% if you are a US allopathic graduate. This means that you may need to have a back-up plan when you rank your programs and this back-up plan is particularly important if you are NOT a USMD.

By now you know what field you like and hopefully you know which geographic region you would like to be in. If the field that you are interested in is a competitive one then you should definitely have a contingency plan. Like we discussed earlier, pick a number of programs; let us say 5-10 in one of the competitive fields, but you should also choose few other programs as your back-up such as internal Medicine, Family Medicine, or a transitional year, so that comes the match day in March you have at least matched to a program and you have a job for the next year.

## Unique Residency Programs

There a number of residency programs that consist of a combination of residencies but you can complete them in a shorter period of time compared to if you did each residency alone. Some examples are as follows:

- **Internal Medicine/Pediatrics Residency:** You train in both Internal Medicine and pediatrics. Instead of doing two separate residencies (each of which is 3 years for a total of 6 years) you go through a combined internal medicine/pediatric residency (commonly referred to as "med-ped") and you finish your training in 4 years. Because med-ped residency programs require that all candidates meet all the inpatient and intensive care (ICU) requirements of both the American Board of Internal Medicine (ABIM) and the American Board of Pediatrics (ABP), the training is heavily weighted towards inpatient and ICU settings. However, this training allows med-ped graduates to sit for both ABIM and ABP boards. This seems to be appropriate training programs for candidates who plan to work as hospitalist (particularly in smaller community hospitals) or in an outpatient practice where a physician treats both adults and children. In essence you can treat the entire family with the exception of the fact that you will not be able to practice Obstetrics and Gynecology because it is not part of your training. Being a med-ped graduate (approximately 300 physicians graduate from med-ped program every year in the US), poses certain challenges, which requires extra attention to scheduling, salary, and benefits.

For a physician who would like to be a hospitalist, the dilemma is whether to concentrate on adults or pediatric population. Most of the hospitalist (a physician who exclusively practices hospital-based medicine) positions are either for adults or children, however there are an increasing number of positions for med-ped hospitalists. One approach that has been suggested is for med-ped physicians to seek knowledgeable department heads and knowledgeable administrators and following other med-peds graduates who followed this path and have experience practicing both adult and pediatrics. Anecdotal reports from med-ped graduates are mixed at this time.

In academic settings; some have been able to strike deals with employer so that their time is equally split between pediatrics and adult medicine; others have faced obstacles. In academic settings, a med-ped hospitalist position tends to be crafted between two distinct departments offers some advantages: these are usually larger medical centers with affiliated community hospitals, which means more hospitalist physicians. This is conducive to more flexibility with scheduling of patients and call schedules. The possibility of a med-ped residency program at the same site with the ability to get involved in teaching is an additional advantage in academic programs. However, there are multiple barriers to an academic med-ped hospitalist job. Determining who will pay the hospitalist salary and benefits, how the schedule will be coordinated, and to whom the hospitalist reports to can be tricky, especially because an internal medicine department and a pediatric department are not used to working together. Serving as a member of various committees in two distinct departments is another challenge. Furthermore, it is often not clear who should take the lead in the promotion of a med-ped academic hospitalist. In community-based settings; the challenges have included the lack of understanding by administrators as to what is a "med-ped physician" and what he/she is capable of offering to a medical center.

If you decide to choose this residency, following graduation, it is critical that the hospital administrators or the health care system in your area are educated about med-peds physicians and the role they could play in patient care. It is not uncommon for a med-ped physician to work full-time in one discipline, often internal medicine, and "moonlight" or work part time in pediatrics. In general, the compensation is higher for an internal medicine hospitalist (median annual compensation $215,000.00 for 2009) compared to a pediatric hospitalist ($160,000.00 for 2009). Therefore, it is expected that a med-ped physician compensation may suffer if she/he devotes more time to pediatrics.

- **Internal Medicine/Emergency Medicine:** This is usually a combined 5-year program in which the physician is trained in both Internal Medicine and Emergency Medicine. This combined residency program may be suitable for someone who is planning to work harder early in her/his career and practice Emergency Medicine with its intense work and erratic call schedule. In the later parts of his/her career she/he can gradually switch to office practice in Internal Medicine. The numbers of programs are very limited and therefore, these programs are competitive. Again, good planning on your part will certainly go a long way towards increasing the probabilities of securing a position in one of these programs.

- **Pediatrics/Physical Medicine and Rehabilitation (PM&R) or Internal Medicine/PM&R:** These are usually 5- year programs in which physicians are trained in both Pediatrics or Internal Medicine and PM&R. These programs provide the candidate with a good background and skills in general internal Medicine or General Pediatrics in addition to PM&R. You could practice both fields, however if you decide to practice in an office setting referral may be problematic. You will not be able to refer patients from your own Pediatric or Internal Medicine to your PM&R practice because this may be construed as a violation of the anti-kick-back law. Therefore, referrals for your PM&R practice will have to come from other physicians in the community.

Other combined residency programs include:

- Internal Medicine/Emergency Medicine/Critical Care Medicine

- Family Medicine/Preventive Medicine

- Pediatrics /Child and Adolescent Psychiatry

## Cheap accommodation for the Residency interview, where do you find one?

One of the financial burdens associated with the residency interview is the accommodation. Some programs will provide you with accommodation for the night prior to your residency interview, however others do not and obviously you will have to find your own accommodation. In most larger cities in the US and Canada accommodation can be very expensive and this can eat up your residency program interview budget. One option is to stay in the so called "hostels". In most countries in the western hemisphere, hostel refers to sociable accommodation where the guest rents a bed and shares bathrooms, showers, a lounge and sometimes a kitchen. The word hostel refers to other things in some countries ranging from boarding schools, to accommodation for nurses, drug addicts, or defendants on bail. In some countries, hostels are also called backpackers' hostels.

*What is the difference between a hostel and a hotel?*

Hostels tend to be budget-oriented; rates are considerably lower, and nowadays many hostels have programs to share books, DVDs and other electronic items that you may need in preparing for your interview. For those who prefer an informal environment, hostels do not usually have the same level of formality as hotels, however, for those who prefer to socialize with their fellow guests, hostels usually have more common areas and opportunities to socialize. The dormitory aspect of hostels also increases the social factor. Also, hostels are generally self-catering and are more - "adventure travel" oriented than "leisure travel" oriented, thus attracting a younger, more venturesome crowd. Also, you need to recognize that there is less or at times no privacy in a hostel than in a hotel or motel and sharing sleeping accommodation in a hostel is very different from staying in a private room in a hotel or motel and hostels encourage more social interaction between guests due to the shared sleeping areas and communal areas such as lounges, kitchens and internet cafes. Noise (from talking, snoring, or even sexual activities) can make sleeping difficult on occasions. This may be mitigated by carrying earplugs.

Care should be taken with personal belongings as guests may share a common living space, so it is advisable to secure guests' belongings. Most hostels offer some sort of system for safely storing valuables, and an increasing number of hostels offer private lockers; there are other things to consider as well when choosing a safe hostel, such as whether they have a guest curfew, uphold fire codes, 24-hour security, and security cameras.

There are many sources on the internet to find hostels in the cities that may be your destination including: hostel international, which has a general website, which can direct you to specific country and state. Some resident physicians have continued to use hostels when attending conferences during their residency in order to stay within the budget. For instance you may spend a night at a hostel in New Orleans for under $ 25.00, now that is a bargain! If you decide to travel through Europe on a budget, hostels are an attractive option.

## The Residency Training Program Interview

There are books written on how to prepare and conduct yourself in an interview in general. However, we are talking about interviewing for a residency program in one of the specialties in Medicine, which is very unique for a unique group of professionals who have very high standards. You are invited for an interview because the leadership in that particular program believes that you are a good candidate for their program. It is your responsibility to take this opportunity seriously and attempt your best to present the best image of yourself. Here are some suggestions for your interview.

Be prepared: Gather information about the program, the program director and other leadership figures in the program. You may be able to "get away with not knowing much about an average program", but if you are applying for a competitive program being knowledgeable about the program can impress the leadership in that program, and this in turn may help you in being ranked high on the match list for that particular program.

Individuals who are in leadership positions in a program may be known for their accomplishment in their communities, nationally or internationally. For example a physician who is interviewing you may be the chairman of a department or a particular committee in that hospital, or she/he may be the head of a coalition in a community. It also helps to know their clinical and research interests. If they are into research, it is worth knowing their area of research and expertise. If they have published articles in medical journals you may consider reading them ahead of the interview in case a discussion related to the topic of their research comes up. You will be prepared and the physician who is interviewing you will be impressed. Human beings like to be appreciated and showing appreciation for what they have done is ego boosting. One way to appreciate them and give them importance is to know about their accomplishments.

In some programs you can request to be interviewed by particular individuals. If you have done an elective in that program and you believe that you have established rapport with certain individuals in that program, it is perfectly fine to request that you would like to be interviewed by one of them. If you share clinical or research interests with certain faculty members in a particular program, that may be another reason for you to ask to be interviewed by these individuals. Even if you believe that you share certain hobbies with certain faculty members, that may be a good reason to ask the program to be interviewed by those physicians. It does not hurt to ask. Remember when we discussed earlier that administrative assistances are important people and that you have to be nice to them with every type of communication. It comes in handy here too. If she knows you and you have been nice to her, she my go the extra mile to arrange for an interview with the physicians of your choice in the program. This certainly will be very helpful towards your applications in a competitive program provided that you have all the other competitive qualifications. So, the bottom line is that it pays to do your homework and make every extra effort to increase your odds of getting into a competitive program of your choice.

Dress appropriately: It is understandable that as a medical student or a resident your resources are limited, but you can still dress appropriately without spending thousands of dollars. For male candidates, a two-piece suit with a matching tie would be appropriate. Since most interviews are conducted during the months of November through February a suit is appropriate for most programs in most states in the US. Make sure your shirt is ironed and your tie matches the shirt and the suit. As you can see it does take some preparation if your resources are limited. You may have to borrow or rent a suit and/or borrow a nice tie from a friend. If you want to go an extra mile you should shine your shoes, make sure your sox match either your pants or your shoes and your hair is tidy. For female candidates a nice conservative suit is appropriate.

Dressing appropriately for the interview shows that you care and that you are taking the interview and the program seriously. Trust me we have seen physicians wear a Hawaiian-type shirt and a pair of jeans for a job interview (not a residency). We have also seen candidates (who were sons of physicians) show up for an interview for a residency with wrinkled and untidy shirt. That is inappropriate and gives the impression that you are not serious about the process. You may want to make sure the motel or hotel that you are spending a night in has an iron in the room or you can borrow one from the front desk, in case your shirt gets wrinkled during the packing.

Communicate effectively: It is important to communicate well with everyone you meet during your interview in search of a residency position. Shake hands, exude confidence, make eye contact, and engage the person who is interviewing you. You want to give the interviewer the impression that you are interested. Interviews for residencies and especially for fellowships are often long and you may have to meet 4-6 people during the day. Continue to maintain your enthusiasm as the day goes by. It is very easy to get bored with the same process and sometimes the same questions beings asked over and over, but maintain your focus, be patient and continue to show interest, otherwise the interviewer may get the impression that you are disinterested.

Over the years physicians (who have recommended applicants) have received calls from program directors (residencies and fellowships) regarding candidates with the complaint that he or she appeared disinterested and was not engaged. Sometimes you may be tired from a flight across the country with time-zone changes which may lead to a little bit of jet lag. If you feel that way find the nearest restroom, wash your face and grab a cup of coffee or tea and walk into the next interview with enthusiasm and energy. However, make sure you leave your cup of coffee behind and not into the interview room. Same goes for cell phones or any other electronic devices. If you decide to take them with you, please turn them off. Trust me it happens, your phone is in your pocket and you receive a call. That would be very distracting and disrespectful to the interviewer.

When answering questions be pleasant and don't limit your answers to "yes" or "No" so that the interviewer does not feel that he/she is pulling teeth to get an answer out of you. Follow either with a short sentence or two and make your answers interesting. At the same time don't go on and on answering a question. The interviewer does not need to know your life story. Keep your answers succinct and to-the-point. Use proper words and avoids slangs. On several occasions an interviewer came to us very disappointed because an applicant said something like " It pisses me off to see...." Now that is an inappropriate use of vocabulary in an interview for residency. She could have said something like " I don't appreciate it when ...".

Make sure you have your facts correctly including your graduation dates, previous experiences including employment, volunteering,
research training and the names and positions of people you have
completed these activities under. Listen carefully to a question and
take a moment to gather your thoughts before you respond. Try your
best to give the correct answers to the best of your abilities. If you are
not sure of the answer it is better to say "I don't know, but I will find
the answer" rather than giving the wrong answer. Do not "badmouth"
your medical school, the faculty there or previous programs you have
interviewed at. Even if you did not like them and it is true that some
of the individuals were "idiots" or "jerks", please don't use these words
during your interview. The world of Medicine is a small world and
you don't know that the person who is interviewing you now may be
friends with some or many people in that other programs.

Don't forget to follow up; whether you think you didn't make the
best impression or you believe your interview went well, be sure to follow up with a thank you note reiterating your interest in the program.
You may do this by sending an email to the program director and
the individuals who interviewed you stating how much you enjoyed
meeting them and that you are really interested in their program or
yet better send them and the program director a thank you card. In
order to be able to accomplish this you may want to ask for their business card at the end of each interview.

*I am nervous about the interview!*

Some degree of anxiety is normal and we all face it in different situations in life and being in an interview for a residency is one of those
situations. However, some of us are more nervous about it than others
and this trait has been shown to have some familial pattern in studies
using Positron Emission Tomography (PET) scans. In people who
are superanxious, the basal ganglia tend to light up on PET scans,
so there is a physiological explanation for it. Some people have more

anxiety than others, but you should be able to deal with it with simple strategies. If you used to (or still do it) to bite your nails when you are anxious, that means you are more prone to anxiety and you may have a more difficult time dealing with anxiety-provoking situations. Here are some suggestions:

1.  While you are sitting and waiting for the first or next interview, try to focus on "good thoughts"; remember those situations where you were most competent and successful and focus on them, this is likely to lead to more positive thoughts.

2.  Avoid the so called "automatic negative thoughts or ANTS" such as ".. this interview is going to be a disaster', "I am probably going to make a fool of myself"

3.  Use relaxation techniques, while you are waiting for your next interview by using abdominal breathing relaxation techniques. Take a deep breath through your nose, hold it for few seconds, then exhale through your mouth slowly while focusing only on your breath and forget about everything else around you. Come on, do this technique few times while you are reading this page and see how much more relaxed you feel!

4.  Most hospitals have a chapel; if you are still very nervous and you have time before your next interview go to the chapel, which is usually a quiet and serene place to apply those relaxation techniques. They are likely to induce calmness in you and make you more relaxed and confident for your next interview.

## What do strong programs look for in a candidate?

*What is something you do better than anyone else? And what is the evidence for that?*

Driven and passionate people leave behind them a wake of results wherever they go. You may use anecdotes to support your claim in being able to get things done against all odds, really impresses most people. Candidates who are not afraid to push the envelope a bit in the name of a job well done are likely to be selected above others.

*Did you come to the interview prepared?!*

As we stated earlier when you speak during the interview it is evident that you have done your homework and you know something about the institution and people who work there. You are likely to impress the interviewer. When you ask great questions about the program, it demonstrates not only your interest in that program, but also your ability to gather data and information. Programs also look for your ability to take on projects and function creatively and somewhat independently.

*Do you exhibit passion?*

Programs want to know why you are truly excited about the opportunity rather than every other opportunity out there. Candidates who are infused with this quality demonstrate an enthusiasm and aliveness that is contagious to their colleagues. It can be harnessed to learn the job to be done and then to do it without having to be constantly encouraged, prompted or micromanaged. Such people are willing to 'go the extra mile' to assure that everything is done and done well. They demonstrate initiative and creative problem-solving skills. Truly passionate candidates are not only likely to excel in their role, but, because they enjoy what they do, they will also remain engaged in their responsibilities and energize those around them. If a resident is not eager to learn, he or she will have difficulties accepting change and bringing innovative ideas to the program. Interviewers can see right through "robotic" candidates who 'say the right thing.' It's those who come specifically prepared to tell you exactly why the position is right for them that impress the interviewer the most.

*Confident but humble!*

Humble confidence shines as knowledge, humility, skilled verbal and written communication, friendliness and appreciation

*Professionalism*

Professionalism demonstrates that you have the right blend of technical and soft skills, mixed with enthusiasm and dedication. As we stated earlier at an interview it is all about how a candidate presents him or herself. Are they showing enthusiasm and motivation for the position? Are they really listening to the questions and answering them accordingly? These are the qualities that are not shown on a résumé and are near impossible to teach

*Body language*

Starts with the hand shake as you walk in to the office of the interviewer. The hand shake: it has got to be strong and firm from the get-go. Candidates usually come prepared to an interview, but competitive programs are looking for individuals who come to the interview with strong statements regarding what they can do for the program and what they can add to the program.

*Attitude*

The most impressive quality is to be a 'high performer,' a package of the right attitude, a passion for doing the work and the skill. 'Attitude' may mean different things to different people, but it boils down to having an 'I can' attitude. Everyone thinks his or her attitude is fine, however, some of these same people believe that is fine to blame, make excuses and declare something cannot be done. Open-mindedness, perseverance and a "can-do" attitude are what competitive programs are looking for in a candidate.

*What are some of the questions that I may be asked in an interview for a residency program?*

The purpose of the interview for a residency training program is evaluate who you really are and to find a good match between you and the program you are applying to. Most physicians who will interview you are not trying to intimidate you or stress you out; they are just trying to find the most suitable candidates for their residency program. There are common themes that are commonly asked during interviews for residency programs. There are no guarantees that you will be asked these questions, but here are some of the common questions you may be asked during an interview for a residency program:

1. *"Tell me about yourself"*: An open-ended questions that is often asked in interviews and certainly may be asked in a residency interview. What the interviewer would like to hear is why make a good candidate for her/his program, therefore you need to tailor your answer along these lines and try to use examples that would highlight why you are a good candidate for this program. While trying to achieve this task balance your answer so that you do not come across as arrogant.

2. *"Why are you interested in this field"* e.g. Internal Medicine, Pediatrics, Surgery etc. Make sure you have an answer that is appropriate for the question and back your answer with examples.

3. *"Where do you see yourself 10 years from now"*: This is also a common one, the number of years may vary, often you are asked "where do you see yourself 5 years from now?". What they would like to hear is that you are determined to successfully complete your residency training (because the percentage of applicant who complete the residency program is one of the strengths of any program and is tracked by the residency review committee) and to hear what do you see as

your contribution to the program and the field that you are applying for. Current leaders in a residency program would like to accept candidates to the program who will be good ambassadors for the program and the specialty in the future. If you can impress the interviewer that you *will be* a great ambassador for their program and you back that with examples of leaderships you have demonstrated in the past you have more than likely have done a great job.

4.   *"What do you think is your strength?"* speaks honestly from the heart about what you believe is your strength and back your statements with concrete examples. For instance your strength may be problem solving; you can state that and back it with examples from the past that have made a significant impact in that place. That could be a high school, a boy scout, a college or University or your community. Emphasize how your strength is likely to contribute to the program and the field.

5.   *"What do you believe is your weakness?"* no one is perfect. We all have our weaknesses. Again speak honestly about your weaknesses. For instance you may say, I am not good at handling sick children and therefore, I would not make a good pediatrician or a pediatric intensive care physicians and that is why I am choosing adult medicine or one of your weaknesses might be scientific writing and you are working hard on improving yourself in this area.

6.   *"Why are you interested in this geographical area?"* Residency program directors and those in position of leadership would like to make sure that they select candidates that are a good match to their program. One of the issues is the location. They want to make sure that you are drawn to the area where the program is located so that you will be content during the 3-5 years of your residency training program. In you are applying for a program in Buffalo, New York where the winter is very

long and harsh, and it snows heavily with snow accumulation from several inches to few feet is not uncommon, then you should be prepared to deal with that issue in the winter. One the other hand in a state like Arizona, the summers are very hot with triple digit temperatures. Do you mind those extremes of weather, or you like them?

7.  *"Tell me about ....."* These are issues that are on your CV and can range from academic achievements or publications to hobbies. Therefore, it is critical that you review your CV thoroughly and make sure you understand every section of it and that you are prepared to answer questions related to every issue. If you have put down that baseball is your hobby, the interviewer may ask you "What is your average batting?". If you put down travel, she/he may ask you about the places you have travelled to, the places or things that you saw and what was it like. The interviewer may have travelled to the same places and be very familiar with a city or a location. If you are asked a question and you do not seem to know what the interviewer is talking about it can be embarrassing for you.

8.  *"Do you have any interests outside Medicine?"* This obviously has to be things that you like to do when you are not learning medicine such as a hobby, volunteering, etc. again be honest and state facts and things that you really like to do and things that you do often outside Medicine. The interviewer may have the same hobby that you like. That would be great, it may make the interview more exciting for both of you and may leave a positive impact on the interviewer. Remember the interviewer are people too, they have hobbies and interests just like you do.

9.  *"Do you have any questions for me?"* The most important issue is not to say "NO". It may be construed as lack of interest or ignorance. However, when you do ask questions, it is very critical that you ask the interviewer relevant and appropriate

questions. Know who is interviewing you, who is she/he, what field they are in, and what is their position in the residency program. Most interviewers do not know details of the working hours, vacations, coverage for holidays, when you will be allowed to moonlight or if there are moonlighting opportunities in the program. Leave these questions for the program director. Ask questions that are likely to be answered by the person who is interviewing you. For example, if she/he is active in a research area that is of your interest, you may ask if there will be any opportunities for residents to get involved with research in that particular area.

10. *Final, but important issues to remember during your interview:* remember that interviewers are human too just like you, the better your level of energy and the more positive is your interaction the easier will be the interview on both of you. Therefore, be aware of your posture: make sure that your facial expressions portray interest, and your posture exhibits positive energy. Pauses are fine, but avoid long periods of silence during the interview. Avoid use of profanity or certain acts such as chewing gum during an interview. Avoid looking at mission statements for the institution and then regurgitating it during the interview. Interviewers like to hear words that are your own and reflect who you are and how you see a particular program or institution. Please remember the names and ranks of people who interview you so that if the interviewer # 3 asks you who has interviewed you so far, you will have the correct answers e.g. John Doe, Director of Pediatric Gastroenterology and Nutrition, instead of mumbling a name!

## What should I bring to the interview?

1. Please know the name and telephone number of the administrative assistance for the residency program. Things happen

in life. In case you are late, you can't find the location of your interview; You know whom to call

2. Bring detailed directions with you: such as Google map, or MapQuest which gives you directions to the location of your interview from your hotel or motel, this may be available on your laptop or your cell phone, but as a back-up bring hard copies with you too. Like we have suggested before, try and stay as close to the place of your interview if that is safe and affordable.

3. Bring multiple hard copies of your CV with updates (if any); just in case someone asks you for an additional copy. You can have it handy. If expense is an issue, bring at least one copy. You may be able to make additional copies in the residency training program office.

4. If you live in an interesting city you may want to consider and bring some brochures from that city in case someone asks for one. If they do and you have already brought few with you, you will earn brownie points

5. Bring something to write on; this could be your iPad if you have one, or the a note section on your cell phone or a paper pad

6. Bring something to read

7. Bring something to snack on especially if you have restrictions with certain types of food e.g. you are vegetarian or you eat only kosher food.

8. Bring with you some basic over-the-counter medications such as acetaminophen, ibuprofen in case you get a headache, menstrual cramps or you twist your ankle on one of the stairs.

9. Some individuals are so nervous that they get diarrhea, if you are one of those, you may want to bring with you Imodium or a similar product.

**THE NRMP rank-list, how to rank programs?**

The National Resident Matching Program (NRMP) is an independent non-for-profit organization which functions to provide an impartial venue for matching applicants to their preferred residency programs and vice-versa. Each year approximately 16,000 US allopathic Medical school graduates and 20,000 so called "independent applicants" compete for the 25,000 positions available in various residency programs in the US. "Independent applicants" include former graduates of US allopathic Medical school who for one reason or another did not apply for the NRMP during their 4th year of medical school, graduates and former graduates of Osteopathic Medical Schools in the US, Canadian Medical School graduates, and graduates of International Medical Schools which are recognized by the World Health Organization as legitimate Medical schools. According to the data from the NRMP, in 2010, a total of 37,556 applicants participated in the Match. Of those 16,427 were graduates of US accredited Medical Schools and 21,129 were independent applicants. The NRMP also conducts matching for 38 fellowship programs in various sub-specialties. Remember, a fellowship is the additional training that some physicians undertake after they complete their residency program if they wish to become an expert in one specific field e.g. Adult Critical Care.

The matching process begins in mid-august of every year. That is when you apply to the NRMP for a position in a residency that starts July 1 of the next years.

You apply online by accessing the NRMP website at: www.NRMP.org as follows:

- Register and obtain an Identification (ID) number
- Enter your personal and professional information
- Agree to the terms and conditions of the match. What does that mean? The NRMP will verify all the information that an

applicant provides during the registration. If an applicants and a program match then it is legally binding, which means that you are obligated to join that particular program and the program is obligated to give you the position for July 1, of that cycle.

- Pay the fees: The only method of payment acceptable to NRMP is credit card (VISA or MasterCard) and "Telepayment". Other methods of payment are not acceptable. So, you need to have a credit card or pay by "Telepayment". Checks and cash are not acceptable methods of payment. If for one reason or another you do not have a credit card then you need to plan ahead to pay the fees, otherwise you may not be able to participate in the match.

- In mid-January of the following year, the ranking list opens and remains open until mid-February.

- Neither the program nor the applicant should give a commitment to the other party with regard to how they will rank each other on the rank list. Either the program or the applicant can show a great deal of interest, but the final commitment is revealed only on the match day.

- The final result of the match will be available to the residency program directors and applicants on the match day which is usually in mid-March for a position on July 1st.

## How to rank the programs of your choice?

- Select about 5-10 programs that you believe you would be a competitive applicant for, based on your USMLE scores, your medical school ranking nationally, your Medical School GPA, your research experience and publications, and how well your interview process went in a particular program. Often, you get a sense from the program director that a particular program is really interested in you. The program is allowed to show a great deal of interest in you and if it does, this should be one factor in deciding how to rank programs on your rank list.

- Once you have selected these 5-10 programs you would like to join, rank these programs in order of your preference.
- If you are applying to very competitive residency programs there are always the possibilities that you may not match to one of those competitive programs even if the program director has shown a great deal of interest in you. So you need to have a back-up plan.
- The back-up plan would be to apply to programs in other less competitive fields (in addition to your programs of first choice) that you are almost sure you will match with. This is important if you would like to make sure that you have a position (which is equivalent to having a job) on July 1st. The options are as follows: a Transitional year, Internal Medicine, Family Medicine, Pediatrics etc.
- The transitional year residency program (as the name implies) is for candidates who would like to start a residency in a field which requires one year of post-graduate training before joining the program such as radiology. If you don't match with your preferred program the first time, you do one year of residency in a transitional residency and apply again to your favorite field next year.
- If geographic location is important to you, then think about where you would like to spend the next 3-5 years of life going through a residency program. Is being close to family and friends more important to you, or it is more important to you to live in a beautiful and popular city for the next 3-5 years and you plan on visiting the family/friend on holidays?

**The NRMP results are in the Spring, where are you going ?**

North America is one the most beautiful parts of the world. The US consists of 50 states and the District of Columbia. Each state functions independently like a separate country, but there are Federal laws and regulations that unite these states. There are many beautiful and interesting cities that you can live in during your residency. It has been shown that 70% of graduates end up practicing medicine in the same geographical area where they completed their residency training programs. Therefore, it is imperative that you give this factor some thought when selecting a residency program.

If you are considering settling in a particular state following completion of your training, you may want to give consideration to the geographic location of the residency or fellowship you are considering. However, there are few important factors to consider when choosing a location or a State to conduct your residency or Fellowship training in. Some of the relevant factors are: Financial health of the state, taxation and climate. We will discuss each of these issues separately.

*Climate:* States that have a good climate attract more people from all walks of life, including people who hold full-time jobs and professionals who contribute to the growth of the state and the country. These states tend to be more densely populated and therefore, you are likely to come across more opportunities in your career. People are more likely to want to live in states which are characterized by a modest temperature all year around such as most places in the state of California. Some people prefer not to live in a places where the winter is very long and harsh such as Milwaukee, Wisconsin or Buffalo, New York, where the average temperature in the protracted winter months is around 24 degrees. Climate becomes more important as you get older and approach the age of retirement. You may not want to live in a state or city where the winter is very cold and harsh with several inches of snow most of the days of the protracted winter months. On the other hand you may be an avid skiers and may like this kind of climate. If you do that is great, then you may want to be in places where winter are cold and plenty of snow all winter to enjoy skiing. Sometimes, if you really want to get into a competitive residency training program and your choices are limited, you may have to sacrifice this issue and go ahead and accept a position wherever you are given the opportunity to conduct the residency of your dream, but the climate is not to your liking.

*Financial Health of the state:* The economy of the US is a dynamic one and economies of cities and states are constantly changing. There are numerous cities in the US that were affluent at some point in the past, but are now (in 2010) suffering from very high unemployment and are barely able to sustain themselves. The financial crisis of 2008 has left many states and cities in financial turmoil which is likely to continue into the distant future. This would translate into higher unemployment (which means there will be less insured people), poverty, higher crime rates, and inability to continue various programs including some related to health care. As of 2010, there are a number of states which are in "financial trouble". Take for example the state of Illinois; it was reported by pew's analysis that the state borrowed money to fund its pension program. California's economy is also in a state of disarray and it has been facing difficulties funding its programs. Others states in the Pew's report that were considered to have financial problems include: Florida, Arizona, Nevada, Michigan, New Jersey, Oregon, Rhode Island, and Wisconsin. These states along with California and Illinois are the top ten most troubled states financially. In addition to the overall financial health of states, there are financial issues that are directly related to health care and to you as a physician who will provide health care to patients in a particular state. There are a number of states (as of 2011) which are facing financial shortfalls when it comes to Medicare and Medicaid (the two major government-funded health insurance programs in the US). With the recent focus to control the spiraling costs of these health care programs and in an effort to restrain government spending, the result may be significant financial changes to these programs. However, the economic crisis of 2008 and the protracted recession has meant that more people have been and will be unemployed, which translates into more families applying for and needing Medicaid as their primary insurance. According to data published by Kaiser Family Foundation, Medicaid spending increased by close to 9% in most states in 2010, compared the projected spending of close to 6%. This was partly related to the ballooning of the number of families joining Medicaid as their primary insurance during the period of economic recession.

Some states may be affected more than others. For instance in September 2010, the state of Washington, announced that it will cut $ 113 million in Medicaid funding because of financial shortfalls. This significant cut was described by the Director of Medicaid in that state as "devastating". Due to significantly more enrollment the state of Kentucky Medicaid program is expected to face a budget shortfall of close to half a billion dollar in 2010 and for Arizona the figure is double of that of Kentucky. The state of Main still owes close to $ 400 million to those hospitals in the state which provide care to Medicaid patients. Louisiana cut Medicaid inpatient hospital reimbursement by 3.5% for 2009, has already cut this further by 12% in 2010, and is planning to cut an additional 4.5% in 2011. Hospitals likely to be affected the most by these financial issues and budget cuts are the so called "safety-net hospitals", hospitals which cater to the underprivileged population who have Medicaid as their primary insurance. In 2008 the American Recovery and Reinvestment Act included Federal Government funding to states of up to $ 87 billion to help with Medicaid payments from October 2008 through the end of 2010. The main purpose of this funding was to boost the so called "Federal Medical Assistance Percentage", a program which boosts the Federal Medicaid Matching rate for states. In August 2010, Congress passed a legislation which will provide $ 16 billion dollar in additional funding to this program which is likely to continue through June 2011. June is the end of the fiscal year for most states and it is not clear what will happen then. There is increased demand for Medicaid as the economic recovery has been slow and states are strapped for cash.

Another issue is that new federal funding will become available in 2014, when the new health care reform rules is likely to be fully enforced. It is not clear how these funds will be disbursed, but will likely be either through direct payments to Medicaid or through subsidies to state administered health insurance exchanges. However, during the same year "safety-net hospitals" may begin to see cuts in Medicare Disproportionate share payments, which helps these hospital with the costs involved in treating the uninsured or underinsured patients. With the new health care reform most people will have some form of insurance; but it is projected that about half of the currently uninsured patient will have Medicaid, which means that significant financial cuts could have adverse effects on those hospitals which serve these patients. So, whether you are applying for your residency, Fellowship or a new job following your graduation, these financial issues are relevant to you and you may want to ask appropriate questions related to the health care reform, Medicaid, and Medicare. Is the hospital you are applying to is a safety-net hospital? What are the implications for you and your future?

*Taxes:* which include property taxes, sales taxes, city and local taxes will take a significant chunk out of your income and are therefore important in your life, particularly when you start going into practice and become a high-earner as an independent physician. New Jersey, for instance has the highest property taxes. The problem with property taxes is that as you graduate and your income goes up, the tax benefits that you receive from paying property taxes phases out according to the Internal Revenue Service (IRS) rules. You probably have heard that it is a good idea to own a big and nice house because you can ride off the interest you pay to your lender (for your mortgage) and the property taxes you pay to your city. It is true that the interest rate you pay to your mortgage company is fully deductible to you, but the property taxes you pay are not fully deductible. This is because the tax benefits from paying property taxes phase out as your income increases and for most physicians only a small portion of what you pay is deductible.

States with the highest tax burden following New Jersey are New York (it has been reported that it is probably in the top 5 in terms of per capita tax burden), Connecticut, Ohio, Maryland, Hawaii, California, Wisconsin, Rhode Island, District of Columbia, and Vermont.

For instance, Ohio may not be desirable to some because the climate is harsh with very protracted, cold and long winters with the average temperature of 24 degree Fahrenheit in Cleveland, has high unemployment rate, and a high tax burden. Massachusetts and Connecticut both have harsh and long winter months and very high tax burdens. In fact, Connecticut was reported to have the third highest tax burden after New York and New Jersey. Besides cost of living in the New England states, New York and New Jersey is very high. That is why you will notice that the stipend for Post-Graduate Year (PGY)-1 is much higher in programs located in one of these states compared to states located in the Midwest and the southern states of the Union, because of significantly higher cost of living.

The shifting demographics in the US will make this issue more and more important in the next decade or two (as of 2010). You have heard of baby boomers, generation X, and generation Y. Who are they and what do they mean to you as a physician who has to provide care to people and at the same hoping to make a decent living?

1957 through 1964 was a period of peak birth in the US, when the live birth exceeded 4 million babies per year. Those who were born during this period and who are now in their 50s and early 60s are called the baby boomers. Meanwhile, the Bureau of Labor and statistics of the US has suggests that the peak age for productivity is around 50 years of age, when our income and consumption is at its highest. It is logical that the Internal Revenue Service (IRS) depends heavily on this age group (45-55) for its major source of revenues, the taxes!. The same would follow for states which depend on sales taxes and other consumption taxes, and the local municipalities which depend on property tax revenues from large number and size of properties by these large numbers of baby boomers. Therefore, the current years (around 2010) have been the most productive tax-paying years in a generation for federal, state, and local governments. We are probably, as a nation, lucky that the financial crisis of 2008 coincided with the most productive tax-paying years, when the large numbers of baby boomers were here to pay the taxes into the system and bail the nation out. As the baby boomer age out of their prime and most productive years and the tax revenues that are generated from them decline, the next generation; generation X will have to carry the torch. But will they be up to the challenge?

Generation X, are those individuals born between 1965 and 1984 and are now in their mid-twenties to mid-forties. They were born during a period when there was a low fertility in the US compared to the previous generation and accordingly generation X is smaller than the baby boomer generation. As a result, generation X does not have the critical mass of the baby boomers because this generation is at least 9 million smaller than the baby boomer generation. Accordingly generation X does not have the same ability to produce and consume and pay taxes at the same level as the baby boomers did. Federal, State, and local taxes will fall in the next 10-20 years. States which are strapped for cash are likely to be affected the most and states which have high taxes will probably continue to have high taxes and the taxes in these states may actually increase to close the gap. The various programs including some are related to health care delivery may have to be closed. This may mean less for your bottom line as a provider of health care in these states.

Other issues

*Does that mean you should not consider joining a residency or fellowship program in one of these states?* NO.

Each individual has to consider her/his criteria when applying for and selecting a residency program. The issues of climate, fiscal health of the state or the tax burden may not be as important to you, but it is brought up in this section of the book for you to think about these issues as factors in selecting a residency program. For example, data published in 2014 by the Mercatus Center of George Mason University showed that

Alaska and the Dakotas were the healthiest states financially, but some people may not want to live in these states because of their climates. There is a positive aspect to the changing demographics in the US, which have positive implication for the future. First, there are millions of Latino-Hispanics who have come and continue to come to this country to fill unskilled jobs. A significant number of them are in the same age group as generation X. If they advance economically in the next 10 years, they could fill the gap created by the lower mass (compared to the baby boomers) of generation X. Second, data published by Pew Research Institute show that African-Americans as a group have made significant economic advances and if this continues, their economic success could be a source for local, state, and federal government revenues in the future. And lastly, a very high percentage of Generation Y (born between 1984 and 2004) are unemployed and are embarking on establishing their own businesses. Small businesses are the back-bone of US economy and if these businesses succeed it could have significantly positive ramifications for the US economy in the future.

## Preparing for or enhancing your career

### Learn and acquire good habits early in your career, it is one of recipes for success:

#### Communicate effectively with people around you:

When talking to people around you be polite, concise and use proper language. Thomas Jefferson once said "it is a crime to say something in two words if it can be said in one word". Get your message across with minimum words. Avoid use of profanity, shouting or throwing tantrums every time *everything* does not go your way. Because of the advent of Health Insurance Portability and Accountability Act (HIPPA), you should not discuss any patient-related matter in public places in a manner that can be heard by others.

Apply the same principles with the use of various electronic methods of communications such as cell phone, text messaging, and email. Do not use the hospital or clinic email for personal purposes. You should have our own private email account for personal purposes. Avoid sending outrageous texts and emails to colleagues or patients. Also, be careful with what you put on your Facebook .

**Avoid Tardiness:**

Attending clinics, conferences, and meetings are part of your life as a physician. When you are on time, you are sending a message to the others that you care; you respect their time and you are eager to be there. Consistent tardiness suggests otherwise. Arriving late once in a while is understandable, but if you are a perpetual late arrival, it suggests your lack of desire to be there. If you are always late to a certain function, you may want to explain that to other people involved at some point, why you are always late.

**Be productive:**

When you are at work whether you are a resident, a fellow or a full-fledge physician you are there to serve a purpose. Therefore, refrain from using the time you are there towards your personal needs such as making personal phone call, sending and receiving personal emails or texts. These are very distracting habits; they interfere with education if you are still in training and with your work: seeing and caring for patients if you are an attending physicians. It may also interfere with other activities such as teaching or conducting research.

**It is difficult to get a hold of you!**

When you are unavailable when needed, it demonstrates utter disregard to your patients and your colleagues. Common examples are turning your cell phone or your pager off. It is acceptable to turn them off after an on-call night to catch up on some sleep, but if you decided to do that, make sure you leave your pager or cell phone on vibrate and keep them away from you (while you are sleeping) so that if someone would like to reach you for an important issue she/he may either leave a message, a text or a phone number for you to respond at a later time. As physicians we deal with human-beings who are facing a crisis because they are ill. Your colleagues, may have an important question to ask you about an important issue regarding a patient and therefore, it is imperative that you return their call as soon as practical. When you go into practice other hospital departments, a colleague who is taking over the call from you, or one of your patients may have a question, again, it is imperative that you return the calls within a reasonable period of time.

**Omnipotent:**

*You are not!* This is the opposite of "not available". Some physicians work very long hours accepting responsibilities without questions. They are everywhere all the time. It has been clearly demonstrated that extended hours of continuous work (> 24 hours) has negative effects on the performance of physicians and their ability to deliver high-quality care to their patients. Residents and fellows particularly in high acuity fields are susceptible to this pattern. To protect against this pattern of practice the Accreditation Council on Graduate Medical Education (ACGME) has restricted the total weekly hours worked by residents to 80 hours per week averaged over a 4-week period. Furthermore, a new amendment to this guideline took effect in July 2010, in which first-year residents can work continuously for only 16 hours and with more close supervision. At this time, there are no rules or regulations for restricting to the total number of hours worked by attending physicians, however, if you are an attending physician, you may want to apply some principles that are conducive to your wellbeing and to providing quality care for you patients: get your job done and go to your home and your family, get enough rest and sleep between calls and if you need help do ask a colleague to help you out. Otherwise continuous pattern of long-hours of work will lead to the next issue which is:

**Burnout.**

*How does burnout manifests itself?*

The majority of physicians who are experiencing burnout may exhibit any of the symptoms below for an extended period of time. However, physician burnout may reveal itself in the interactions of the physician with patients; this may take different forms including violation of boundary between the physician and her/his patients, which may include having a relationship with a patient (sexual or otherwise), breach of patient confidentiality through discussion of patients' issue in the hallways, in physicians' lounge or in other public places, prescribing for self and/or divulging personal information. Burnout also may affect physician's professional performance such as showing less or no empathy towards patients or their families, substance abuse and even suicide. Substance abuse and suicide account for demise of up to 700 physicians annually in the US.

**Be patient with your career:**

Early in your career while you are still a resident or a fellow, you have to learn to adjust to your environment and adapt to it. It is emotionally and financially draining to have to change residency or fellowship programs. If you have a family with children it will affect them emotionally too if you spend only a year or two in one city and then you are on the move to another city because you disliked certain people in the program, you do not like the patient population or the hospital or the city. You should have evaluated these issues during your application process (see pervious chapters), your interview and when you were making a decision about ranking your programs on the **NRMP**. If you decide to move, you may have to spend up to 6-9 months searching for programs and applying and interviewing, all of which are financially and emotionally draining. Apply the same principles following your graduation when you get a real job.

## Best ways to have more energy throughout the day

Despite the 80-hour/week limitations for residents and fellows, the residency and fellowship are very demanding times. You can always use some means that will increase your energy level so that you can function well, learn a lot and graduate with success. As of 2014, following graduation from residency and/or fellowship, there are not weekly limitations to the number of hours you work. You may have to work harder in the first few years in order to establish yourself in the institution or the practice group you join. Here are some tips on how to increase your energy level as a health care provider:

### Have a breakfast of Champions:

In order to get your first energy boost of the day, make sure you eat something early in the morning. Studies have shown that breakfast-eaters enjoy more energy and stay in a better mood throughout the day than their breakfast-skipping counterparts. But we are not talking just any breakfast. Make sure that the breakfast that you eat has a good mix of high quality carbohydrate, lean protein and healthy fats. Egg white is an excellent source of protein. Each egg provides about 6 grams of quality protein. Combined with a bowl of oatmeal with some nuts and a side of fruit such as berries should provide you with the excellent level of energy you need for your day. Try to avoid refined sugar. They may give you energy immediately, but two hours later you may be looking for a couch for a nap. No wonder many physicians fall asleep during rounds and educational sessions.

**Get small hits of caffeine to get you going after a call night:**

Instead of drinking one giant cup of coffee in the morning, drink smaller amounts, let us say 4 Oz every few hours to get you going. Studies suggest that low doses of caffeine throughout the day are more effective than the traditional large cup in the morning. Researchers found that shift workers, medical residents, truck drivers, and others who work odd hours not only got a better boost from caffeine when they drank it in small portions, but they also performed better on cognitive tests. You may read more on this topic at Health.com

**To find the energy to deal with conflicts at work be kind to others**

Yes, and that includes telling the truth to everyone the way it is. Making up stories, even if you consider them "white lies" takes more psychic energy than simply telling it like it is.

When you withhold information and you are not forthcoming, you're constantly thinking about what you're saying and how you're saying it in order to avoid "blowing" your cover. However, how you deliver the information is important too!, try your best not to unload your honest thoughts in a harsh way. Try wrapping the truth in something positive. For example instead of telling a physician who is junior to you or a nurse "your idea is terrible", you could say something like "you always have great ideas, but I do not believe this one works in this situation".

**de-clutter your surroundings?**

Cluttering could be at your place of work (your cubicle, your desk or your office) or at home. Physicians are always busy, and often are short on time to make their surroundings tidy. Cluttering can give you a sense of helplessness and may be a great drag on your daily energy. Most of what ends up as clutter are tasks that we have not finished or obligations that we have not been able to meet and who wants to be in a space where there are constant reminders of issues you should be doing or aspiring to completing; To deal with this issue, do some mind mapping to get yourself motivated to completing these tasks. Write down words that describe your goals. Examples: "I want to organize the office so that it is presentable to my colleagues". I want to clean the basement so that I can invite friends over for the 4th of July party". Make clips of these statements and stick them on your PC or your refrigerator.

**Try and change your daily routine often**

Doing the same thing over and over can get boring and can drag you down. When you switch things around, dopamine is released in the brain which prepares the body for actions. When you are constantly changing your routine, the brain perceives it as if something new and a you get an opportunity to learn something new. It gives you energy and gets you going. This is likely to occur even when you make simple changes in your life. Such as taking the train, or the bus to work instead of driving, or taking a different route to work if you are driving. Other examples are trading swimming for jogging or soccer for basketball in your spare time and so son and so forth.

**Turn your emotions into positive energy**

Which means, substituting the thoughts of what you have in your life for thoughts of what are missing from your life. Whenever you get into a bad mood, stop and ask yourself "what was I just thinking that put me into this bad mood?" focus on the problem and replace it with something positive and centered around your gratitude for what you have in your life. For instance, I am grateful that I am healthy and have a wonderful family. I am glad I had that argument with Dr. John Smith (who is not nice), It was a good reminder that I am not a door mat. This method of redirecting the energy will keep you from wasting your energy throughout the day.

**Sip on a cold drink to stay alert while you have to attend a long meeting**

This will keep you hydrated, which will put you in a good mood and gives you more energy. Obviously, water is always a good drink, but to get an extra boost you could make it an iced tea. The combination of caffeine and theanine in this beverage have been shown to be associated with alertness.

**If you get upset, do not forget to breath**

Most of us will have days when we get upset about an issue and that is fine, but do not stay worked up about it all day. That is just a waste of energy. Try and use the breathing technique recommended by Dr Andrew Weil (The Harvard trained physician who is a leader in holistic medicine) as follows:

Place the tip of your tongue against the ridge behind your upper teeth and exhale completely through your mouth so that you make a whoosh sound. Then close your mouth and inhale deeply through your nose for a count of 4, hold your breath for 7 counts, then exhale through your mouth for a count of 8; repeat three more times.

These deep breathing exercises (unlike the shallow breaths, which we tend to do when are
Stressed) allow more oxygen into your cells, slow your heart rate, lower your blood pressure, and improve circulation, ultimately

resulting in an energy boost. The trick is to let the belly expand with each inhale. Over time, this pattern of breathing improves many aspects of our physiology.

**To avoid an afternoon energy slump: Get moving, exercise and stay hydrated**

The more active you are, the better your circulation is. And the better your circulation is, the easier it is for blood to transport oxygen and nutrients to your muscles and brain. So go for a walk. If the weather conditions does not allow you to go outside, walk or run up and down a few flights of stairs. A brisk, 10-minute walk is enough to boost your energy level for up to two hours, according to research from California State University. Where dehydration goes, fatigue follows. But staying hydrated involves more than drinking lots of water. You also need potassium. To stay hydrated, besides drinking water and eating water-based fruits and vegetables throughout the day, aim for at least one serving of a potassium-rich food or drink -- such as avocado, coconut water, banana, and white potato (unless you have renal failure, in which case you should consult your physician).

**You still do not have enough energy: Fake it!**

Put on a nice smile even if it is fake! If you are a female put on some bright lipstick. Wear an outfit that is clean and crisp instead of scrubs. It has been shown that if you fake energy until you feel it, soon your brain and body will catch on. Research also suggests that simply smiling, for instance, releases endorphins and boosts serotonin, which actually lead you to feel the emotion you are projecting.

## How to be a successful leader

### How to motivate people around you when you are a leader?

As you move into a new role, from being a medical student to a resident (or you may be given the task of being a chief resident) or a fellow to becoming an attending physician it is inevitable that you will have some people who support what you are trying to do, some who resist it and some who will sit on the sidelines and watch what you are trying to accomplish. Let us label these three types of individuals as *contributors, detractors, and watchers* respectively. Let us discuss some of the ways to deal with each one of these in a constructive fashion so that your efforts are rewarded and your goals and objectives are more likely to come to fruition.

**Contributors:**

Contributors are individuals who would like to contribute to your progress. They share your vision and have been working for change. Often contributors are relatively new to the organization and therefore they see that there is more to gain by going forward with new leaders than by holding on to old ideas.

**Detractors:**

Detractors are people who have been in a position for a long time in an organization. They fear that major changes may have negative consequences on themselves and/or their allies and therefore, they tend to be comfortable with the status quo.

**Watchers:**

Are on the fence and are generally the silent-majority. Note that people with high levels of personal or resource-based power have a bias to resist change, because they have more to lose than to gain from any major changes in an organization. It is not always true, but often you will have to be careful in dealing with this group and with individuals within this group. Here are some steps that you can take to get them off the fence and move them into your camp:

Move every influencer one step at a time in the right direction. Do not try to turn detractors into contributors too quickly or in one step, do it gradually

In general, start by turning your contributors into team leaders, then move the convincible watchers into contributors, and get the detractors out of the way.

Actively change the balance of consequences and make it less risky and more rewarding to follow you, while at the same time more risky and less rewarding to resist your vision.

Increase positive consequences of good behaviors and increase negative consequences of bad behaviors.

Additional steps that you may take to lubricate the wheels to get the team moving in the right direction include:

Change the balance of incentives including recognition and rewards to support the desired culture in light of the context and make sure that everyone understands the changed balance of consequences.

. You can also change the organization and/or resource allocation to support the desired culture in light of the context.

For example, you can handle someone who is resisting change by moving him/her from leading a big team to working as a solo practitioner. In this way his/her impact is minimized. Over time, this person may choose to go along with the change and if he/she does not, you can remove them with minimal disruption.

Always drive your message by setting up action-forcing events such as regular meetings, updates and when you achieve something call it a milestone. Additionally, leverage small commitments into larger ones, most likely starting with contributors who step up and then expand the issues to convincible watchers.

Many leaders simply hope that people will eventually move in the right direction. Hope alone will not get the job done. Actively manage the people and you will see better results.

**Personalities of Leaders:**
**Are you an "Introvert" or an "extrovert"?**

Extroverts thrive on constant stimulation, being the in the spot light and just being a "bull" and they demand to be the center of attention. Introverts on the hand feel more comfortable in an environment of serenity and quiescence. They can think and reflect better being in a quiet environment. Most people think of a "leader" as someone who is dominant, outgoing, who stands up and speaks out, gives orders and makes plans. These are the traits of an extrovert. For a long time people have believed that extroverts, make leaders or that extroverts make better leaders than introverts. However, most recent research from Wharton College of Business, Harvard School of business and the University of North Carolina, suggest that this assumption may not be true and that the personality of a good leader depend s on the type of people they are leading. For instance if you pair subordinates who like to speak out and want their opinions heard and who take initiatives with an extrovert leader, it can lead to conflicts with an extrovert leader who wants to be the center of attention and who may feel threatened by the proactive nature of such employees or subordinates. On the other hand these same subordinates or employees may thrive under the leadership of an introvert leader who does not command to be the center of attention and is willing to listen and reflect on the suggestions of her/his subordinates. The tendency is for people to believe that as a leader you need to be always excited, talkative, and constantly motivating your subordinates or employees to "get them on board" on issues, but research shows that there is also a lot of wisdom in (an introvert leader) in being quiet and reserved in order to give the employees or subordinates some breathing room to enter the dialogue, share their ideas and show their creativity. Prominent examples of introverts are Bill Gates of Microsoft and President Obama. Even Albert Einstein is believed to have been an introvert. It has been said that introverts have been taught over the years "to fake it" so that they are accepted by the main stream. So, if you are that quiet person (introvert) and find yourself surrounded by a sea of extroverts, find yourself a quiet place and reflect on what is inside you and you are likely to be a good leader, as good as an extrovert!.

## How to be an efficient perfectionist!

We as physicians have this relentless desire to appear skilled, and to be competent in everything we do, day in and day out. It is a human nature to want to avoid appearing clumsy or out of depth with any issue because we are trying to avoid feeling embarrassed. After all, which human being does not want to appear to others that she/he is intelligent, musically talented, or athletic. However, we as physicians often insist that we have to excel at everything we try, partly because of the perception by many of us that if we are not trying our best, then we are agreeing to lower the bar or even worst we may be perceived as lazy.

If you take a step back and think about it, you will promptly recognize that trying to do everything very well may leave you feeling stressed and exhausted all the time, and as though you never get to work on what is most meaningful to you. You do know that there are time and resource constraints. However, some of us physicians often forget these constraints and forge ahead when we are operating on cruise control, but only to realize that we ran out of time at the end of the day, week or month with a still-long to-do list while wondering what just happened. In other words, you have to actively and regularly remind yourself that you have both limited time and resources.

Therefore, it would be prudent to step back and ask yourself an important "What do I want to do with my life and what do I want my life to stand for?" pick your fights and build strategies about when to give your complete and best efforts rather than waste these exceptional efforts on less important issues in life. Consider the following strategy:

1. Your "A list" tasks: pick few items that are most important to you and consider them the tasks that you would like to excel at. These are the tasks that will leave you most satisfied and for which you would like to give your 100% effort all the time. Then create

2. Your "B list": These are aspects of your profession to which you would not give 100%, but let us say 75% of your best efforts. These are the tasks that are likely to turn out fine, even if you did not complete them in a flawless manner.

3. The "C list": These are the tasks that you could perform with an average performance. These are tasks you can complete as efficiently as possible and then move on to more pressing issues. In other words, sometimes it is more effective to "lower the bar." And finally, are there tasks that are time-consuming but that, in reality, don't matter to your career or your life? You may refer to these as the D tasks. These endeavors do not give you any satisfaction once you complete them, nor do they garner you any recognition when finished. However, to this point, you have assumed that you still needed to work hard at them. The point to recognize is that you as a physician have a busy life, (both professionally and in your private life) and you have limited time, energy and resources. Be strategic about where to excel and devote the lion's share of your efforts. Redistributing time and attention from less important, less valued tasks to more important ones will pay off!

## Speeding tickets/Traffic violations

Physicians lead a busy life (whether you are still a resident or a fellow or already in practice your schedule is usually very busy), but they are also highly intellectual and some have big egos. Because of the latter two factors, often they are determined to fight a speed ticket, sometimes driven by the way the ticket was issued, or the way they were treated by the police officer writing the ticket. However, the question is, is it worth your valuable time and effort to fight a ticket. We present this topic in this section of the book because with your busy schedule as a medical student or a resident, you are likely to have an encounter with the police because of traffic violation.

*What have been driving lately?*

**Does the type of care you drive when it comes to how many traffic violation tickets you get?**

It appears that the type of vehicle you drive does have an impact on the number of traffic violation tickets you are likely to receive. Quality planning is an analytic company that collaborates with auto insurance companies to compile data on the relationship between the type of vehicle and traffic tickets. The results are expressed as the number of violations issued for each 100,000 miles driven. Here is a list of the vehicles which have the highest rate of traffic violation tickets per 100,000 miles driven and then expressed as a percentage of the average vehicle:

| Car type | % violation | average driver age | % Male |
|---|---|---|---|
| Volkswagen GTI | 178% | 40 | 44 |
| Mercedes-Benz CLK 63 | 179% | 47 | 44 |
| Pontiac Grand Prix | 182% | 40 | 41 |

| | | | |
|---|---|---|---|
| Acura Integra Coupe | 185% | 33 | 60 |
| Mercedes-Benz CLS-63 | 264% | 46 | 48 |
| XB Hatchback | 270% | 37 | 40 |
| Hummer H2/H3 SUV | 290% | 46 | 73 |
| Scion TC Coupe | 340% | 30 | 40 |
| Toyota Camry-Solara Coupe | 350% | 50 | 40 |
| Mercedes-Benz SL-Class Convertible | 400% | 53 | 40 |

Vehicles with the least traffic violation tickets include the following:

1. Buick Ranier SUV
2. Mazda Tribute SUV
3. Chevrolet C/K 3500/2500
4. Kia Spectra sedan
5. Buick Lacrosse sedan

**States and traffic tickets:**

When it comes to traffic violation tickets, it does matter where you live or where you drive. You may be driving in one of these states or cities for an interview for residency/fellowship or for a new job following completion of your training. It would be very anxiety-provoking to get a traffic violation ticket on your way to such an important interview. The information we discuss in this section may be helpful to you in lowering your chances of getting a traffic- violation ticket.

Here is the list of cities/states and the pattern of traffic violation tickets:

Los Angeles, California:
Most of the speeding tickets are issued for drivers driving on bou-levards where the speed .limit could be as low as 35 or 40 miles per

hour. If you are caught driving above the speed limit, the fines are considerable and it is very difficult to fight speeding tickets in the LA courts. The city has financial problems (as of 2011, but improving as of Jan 2014), and therefore, any extra cash comes in handy for the city's budget. So, your best bet is to hope that you will never get a speeding ticket, but if you do, it is probably not worth your valuable time as a physician to waste the time trying to fight it in LA courts.

Chicago, Illinois:
The city of Chicago uses cameras to document motorists driving above the speed limit or driving through a red light. This is likely to increase the city's ticketing power, because the camera may catch you even if the light is orange as you approach the traffic light and by the time you are just past the light, the light may have turned red and "you are caught running a red light". The problem is that most of the traffic lights are very old and the original studies that were done to determine the safe speed limits based on engineering data are close to 20 years old. Another interesting piece of information that the CNBC financial channel reported in 2011 is that the speed limit in some locals are determined by politicians and not engineering data and that often a short strip before, entering a high way is " a speed trap" for motorists. So, in some areas of Chicago, be careful to observe speed limits particularly in zones that are low speed limits, but which lead to a high speed boulevard or a highway.

The great State of Texas:
They say "everything in Texas is big" and so are the traffic tickets. Some drivers describe Texas as the "Police State". However, it appears that in some locals documentation of traffic violation may be poor. One driver in Texas had to undergo a driving education course in order to eliminate a speeding ticket. She reported further, that about a year later she was contacted by the traffic department and was informed that the speeding ticket that was issued a year earlier (which

was supposed to have been eliminated because she took the driving education course stated above) was now a warrant i.e. there was a warrant for her arrest. Luckily when she received the notice, she had the documentation for the courses she had successfully completed to eliminate the ticket. The top cities in Texas that are considered worst cities to receive a traffic ticket are: Austin, Dallas, and Houston.

Austin (the capital city), Texas:
The capital city like most other cities in Texas can enforce local laws and not follow federal and state laws (usually for driving > 5 miles above the speed limit). This is how the city can "get the drivers" who may be driving few miles above the "speed limit" in a school zone, or less than 5 miles above speed limit on other areas. The northern and southern ends of the city are particularly notorious for the drivers to get speeding tickets. So, if you happened to be driving in Austin, Texas you may want to be extra careful when you are driving in these zones.

Dallas, Texas:
Like other cities in Texas, they may elect not to follow federal and state standards and instead have their own local laws. What is unique about this area of Texas is that the speed limit on the same highway may changes 2 -3 times. Most highways in the US have a set speed limit e.g. 65 mph, or 70 mph, but in Dallas, this may not be the case. So, when you are driving in this region of Texas pay extra attention to changing speed limits in a highway or other streets. This is particularly important because they may issue you a ticket for going few miles over the limit. Whereas in most other parts of the country, it is uncommon for the police to issue you a speeding ticket unless you were driving > 5 mph over the speed limit. Another criticism of the city is that the speed limit may be changed based on the opinion of a city council member instead of relying on traffic engineering and/or law enforcement officers. This is partly because of shortage of traffic engineers in these locals.

Houston, Texas:

Drivers' note on Speedtrap.org that there are traps set at the Houston city limits and near attractions like the Astrodome, and the speed limit can change rapidly and dramatically (as we discussed above in Dallas). One motorist wrote that entering the city on Highway 59 North, the speed limit dropped suddenly to 55 from 70. Just as the motorist noticed the speed-limit change on his GPS, BAM! There was a speed trap. The number of tickets was even more staggering when the economy got bad in 2008. One of the local TV stations in the Houston area (KTRK Channel 13) reported in March 2010 that Houston police officers wrote about 3,000 tickets per day, or 147 an hour.

Florida:

Florida is *the state* where drivers are most likely to receive a speeding ticket. You are more likely to get a ticket when you are on vacation and in an environment that you are not familiar with. One driver remembers getting a ticket for "going through a stop sign" at night. When he went back to the intersection the next day, there wasn't exactly a clear stop sign. Experts in the field have also stated that Florida street signs do not meet even Florida state standards in terms of size and locations.

Jacksonville, Florida:

Jacksonville, in particular, is known for speed traps where multiple drivers are pulled over at once, often by unmarked police cars, and motorists can be charged for going 5 mph over the limit, partly because of the limitation of signs mentioned above.

Orlando, Florida:

Orlando, home of Disney World and Universal Studios and Sea World, benefits from a steady stream of tourists and revenues from speeding tickets. Orlando definitely has speed traps. Some of the worst ones are Colonial Drive (State Route 50), where the speed limit constantly changes, the Beach line (State Route 528) as motorists drive west from the airport (That's right, they get you straight from the airport!) and I-4, especially downtown near the Millennia Mall. In addition, Orlando was one of the early adopters for red-light cameras and it was using them even before state laws allowed them to. In the first three months of installation of these cameras they generated 700 tickets. The Orlando police are also very tough on motorists. One motorist noted on Speedtrap.org, that police officers on motorcycles often snag motorists in a short school zone for doing three to four miles over the speed limit.

Denver, Colorado:
Like some cities in Texas, Denver has "home rule," where cities do not have to comply with state laws. A local TV station (7News at ABC affiliate KMGH) has reported that officers will even wait for drivers riding in the exit lane who dart back into other lanes at the last minute, and nab them for crossing a white line!.

Springs Lakes, Colorado:
Colorado Springs takes full advantage of the "home rule," where municipalities do not have to follow state laws, However, unlike other cities, Springs Lakes does clearly disclose that drivers will be penalized if they drive 1-4 miles over the speed limit. They also state that "one's intent is irrelevant," which means they don't care if you didn't mean to speed; you had to speed because you had an emergency case at the hospital, had a broken speedometer or have oversized tires. Drivers write on Speedtrap.org that often police use unmarked vehicles to catch drivers who may be speeding and like Denver, wide roads are often slapped with a 25 mph limit and entering the city from the southeast, one motorist notes, the speed limit drops quickly from 55 to 25.

Las Vegas, Nevada:
Speed traps are common on the highways heading into and out of Las Vegas. The Department of Transportation records indicate that the

traffic could handle 80 mph but a 70 mph zone is strictly enforced. Even side streets have traffic stops, one motorist noted on Speedtrap.org. It has also been reported that anytime there's a budget crisis, the number of tickets written out seems to go up and your chances of successfully fighting them are slim when the city is still struggling financially.

You may find more information about traffic tickets for other cities in the US at www.speedtrap.org

## Contract Negotiation

**Not it's not too early; you need to learn about contract negotiation early in your career!**

**If you have decided that you would like to be employed (and most physicians will be initially employed), here are some tips on how to negotiate your contract:**

A contract has multiple components including hours of work, call schedule, compensation and benefits, vacations and many other issues. However, the primary component that is often negotiated the most is the salary. The employer wants to pay less and the employee, in this case you the physician, wants to get paid more.

Unfortunately most physicians do not have the training in the art of negotiation and few have the innate skills in this art. If you negotiate harder, it may result in more pay, less call nights or weekend calls, which may be conducive to better job satisfaction. Since most physicians are not good at negotiating this critical element of their career, you will have to try your best to identify your prospective employer's negotiation techniques because this may provide you with the insight to succeed in the negotiation. Here we discuss some tips you can apply to accomplish these goals. First listen to what the employer has to offer, often the offer in its initial stages is verbal and not in writing. Then analyze the offer by talking to friends and colleagues, doing research on the subject and then make a counter offer.

Example: You are negotiating a contract to work as a critical care physician for a pediatric institution. During your interview the discussion of salary came up and you were told that the annual salary ranges from $ 180,000.00 to $ 200,000.00 . You feel that you have few years of experience and that your salary should be $ 200,000.00. The employer offers you $ 180,000.00. You respond by stating that you believe that with your experience you are worth $ 200,000.00. A week goes by and an administrator from your prospective employer calls you to follow up with the contract negotiation and he states that "we have looked at the MGMA survey for physician salaries and have discovered that the offer of $ 180,000.00 was based on the salary from a different state and that the appropriate salary for their state is closer to $ 170,000.00". You think about it for few hours and call the administrator back and state that you will take the offer at $ 180,000.00.

*What is happening here?*

Your prospective employer offered you $ 180,000.00 which you refused. Instead of increasing the offer, your potential employer lowered it to $ 170,000.00. In doing so the employer is forcing you to compare the $ 180,000.00 to $ 170,000.00 instead of comparing it to $ 200,000.00. If you decided to accept the offer at $ 180,000.00 you will feel that you are the winner because you will be making $ 10,000.00 more. Here is one analysis for this situation: your prospective employer is using a technique called "offer withdrawn".

*What should you do?*

So, now you recognize that your prospective employer is using a specific negotiation technique. Be calm and rational and give them a counteroffer.

You could say something like " Will you honor your initial offer of $ 180,000.00?" "I believe that with my experience, the market supports a salary of $ 180,000.00". This may force your prospective employer to come back with a reasonable counteroffer.

However, also recognize that your potential employer may be at a point very close to walking away from the table if they have other candidates. So, you may want to consider settling somewhere in between if there are other candidates (continue to read below). Also, remember that with this type of potential employer it is possible that they may put you in a "like-it-or-leave-it" situation too, again if they have other candidates.

*What else you can do in this situation?*

You could bring in other elements of the contract such as call nights, vacation days and other additional services that you will have to provide. In this case, let us say that it was stated in the contract that you will have to provide one day per month of sedation for pediatric patients who need diagnostic imaging. Many pediatric critical care programs offer sedation as an additional part of their service to the hospital. You could say something like "When I indicated that I will be willing to do one day per month of sedation, I assumed that I would receive additional 6 weekends off in return". Since these additional days of sedation will take my time away from my family, I will not be able to take the added work", I am sorry if I made the wrong assumption".

Another technique that is often used when negotiating a contract is the so called "Appeal-to-a-higher-authority". In this technique, the administrator that you are negotiating with, may say that he will have to run your contract by the Chief Executive Officer (CEO). This is a technique that you may have seen often used by car salesmen. Let us say that you are at a car dealership and you have offered $ 30,000.00 for a new 2012 Dodge Durango, but the salesman says he will not budge from $ 34,000.00. You go up on your offer to $31,000.00, but the salesman is not impressed. He says he would like to help and he is willing to speak with his boss. He goes into his boss' office and comes out mildly shaking his head and tells you that "The boss says he is not allowed to sell it for less than $ 34,000.00". You increase your offer to $ 32,000.00 and "BAM", the Durango is yours. The Sale's person was using the technique of "Appeal-to-a-higher-authority".

*What else was happening here?*

The salesman was also using the "good-cop-bad-cop" technique. In this case he is the good cop and he is negotiating with the bad cop, which in this case in his boss. The same thing could happen when you are negotiating your contract. The recruitment officer in the institution may say that that I will have to negotiate your contract with the CEO and see what she/he thinks.

In the case of the car salesman, another strategy that he was using was that he was trying to tire your out. And apparently time constraints (as most physicians are very busy all the time) and fatigue, perhaps led to frustrations on your part and made you concede. With this concession you gave him $ 3000.00 without getting anything in return. The same thing could happen to you with contract negotiation for employment. The lesson to learn from this example is, do not make a concession without receiving one. Make sure you are negotiating with a person who can receive and GIVE concessions. In the case of the car salesman you were negotiating with a person who can receive concession, but cannot give one. Therefore, next time remind the other party that you are aware of the "appeal-to-a-higher-authority" technique. You may even say "are you going to use this technique on me?". Next, you ask the person you are negotiating with "Are you able to negotiate this deal with me and sign a contract? if you are not able to do that I would like to speak with the person who can". This may include the CEO who makes the final decisions on a physician contract.

***Always make sure that you get a concession when you give one.***

*How can you use your own "appeal-to-a-higher-authority"?*

You can say something like "I would need some time to have my attorney look at my contract ".

Other negotiation techniques used by negotiators:

"Not-my-fault, Not-my-problem"

Sometimes when you are at a car dealership the salesperson will tell you, I cannot possibly sell this Durango for less than $ 35,000.00, I paid that much for it. What he/she is trying to do is to get you to accept his/her position as your own. She/he is saying that you would not sell something for less than what you paid for because it would not be fair. However, the real issue here is not how much the dealership paid for the car, but rather how much the Durango is worth. You could say something like "I am so sorry that you paid that much for this Durango, but I am willing to spend only $ 30,000.00".

When you are negotiating your contract, you could add in factors such as your experience, your previous salary, the extra amount of work and calls you will have to do, and any excess cost of living in the new location. You can include all these factors in your reasons behind the compensation and benefits you are asking. You could say something like "I made $ 170,000.00 at my previous position, this position calls for more responsibilities, longer hours, more weekend calls, and the cost of living is 20% higher compared to my previous location,… anything less than $185,000.00 would be a step backward for me".

*Cautions with the use of these techniques:*

Be careful not to let your prospective employer know your walk-away point, and do not mention any amount less than what you are willing to accept. Furthermore, this negotiation technique will work against you if you come across sounding as if you are trapped by a bad decision you have made in the past. In general, use this approach only when you are very close to your walk-away point and cannot give much more. Finally, be prepared to walk away.

"Can we split the difference?"

Experts advise against this approach, if you have made a concession and have not received one yet. In the case of the Durango, if the salesperson says "We are only $ 1000.00 apart, let us split it" you are really being offered a $500.00 concession for a $ 500.00 concession. If his offer is $ 33,000.00 and yours is $ 32,000.00, you can counter by saying "now we are only $ 500.00 apart, I could pay $ 32,250.00 for the Durango". The same would apply to the contract negotiation for employment.

There are many negotiation techniques in use today. Those presented here are among the most commonly used one. We hope that by reading this section will help you gain confidence, get better results and even have a little fun the next time you are in a situation that requires negotiation because successful negotiation often depends on recognizing the games other people are playing and how you will react to them.

Now that we have discussed some of the aspects of the art of negotiation, it is time to tackle some of the issues related to the actual contract that you will eventually sign. Take your time in doing so. Avoid, intentional tardiness and be honest with your prospective employer and tell them that you are looking at the offer and discussing it with your family.

In the early stages of contract negotiation the focus was on defining income, benefits, and working hours. However, you must also recognize the importance of other business-related stipulations because physician employment contract have been very complex and you will need to pay attention to every page and section of the contract. These include issues such as the exact date of start, termination clauses and non-compete agreements. For physicians who will be joining a medical group, partnership requirements are also important.

Restrictive covenants (where there is a clause in your contract that in the event that you depart you current employer, you will not be able to open a practice and compete with your current employer within a certain mile radius, usually 25-60 miles, from the current location of your employment) and conflict resolution procedures are becoming more physician friendly, but deserve the scrutiny of legal counsel. It may also be beneficial to seek the advice of an accountant in order to fully assess your and your potential employer's financial situation. The bottom line: physicians entering into employment contracts should seek the advice of qualified professionals.

Reviewing physician employment contracts is not an easy task and can be emotionally draining. However, physicians who do not take the time to understand the written contract could set themselves up for problems, which may lead to serious financial problems later on, particularly if the position does not work out or personal circumstances dictate a move.

We are not trying to suggest that prospective employers intend to put newly hired physicians in a disadvantageous position. Rather, it is that failing to fully understand contract terms' ramifications and engaging in what-if scenario planning could result in costly surprises later.

In real life sometimes, physicians take jobs that sound terrific but turn out to be not exactly as advertised. Health care contracts lawyers report that the most common reason physicians leave is workload, either unevenly distributed call duty or punishingly long work weeks for the new physician. Unfortunately, problematic contract provisions still apply, even when the physician has defensible, understandable reasons for leaving. There are many anecdotal reports about physicians where the physician said " I'll take this job even though it is not my dream job". I need to work to get the experience and in the process make money to pay my loans and bills and support my family". Then soon after she/he takes the job another opportunity opens up in the same city or a nearby city and now the physician feels that she/he is caught in a number of problematic situations because of the clauses in the contract ranging from covenant not to compete to termination clauses. Some experts advise that you should not take a job that you do not want.

A basic understanding of the main elements of employment contracts will help you, the physician (young or old), navigate through what is often a multipage document replete with legal terms.

It is true that that you will have an attorney go over your contract and provide you with an advice, however you have to be well informed so that you can be your own advocate. Here are some elements of a physician contract that you need to pay close attention to:

The physician employment contract should address the following issues:

- **What is your scope of work and your employment status:** These sections define a physician's status as independent contractor, employee, or shareholder. Although employers sometimes hesitate to include specifics about the scope of work because workload and patient volume are not always predictable, the contract should stipulate basic expectations and, in the case of specialists, should include estimates regarding numbers of procedures expected to be performed annually or the number of patients seen weekly or monthly.

  Employment status can affect both your tax burden (see the section: W2 or 1099) and potential liability in the event of a malpractice suit, so make sure you understand the difference between contractor and employee or shareholder status.

- **Covenant not to compete.** These "non-competition" agreements typically prevent a physician from working for a competitor located within a specific geographic area for a certain period of time; these covenants thus thwart a departing physician from "stealing" patients. The contract might state, for example, that the physician cannot practice medicine within a 10-mile radius (or up to 60 mile radius in rural areas) for a period of two years. Despite widespread physician opposition, these clauses continue to appear in many contracts. In some states these non-compete clauses are illegal while in other states they are enforceable only if deemed "reasonable". An attorney versed in the particular state's contract laws should review such clauses.

  *How flexible you should be?* The more specialized you are, the more geographically expanded you can expect the covenant to be. Experts also recommend talking to other physicians in your specialty and in the region to get a sense of the prevailing practices regarding covenants.

- **Compensation.** Generally, a physician's compensation is structured in one of three ways:
    - as a guaranteed annual sum or salary
    - as a variable amount based on "production" (usually calculated from billings or collections)
    - as some combination thereof

  If a production formula is used, the contract should provide specific details on how compensation is calculated, when you will be paid, and in what increments. Multiyear contracts should spell out the specifics of annual pay increases. The contract also should clearly delineate terms regarding any money you might be obligated to repay under certain conditions such as signing bonuses, loans, salary advances, or recruiting fees. Also, the contract should address total compensation, including malpractice premium payments; coverage for malpractice claims arising after you leave the practice; health, life, and disability benefits; and vacation policies. Production formulas can get complicated and take several factors into account. What is important than grasping the formula's intricate details is that you understand what your personal compensation will amount to from XYZ dollars in collections from patient care and procedures.

- **Work hours, schedule, and call duty (weekdays and weekends).** The contract should stipulate the maximum number of work hours each week or month and should define call-duty expectations. It also should address whether Continuing Medical Education (CME) can be acquired during work hours or must be completed on the physician's own time.

  Make sure the contract describes in meaningful detail the practice's approach to call duty and coverage for other physicians. For example, a contract that states "call days will be shared on a fair basis" is ambiguous. It is clearer when the contract states that "call days will be shared on a substantially equal basis."

- **Termination.** There are two basic types of termination provisions:

  - with cause" (with good reason) provision allows the employer to terminate the physician for reasons such as loss of hospital or prescribing privileges or inability to meet patient-care obligations.

  - without cause" provision enables the employer to terminate the contract with no stated reason by providing written notice in advance, which is typically from 30 to 180 days. Fair contracts allow the physician to do the same. In "without cause" terminations, the notice period should be long enough to allow the physician to secure other employment. If the physician is permitted to initiate a without-cause termination, he or she should make sure the termination clause does not conflict with the non-compete clause.

*What are some of the pitfalls that you should try and avoid?*

**Poorly or vaguely worded provisions in the contract can create problems down the road.**

Following completion of your residency or fellowship you may get an offer that looks like the perfect practice opportunity for you and you will be very tempted to sign the contract and start packing to move to that particular city. But remember as they say the "devil is in the details". The contract you sign today will dictate the professional and practical aspects of your life for the next several years. Therefore, it is of paramount importance that you read and review the contract thoroughly and have an attorney also review it for you (for a fee) so you do not leave out any issues that have the potential to turn this perfect offer to a bad deal few years later. Experts in this field provide the following advices on how to avoid some of the most common contract pitfalls:

- **Request a "letter of intent" before you receive a contract:** A "letter of intent " is a letter from prospective employer which outlines the fundamentals of the offer including: salary, your obligations as a physician towards the position and termination provisions. This can save time and unnecessary attorney fees. It also will ensure that whatever was agreed upon verbally ends up in the final contract. With a letter of intent, you can make sure you and your prospective employer are on the same page before a contract is drafted.
- **Always negotiate:** Do not be afraid of negotiating and do not worry about losing the offer if you do not sign the contract the way it is handed to you. Health care organization are very familiar with negotiation and in fact they expect you to

negotiate. By negotiating you set the tone and you do not sell yourself cheap. Remember, that this is a business proposal in which the prospective employer is hoping to make money for your services. Therefore, do not hesitate to ask for what you want, especially if you feel strongly about it.

- **Remember that most contracts are written in a way to fit everybody!** But as you have learned by now that medicine is such a vast field and a contract that written for a neurosurgeon is different than a one written for a psychiatrist. Therefore, make sure the contract reflects actual position offered to you and that applies to you. Make sure it contains the scope of work that applies to you and that it does not contain unreasonable provisions. For instance, a clause with regard to covenant not to compete that prevents a physicians from working within a 50 mile radius for two years following termination of a contract may be reasonable for rural areas, but it may not reasonable for a large metropolitan area. The same thing would apply for a subspecialty: remember the more specialized your are, the wider could be the radius of non-compete following termination of your contract.

- **Make sure the guaranteed compensation is adequate.** This implies that it is adequate both in terms of the annual salary and the length of the guaranteed salary. If you are starting a new practice it will take time for you to build a practice. Therefore, make sure the guaranteed salary is for a period of at least 2-3 years because the employer expects you to be able to support yourself or make money for them as soon as possible. The same thing would apply if you will be working shift work such as anesthesia shifts, emergency medicine or urgent care shifts: make sure that you will be given enough shifts per weeks to make enough money to pay the bills (unless you have other sources of income and you do not mind working less hours).

- **Look at the total compensation package.** That means you do not look at salary alone. What other benefits you will receive. Health, dental insurances, malpractice coverage, CME days off and CME stipends are obvious ones, but the more important ones are path to partnership (if you are employer by a medical group), profit sharing and retirement matching. These may amount to millions of dollars over your entire career. When it comes to the potential partnership, beware of nonspecific wording such as "the physician could become a partner at some point in the future". Make sure there are specific provisions on how and when you will become a partner in the practice. For example one provision could state that the price of a share in the partnership is $ 100,000.00 and that you could pay off this amount over 5 years and then you are a partner in the practice.
- **Do not accept a verbal offer or pack and move solely on the basis of a letter of intent.** Do not make a physical move before seeing and signing the actual contract. The contract may be unacceptable or worse, may not materialize at all.

There have recent developments in employment contracts which are both good news and bad news in these situations. The basic problems for the newly employed physician including, unreasonable restrictive covenants, unrealistic work hours and calls, higher expectations to perform, and difficult paths to partnership (for physicians employed by medial groups) still persist, some softening of the stance has also occurred. For example, the non-compete clauses are becoming more fair and representative of actual markets. There are now case laws where the physician prevailed and the employer lost in the issue of covenant not to compete. In some states it is illegal to include this clause in the contract. Furthermore, when a dispute arises, it is more common nowadays to go to the path of alternative dispute resolution instead of litigation. This tends to be more physician friendly and is less costly for both the employer and the employee. Also, today employers are drawing a much smaller radius when it comes to non-compete clause. This is partly because most prospective employers do their research and assess where they drive most of their patients from and then draw the line accordingly. Prospective physician employee could utilize the same strategy as they negotiate their contract.

Contract partnership buy-in provisions and terms continues to be a source of confusion for newly employed physicians. The main questions that must be answered are usually how much it costs to buy a partnership and after how long. Some of the arrangements make sense, and some are absolutely senseless, almost a disincentive to partnership. *Because of the long-term career importance of such deals, physicians eyeing a position with partnership potential should seek legal counsel early in contract evaluation.*

**What is the cost of leaving if you don't like your job? Could be a lot!**

Because of the changes in health care this area is getting sticky by the day. Each party (the employer and the employee) is trying to protect itself from financial losses. For example, if the employer offers a hefty bonus to a newly hired physician, but the physician decides to leave the practice after a short period, chances are the employer will want the bonus paid back.

Likewise, employers are looking to their new hired physicians to carry some of the liability burden, and the associated insurance costs. This is occurring in such areas as general liability for non-medically related incidents that occur or clinical staff actions, where employers are requiring new physicians to indemnify them against such claims and incur the associated coverage costs. You should avoid contracts that require you the physician to indemnify the employer from liability, by essentially forcing you to assume liability for and insure against situations beyond your control. If you see the word '*indemnification*' in an employment contract, you should bring that to the attention of your attorney and discuss it in details before signing a contract. This issue has also been surfacing in the malpractice "tail coverage". A malpractice "tail coverage", is the additional insurance that will cover you for any liability that may arise in the future for care you rendered in the past.

Malpractice premiums have been increasing exponentially over the past several years and employer do not want to pick up the whole tab. The "tail coverage" is expensive, sometime as high as three times the annual premium (unless you carry the same liability insurance for at least five years with some carriers). Consequently, when a new physician who was hired decides that she/he does not like the job and would like to pack and leave prematurely, the employer may refuse to pay for the "tail coverage".

*What are you options if this happens to you?*

Because the cost of tail insurance is going up, more employers are trying to shift the cost to you (the employed physician). There are multiple options on how to deal with this issue. One option is to divides the bill for the tail coverage in a range of ways depending on the circumstances. Some employer contracts state that if we fire you without cause, we will pay the tail, but if you quit, you pay the bill for the tail coverage, while others state (of course in complex legal language) that if we fire you for cause, you pay the bill for the tail.

A physician friend of ours went through this issue. He accepted a position following graduation and things were going well for him for several months, but then his wife developed a terminal illness and he decided to move back to be closer to his wife's family. The contract stated that he assume responsibility for tail insurance if he left before a specified period, but he paid scant attention to the clause. Although he left the practice on very good terms, he still had to pay the tail because he did not rd the clause carefully. This doesn't mean that you should not take a position that involves paying the tail insurance under certain conditions, but it's important to be prepared for that possibility and put money away after you get appropriate legal counsel.

Another issue is the "income guarantee" contract that is offered to an employed physician when she/he agrees to work and stay to serve a community for a specified number of years. For instance, the hospital may agree to pay the new physician an annual salary of $ 240,000.00 (that would be $ 20,000.00 a month) plus benefits. Let us assume that the practice generates only $ 16,000.00 a month. What is happening here is that the hospital is giving the new physician a monthly loan of $ 4000.00 (plus whatever the costs of benefits are). If the physicians stays in the community for several years and her/his practice gets busy, then the hospital may eventually make money. However, if the physician decides to leave the community after 2 years, the hospital will lose money. In this case the hospital may demand or sue the physician to pay the difference in monetary losses the employer or the hospital has incurred. So, it behooves you to read your contract carefully, try and understand it and have it reviewed by an attorney and remember that income-guarantee agreements tend to be physician-unfriendly and can be hugely problematic and cost you a lot of money if you sign a bad contract. Some experts in this field recommend that you should look at an employment contract in the same way that you evaluate a divorce decree (see section on Divorce later in the book). If both parties are happy, you may never have to look at it, however, if issues come up and your situations change, that is when the employment contract becomes very relevant and it will be scrutinized to the highest level possible.

Final words on reviewing your contract: Always look at it from two points of view. If you leave your employer in good terms vs. if you leave on not so good terms. This should allow you to put things in perspective. Every issue ranging from your income, to retirement contributions, restrictive covenants or even the data collected on you during your employment are relevant. And finally, no matter how well the contract is written and how thoroughly you and your employers' attorneys have reviewed it, one of the most important factors is if your personality matches that of your employer. If there is a conflict in this area it is unlikely that you will have a successful long-term relationship.

## How about some R & R time? Do them early, once you have children it will be far more difficult to travel to places!

**Interesting places to visit around the world:**

Paris:

Paris has been called the magnetic city of lights. It draws people to some of its unique sites including the Eifel Tower, the Louvre museum, and Notre Dame Place. If you have been to Paris before, its fine, you can still go back to this interesting city, because there is always a new highly-rated restaurant to try, a new exhibit to see at place Pompidou or a new shop in which to buy latest fashion clothing (if you can afford it). It has been said that Paris has a *je ne sais quoi* charm that's unexplainable but also unmistakable. Paris is a very expensive city, but there are ways to go to Paris, have a good time and still stay within a certain budget. If you really want to save money you may want to stay in a youth hostel if you do not have children yet. There are several of them in Paris. These places are usually for students, but others can stay too. If you are still single or have a girl friend or married but you still do not have children you can probably get away staying at a hostel. You get a bed and a locker and usually you sleep with one or more people in a room. Hotels are generally very expensive and range from $ 300 -500 a night. However, if you are traveling with your family you can still find a place in the $ 300 range (as of 2011), which will accommodate you and your family. For example, for a family of two adults and three children you may find a nice, clean hotel in the heart of Paris (within a walking distance from the Eifel tower) for $ 360.00 a night for a family suite which has one queen size bed and three other single beds, a spacious bathroom and two TVs and wireless internet.

Barcelona:

This is the headquarter for the Catalans. Because of its proximity to the Mediterranean Sea, it has a wide variety of things to offer from its Gaudi and gourmet delights, to its buzzing waterfront on the Mediterranean Sea to historic sites which take you back 2000 years. Barcelona is one of those unique cities that has almost everything, from an engaging culture of siestas, Spanish guitar and tapas to an outrageous nightlife scene. And for the shoppers, Barcelona offers vibrant shopping (Las Ramblas) and even some shoreline to relax on after an unreal night of partying.

London:

London is the bright star in the United Kingdom. There are many activities that one can do in London from touring the Tower of London, the Buckingham Palace or joining the London bus tour. In London you will see a variety of travelers, including couples, families and backpackers. London's varieties of attractions fill more than a week of vacation.

San Francisco:

San Francisco has often been called the most European city in the U.S. San Francisco definitely has a different feel from most American cities. Fun and relaxed, while at the same time, progressive and innovative, the city exudes an air of confidence and possibilities. There are limitless ways to spend your time here, from a bus tour of the city, to walking along the harbor, to driving down the crookedest street. Relaxing in a café in North Beach to barhopping in the Mission are all options that you may explore.

New York:

This is a city that never sleeps. If you have a lot of energy you will never be bored in this city. This is an international fashion capital with the hottest dining scenes in the country and some of the best theater options you could ever find. Plus, nearly the entire city is covered in some of the most recognizable icons in the country, including Central Park, The Times Square and the Empire State Building.

Maui

Maui is one of the most visited islands in the Hawaiian islands. This beautiful patch of land in the Pacific Ocean is the most equipped of all the Hawaiian islands for vacation activities. Some of the activities that you can do on your vacation here include sailing, snorkeling, diving windsurfing, biking, and whale watching.

Montreal

This bilingual (English and French) Canadian city is suitable for pretty much every type of vacationer. Montreal has hundreds of shopping venues both above and below ground, a massive park (frozen in the winter for skating) ideal for pretty much any activity and a buzzing restaurant and nightlife scene, fringed by the embellished iron street lamps of the historic district.

Vancouver

A relatively new city which does not have the historic features of Montreal, but this western Canadian city boasts a vast amount of outdoor activities for vacationers. Kayak in English Bay or test gravity on the Capilano Suspension Bridge, then enjoy lunch in Chinatown, which is reportedly the second-largest Chinatown in North America.

Zurich

Travelers are attracted to the city of Zurich, Switzerland all year around. It has varieties of museums, historic churches, and shopping centers. In the summer you may swim the crisp, clean waters of Lake Zurich and in the winter you might ski on the nearby Alps mountains. You can also hit the local clubs and bars for entertainment and fun.

Edinburgh

Renowned for its now world-famous Edinburgh Festival in August, this Scottish city also rates high during other seasons of the year. Nestled in an awe-inspiring setting of green hills, the small city of Edinburgh is known for its medieval buildings, an expansive park, a handful of museums and more than enough pubs and bed and breakfasts to give you an authentic Edinburgh experience.

US Virgin Islands

The U.S. Virgin Islands offer unique features for the visitors. They use the US dollar as their currency, there are no roaming fees when you use your cell phone and pretty much every one speaks English. The Islands have a Carnival season and clear sky blue Caribbean waters for snorkeling and swimming and scuba diving most of the year. For the best deals and more consistent weather, consider visiting in late spring or early summer.

Washington DC

The capital of the US is one of the most visited cities in the U.S.; Washington DC is filled with a large number of monuments (Washington, Jefferson, Lincoln etc.) and historic buildings. The White House at 1600 Pennsylvania Avenue, the Lincoln Memorial and the Smithsonian museums are prominent landmarks to visit. The city also has a variety of eclectic and walk-able neighborhoods.

## Budapest

Budapest is sure to be a highlight of any trip to Central/Eastern Europe. The city has a lot to offer to all types of travelers with all ranges of budgets. And Budapest will keep you occupied with its thermal baths, mellow coffeehouses, ridiculous nightlife and whatever else you can think of.

## Prague

Before it was discovered by everyone, Prague was the backpackers' secret city. However, over the past decade this city has transitioned itself to being the unquestioned capital of tourism in Eastern Europe. It is a beautiful city and retains its gothic mystique. It may take you days to explore the city.

## Crete

If you have to choose one island to visit in Greece, it's easy to make a case for Crete. Its diverse landscape features everything from ancient ruins to gorgeous beaches, and you can spend a day doing anything from shopping in Agios Nikolaos to hiking the Samaria Gorge.

## Miami beach

This Floridian city is one of the most popular for its bursting colors, crazy nightlife, amazing coastline and intriguing architecture. The city is more suited for the younger crowd and so if you do not enjoy the constant noise and being up all night, Miami beach may not be so appealing to you. However, the weather is warmer all year-round so that if you are getting out of town in the dead of the winter from one of the northern states, Miami beach or south beach is most likely to be consistently warm when other parts of Florida may be cold.

## San Diego

San Diego is home to dazzling beaches and the San Diego Zoo. Visitors can beach bum it in the morning, dine on fast food fish tacos at lunch, engage in some retail therapy/take a hike through the Torrey Pines State Reserve, bring the kids to SeaWorld in the afternoon and rest up for a dinner on the waterfront or a night dancing in one of the city's bars.

## The Bahamas

The Bahamas consist of several islands, but they are all beautiful and have nice climate all year. Airfare and hotel rates are generally modest year-round in the Bahamas, but you'll get the best deals and have less crowds if you plan your visit for the summer or early fall. But take note: These islands' atmosphere and activities largely cater to tourists, and you'll be hard pressed to find an authentic Bahamian vibe during your getaway.

## Puerto Vallarta

Puerto Vallarta, Mexico stands out for its outstanding cuisine, eclectic bars and clubs and breathtaking landscape. You could spend just a day exploring the cobblestone streets or boardwalk of Zona Centro, or extend your trip for a few more days to try out the nightclubs and European cafés of the downtown area, as well as the hiking in the nearby Sierra Madre Mountains. Food poisoning is always a possibility when visiting Mexico and so exercise care with what you eat particularly raw sea food and vegetables.

## Saint Martin

One half of the island is ruled by the French and the other half is governed by the Dutch. Therefore, when you visit St. Martin, you feel that you are getting two for the prize of one. The Island offers great dining and dazzling stretches of sand on the French side of Saint Martin, and animated nightlife, buzzing casinos, and some of the best duty-free shopping of the Caribbean in Dutch St. Maarten. Consider visiting in late spring to cash in on the not-too hot weather and discounted hotel rates.

Aruba

Limestone-carved Aruba will appeal to the adventurous traveler better than any other destination. You could Scuba dive into the depths of Hadicurari Beach to explore the island's many shipwrecks, or experience the Aruban rattlesnake on an ATV tour of the Arikik National Park. However, just a gentle reminder that a trip to Aruba is also one of the pricier vacations!

Los Angeles

The Entertainment Capital of the World; Los Angeles truly needs no introduction. However, be prepared for facing the traffic jam every day. The traffic on the route 101 will tire you out just as much as an evening at a lively West Hollywood club; your enjoyment of a sunset overlooking a beach in Malibu will pretty much equal your disgust at the thick smog blanketing a breezy day.

**Travelling by Air: Are all airlines created equally?**

Travelling by air can be exciting, but it can also become a frustrating experience, if the experience does not meet your expectations. Or worst, if things that were totally unexpected happen as you try to get to your destination.

Operating an airline company is very complex and is associated with significant overhead expenses. However, according to the financial channel, CNBC, 2010 was considered to be a good year for the airline industry from the financial stand point. US based airlines made the highest profits in a decade and with the exception of one Airline company all of them turned positive profits for the year. They have repeated these profits for the subsequent three years. The most likely explanation for this impressive profit is cutting costs in some areas and increases fees in other areas. Some of the fees never existed in the past.

However, consumers did not appreciate the approach that airlines took even though the data show that airline services have improved compared to prior years. Widespread airfare increases, instituting baggage fees (in the past every passenger was allowed to check in at least one bag of less than 20 kg, which is approximately 45 lb.) and later soaring baggage fees were not received well by the consumers. The elimination of free meals on major flights was another factor that led to further dissatisfaction of consumers with airlines. A number of anecdotal incidents also led to unfavorable public relations for the airline companies including incidences of what was perceived as "discrimination" against an obese passenger and another incident with a passenger who was disabled. The respective airlines appropriately apologized, but the damage was done (not surprisingly by the media) to the public relations images of these companies. According to data collected for the American Customer Satisfaction Index late in 2010, four of the major airlines made it on the list of the "18 worst companies in America". The data released by the Airline Quality Rating report in 2011, covered 16 US-based airlines and it involved the experience of close to 15,000 passengers over approximately 29,000 flights. Consumers were asked to rate their experience with these airlines with regard to a number of parameters. Some of these parameters have been published and include: check-in ease, cabin-crew service, cabin cleanliness, baggage handling, seating comfort, in-flight entertainment, flight delays, denied boarding involuntarily, and overall satisfaction. Based on analysis of these data we present those airlines that could use improvements in their services first.

**Delta Airline:**

Few years ago Northwest airline merged with then Delta airline to become one airline under the name "Delta Airline". Delta had the highest customer complaint rate (2.00 per 100,000 passengers) of all airlines in 2010, including regional carriers. If you look at Delta's baggage fees below, it can get expensive for an average passenger if she/he is checking heavy or large bags.

Domestic Baggage Fees
- 1st Bag: $25 ($23 if checked online)
- 2nd Bag: $35 ($32 if checked online)
- 3rd Bag: $125

Overweight/Oversized Bags
- 51-70 lbs.: $90
- 71-100 lbs.: $175
- 63-80 inches: $175

**Continental Airline**

Like most airlines, continental showed improvement in on-time performance and baggage handling categories in 2010 compared to previous years, however significant setbacks included customer complaints (the rate was up to 1.48 per 100,000 passengers versus 1.00 in 2009) and denied boarding (1.82 bumps per 10,000 passengers versus 1.57). Consumers still felt that the baggage fees were too high.

Domestic Baggage Fees
- 1st Bag: $25 ($23 if checked online)
- 2nd Bag: $35 ($32 if checked online)
- 3rd Bag: $100-$200

Overweight/Oversized Bags
- 51-70 lbs.: $200, 71-100 lbs.: Continental will not accept luggage over 70 lbs. as checked baggage.
- 63-80 inches: $100-$200

## Frontier Airline

Frontier's on-time performance improved somewhat with 81.4 percent of flights arriving on time (up from 78.3 percent in 2009), its customer complaint (1.23 per 100,000 passengers versus .92 the previous year) and mishandled baggage (2.58 incidents per 1,000 passengers versus 2.50) increased in 2010 compared to the prior year.

Domestic Baggage Fees
- 1st Bag: $20
- 2nd Bag: $20
- 3rd Bag: $50

Overweight/Oversized Bags
- 51-100 lbs.: $75
- 63-110 inches: $75

## American Airlines

American Airlines has improved in some areas, but customer complaints continued with 1.44 complaints reported per 100,000 passengers. Baggage fees and service cutbacks continue to be an issue for consumers. However, it is important to notice that overall customer complaint rate is very very low. We are talking about 1 or 2 customers complaining for every 100,000 passengers who board these planes. It is a statistical probability for any service that a minute number of customers will complain no matter what was offered to them.

Domestic Baggage Fees
- 1st Bag: $25
- 2nd Bag: $35
- 3rd Bag: $100

Overweight/Oversized Bags
- 51-70 lbs.: $60 (up $10 from last year)
- 71-100 lbs.: $100
- 62-125 inches: $150

## United Airlines

United States and World Report magazine published an article on this subject and the title was " The worst major carrier" and "United had the worst score among major airlines" and "United had the highest customer complaint rate at 1.64 per 100,000 passengers". But as we said before, if you have 1 or 2 customers out of 100,000 complain about the airlines, it is unfair to label a major airline as 'The worst carrier". Is it plausible that these two individuals [who have complained about the airline] are difficult to please and they would complain about any other services provided? However, "high baggage fees" haven't helped the company's image.

Domestic Baggage Fees
- 1st Bag: $25
- 2nd Bag: $35
- 3rd Bag: $100

Overweight/Oversized Bags
- 51-70 lbs.: $100
- 71-99.9 lbs.: $200 (up $100 from last year)
- Larger than 62 inches: $100

Regional airlines:

## 5. SkyWest

Air Quality Rating (AQR) Score: -1.28

SkyWest Airlines has several hubs throughout the United States, including Chicago and Los Angeles. SkyWest received a -1.28 AQR score, an improvement over the previous year's -1.57. One area that contributed to this improvement was mishandled baggage, where it averaged 4.72 incidents per 1,000 passengers in 2010 compared to 5.69 in 2009. SkyWest acts as a regional airline for AirTran, Delta Connection and United Express.

## #4. Mesa

AQR Score: -1.53

Mesa Airlines' AQR score dropped slightly in 2010 despite improvements in some key categories. The customer complaint rate was .53 complaints per 100,000 passengers, down from .61 the previous year. Mesa fared much better than the prior year with mishandled baggage (though still performing worse than the industry average). However, Mesa's rate of denied boarding soared from 1.47 per 10,000 passengers in 2009 to 2.55 in 2010. Mesa acts as a regional carrier for United Airlines and US Airways.

## #3. Comair

AQR Score: -1.56

With a -1.56 AQR score, Comair got the third-worst score among all airlines surveyed for the 2011 AQR rating. Mishandled baggage was a major culprit, with an average of 5.28 incidents per 1,000 passengers in 2010. Comair also had the worst on-time performance of all carriers surveyed in 2010, with only 73.1 percent of flights arriving on time. Comair is a regional partner for Delta Connection. Its airport hubs are Cincinnati-Northern Kentucky and JFK airports.

## #2. Atlantic Southeast

AQR Score: -1.72

Atlantic Southeast serves as a regional airline for Delta Connection and United Express with several hubs, including Memphis and Chicago. It had the second-most incidents of mishandled baggage in 2010 (6.71 reports per 1,000 passengers).

## #1. American Eagle (Worst Regional Carrier)

American Eagle had the unwelcome distinction of having the worst overall score among all national and regional airlines covered. It also had the most incidents of mishandled baggage (7.15 reports per 1,000 passengers) and the highest rate of involuntary denied boarding (4.02 per 10,000 passengers). American Eagle is the largest regional partner for American Airlines and operates out of a number of hubs, including Chicago and Dallas. But again notice the low overall rate: mishandled baggage occurred in only 7 out of 1000 passengers, that is less than 1%!

Airlines that did better included JetBlue and Southwest Airlines, which top the list of airlines in terms of consumer satisfaction. Here is the list of major US-based Airlines from the most favored by consumers to the least favored:

1. Southwest (87)
2. JetBlue (84)
3. Alaska Airlines (79)
4. Frontier (78)

5. AirTran (74)

6. Continental (72)

7. American (65)

8. Delta (64)

9.United (63)

10. US Airways (61)

To put things in perspective, these surveys included approximately15,000 passengers who were reader s of a particular magazine and they expressed their experience on approximately 29,000 domestic round-trip flights in the previous 12 months. Some other measures that received low marks from these self-selected passengers/readers (yes they elected to fill out the survey, there was no randomization of any type) included cabin-crew service, cleanliness, and in-flight entertainment. The proliferation of added fees further contributes to passengers' low opinion of today's flying experience, and even to their decision of whether to fly at all. As a general rule it is difficult to interpret these surveys because the respondent base is self-selected and is permitted to define too many values independently and often idiosyncratically. For example, an issue that one person considers to be an outrage, ma be considered by another person as a mere irritation. Critics have stated that a survey such as this, mirrors broad conventional market wisdom. The majors are bunched up at the bottom of the stack, although they're not all awful every day; US airways is the worst of all, although there's plenty of anecdotal evidence of improvements; This is more like a survey of vague long-term brand perceptions than tangible quality/performance points.

But some carriers have done a better job than others, as evidenced by a wide difference in overall satisfaction scores, from Southwest's lofty 87 to US Airways' lowly 61. Southwest was the only airline to receive top marks for check-in ease and the service provided by its cabin crew. Passengers also gave the airline high grades for cabin cleanliness and baggage handling. The latter might reflect the fact that Southwest is the only airline that lets you check two bags free of charge. But bags three, four, and beyond will cost you $50 each. And like most other carriers, Southwest charges extra for items over its size and weight limits. This survey was conducted before Southwest's well-publicized problems in April, 2011 with questionable cracks in several of its planes.

JetBlue, which ranked second in overall satisfaction, was the only airline to outscore Southwest for seating comfort, possibly because it gives passengers more room than they're accustomed to in this era of tightly packed planes. JetBlue's coach seats are 32 to 38 inches from the seat directly ahead, while coach seats on most other carriers are just 31 inches apart. JetBlue was also the lone carrier to earn top scores for in-flight entertainment; its seatback TV screens offer passengers 36 channels.

The most recent survey of major airlines covered only 10 airlines, due at least in part to industry consolidation. Next time around there might be even fewer airlines. United and Continental recently (as of 2011) merged, although they are still operating as separate airlines for the time being. Southwest and AirTran have also announced plans to merge, pending government approval.

**Airline Ticket pricing:**

On Sunday 9/25/2011, the Sunday Free Press (published in the Detroit Metropolitan Area) published an article titled "Hub premiums cost Delta fliers plenty at Metro". The article was referring to Delta Airline and the passengers who fly out of the Detroit Metropolitan Airport. An example that the article cited was that a passenger flying on the business class from Detroit to Tokyo would pay $ 11,000.00, but if the same passenger booked her/his flight from Flint, Michigan (a city 60 miles north of Detroit), and flew into Detroit Metropolitan Airport to board the same flight to Tokyo, she/he would pay only around $ 5000.00. The explanation for this disparity in the prize was related to the so called "Hub fees". Apparently Delta pays a lot of money for a Hub, but they do not pay the same amount of money for a "feeder airport", which is usually a smaller airport such as the Flint airport. Delta has similar patterns of fees if you board your flight from cities such as Atlanta and Minneapolis. For instance a coach ticket from Minneapolis to Amsterdam was $ 1070.00, but it was only $907.00 if the passenger boarded from La Cross, Wisconsin to Minneapolis and then to Amsterdam. The prize for a business class ticket for the same route was$8400.00 and $ 6700.00 respectively.

To the contrary, other airlines such as US airways, United Airlines, and American Airline, charges less fees if you fly out of one of their hubs. A review of 57 airlines by the same newspaper showed that out of 57 hubs for other airlines reviewed, boarding a flight from a hub was less expensive in 13 out of 19 routes. Fares on flights from Detroit to European destinations rose by 50% between 2009 and 2011 for passengers boarding from Hubs, however, passengers boarding their flights from smaller airport continued to enjoyed lower fares. So, the lesson to learn from this information is that it pays to shop around and to do your research when booking a flight, particularly an international flight. Airlines do not prize tickets based on costs. They prize it based on how much a passenger is willing to pay. They have many different prizes for the 120 seats on a flight: some seats are for business, others are for leisure, while others are for last minute travelers. Airlines are constantly monitoring the inventory of their seats and they change the ticket prizes accordingly and it is a question of supply and demand. When demand for seats is high, prizes go up and when there is less demand ticket prize goes down. That is why it is often difficult to understand airline ticket prizes and even seating arrangements.

**How to stay healthy in the short and long-term if you travel "a lot" as a physician ?**

Most physicians have a steady position and practice in one place, however some of us have to travel more than other physicians. You may travel a lot as a physician because you work in one state and live in an adjacent state. You may travel a lot because you do locum tenet work. Other physicians travel to give speeches in various parts of the US or internationally, while others travel because they are invited to perform surgeries and/or develop programs in other states or countries. As a physician you are acutely aware of the fact that traveling exposes you to more "germs" and consequently respiratory and gastrointestinal illnesses. However, a study from the east coast of the US showed that frequent traveling also has long-term effects on your health particularly higher risk of cardiovascular diseases. This is not surprising since traveling a lot is akin to a sedentary life and is also associated with less sleep and eating unhealthy food while on the run.

We recognize that you probably know all these facts, but it does not hurt to give you a gentle reminder on the some tips that are likely to keep you healthier in the short and long-term.

1. Relax your brain and exercise while traveling: This involves simple preparations and includes bringing some relaxing music to listen to when you have time; while waiting for your flight or in your hotel room. Also, don't forget to pack clothing for exercise, which may not be more than a pair of shorts, a t-shirt and a pair of tennis shoes. If you are traveling during the winter time a track suit may be ideal. So, pack these items before you leave home.

2. Prepare to sleep well: again this involves preparation and packing of appropriate items. A neck role, an eye patch, and earphones to listen to white noise. After all the plane cabin is a noisy place and you need all the help you can get to mask the noise of the plane engine. When you book your hotel room, make sure you ask for a quiet room. You often do not know what kind of a room you are going to get until you get to your destination; when you do get there ask for a room away from the elevator or a club (if the hotel has one) and rooms in upper

levels tend to be quieter. Also, consider using pharmacological measures to help you sleep better.

3.  Eat healthy: it is very easy to eat a lot junk food while you are traveling. Make a concerted effort to eat healthy food even if you have to pay a little more at airports and when you arrive at your destination. Drink plenty of water and try to minimize alcoholic beverages.

4.  Cleanliness: always carry with you wet wipes; women do this often, but guys not as much. Carry it with you so that you can wipe surfaces of your tray in the plane, your ride, your hotel table and bathrooms before using them.

5.  Minimize the amount of time you sit in one place. If you have to read or go over your presentation; dorsiflex your foot frequently and stand up and walk while at airports or at your hotel. Of course going to the hotel Gym daily would be ideal.

## Medical License

### How do I get my Medical License to practice medicine?

Following graduation form a Medical school and following completion of a graduate medical education (residency program), physicians must obtain a license to practice medicine in a particular state or jurisdiction of the US. With rare exceptions, you cannot practice medicine only with your medical degree. You must complete a minimum numbers of years of graduate medical education (GME).

As soon as you match to a residency training program, your institution will secure you an educational license and you will be able to practice medicine under the supervision of physician educators in your residency program. These physicians must have their own independent, full, and unrestricted licenses themselves to practice medicine. However, following completion of your residency training program (or sooner if you plan to "moonlight" outside your residency institution, see below) you will have to secure your independent and permanent medical license from the state or jurisdiction where you plan to practice. That state or jurisdiction could be the same state where you are completing your residency program or another state if you plan to relocate. The process of securing a permanent medical license is a lengthy one. In some states it may take 6-10 month before you receive you permanent license. Therefore, start the process early so that you receive your license on time.

The process for obtaining a permanent medical license requires that the physician successfully pass a qualifying examination, which is currently (as of 2013) the United States Medical Licensure Examination (USMLE) parts I, II, the clinical skill component, and part III. Other examinations that were required in the past include National Board of Medical Examiner (NBME), and the Federation Licensure Examination (FLEX). If you have graduated over a decade ago and you have passed one of these examinations, they may be acceptable by most states. The second requirement for obtaining a medical license is a minimum number of years of GME or residency. Some states require a minimum of one year of GME, while most states require a minimum of two years of GME for licensure qualification. I suggest that you pass part III of USMLE during your first year of GME and apply for your license towards the end of your first GME year if you are in a state which requires only one year of GME.

Another initiative that would be very helpful to you in the future is to apply to Federation Credentials Verification Services (FCVS) an organization that saves your professional information permanently and will submit them to state medical boards whenever you wish to apply for a license in a particular state. This will save the time and the hassles involved in gathering information every time you wish to apply for a license in a different state.

Every time you apply for a license to another state or jurisdiction, you may have to get transcripts from your medical schools, certificates from your residency program, and other professional information stamped and sealed and submitted to the state medical board. This is time consuming and stressful. Applying to FCVS will save you this hassle. You apply to FCVS once, submit your professional information once, pay the fees and your data will be saved permanently.

An advantage to joining the FCVS is that if for some reason your residency program closes and you are not able to obtain verification for your training for a license application (or for hospital privileges), the FCVS already has your information verified and stored and ready to be submitted to a state license board or other entities. This is important because up to 100 residency programs close every year and if you are not able to provide verification for your training, state license will not issue you a license and hospitals will not grant you privileges to practice medicine in case your field does involve caring for patients or doing surgeries or procedures in a hospital.

Another advantage of applying to FCVS is that as of 2010 information you enter on your USMLE step III online application can be used to begin your personalized FCVS physician information profile which contains your primary source verified credentials. This verified information will be available and accessible when you want to apply for your first or subsequent full and unrestricted license to practice Medicine in a state or jurisdiction in the US. The Website for FCVS is: **www.fsmb.org.** We suggest that you take a look at their website for more information. Most states accept information gathered by FCVS for the purpose of licensing. There are a limited number of states e.g. Arkansas which do not accept information delivered to them by FCVS. These exceptions are discussed later in the book under: Getting licensed, state by state.

One more tip on obtaining a license: There are several agencies throughout the US that will do the paper work for your application for a license in a state for a fee. Your prospective employer should offer you to pay for these fees. If they don't we suggest you ask them. One example of these agencies is: **www.physicianlicensing.com**

### Should you get your full and unrestricted license during your residency?

Well, that would depend on what else you would like to do while you are still in training as a resident? Do you plan on "moon lighting"? do you plan to apply for a fellowship after completing your residency in which case you may have to "moon light" to generate more income?

Like we discussed before, during your residency, the institution will help secure an "educational license" for you. With this license you can practice medicine under the supervision of other physicians, only in the parent institution of your residency. You will not be able to practice medicine anywhere else or independently.

If you plan to "moon light" outside your home hospital where you are doing your residency then you will need a full and unrestricted license to practice medicine in that particular state. Many programs do allow moon lighting. Some have a need for residents to moon light within the institution, in which case you do not need a full and unrestricted license to moon light. Your "educational license" is adequate. However, some resident physicians have a need to "moon light" in order to generate more cash that they need for various reasons. These resident physicians often "moon light" in another hospital which could be in the same state or in another (often contiguous) state, in which case they will need a full and unrestricted license.

### What is the difference between working in your residency as a physician and "moon lighting"?

If you 'moon light" within your home residency institution, then there are not that many differences: you can work with your educational license and you are still under the supervision of the attending physicians in your residency while you are "moon lighting". What that means is that, the liability still lies on the shoulders of the attending physicians (on that particular ward or unit) and in general you are unlikely to be named in the lawsuit because you are still a physician in training.

If you "moon light" outside your parent institution with your own unrestricted license, then you are on your own. You are the physician of records and the one ultimately responsible for all the management issues with patients that you treat. You have to carry your own medical liability insurance and if there is a malpractice lawsuit that is filed against you and/or the hospital you are working for, you will be named in the lawsuit and your name will be registered with the National Practitioner Data Bank if the plaintiff prevails. So, before you rush into offering to moonlight we suggest that you take the following steps:

- You will need a full and unrestricted license to practice Medicine in that state
- Make sure that the type of Medicine you will be practicing is within the scope of your training or at least you have some experience in that field before you start "moon lighting"
- Make sure your program does allow "moon lighting"
- Make sure you are provided with a medical liability insurance that is separate from the liability insurance at your parent institution (the latter does not cover any practice outside your parent institution).
- Do not overestimate your abilities. Be honest with yourself. You may want to spend some time with another physician who works at that particular facility before you work independently in order for you to get a good feel for what it is like to work independently.

## Securing a full and unrestricted License, State by State

Licensure Boards in most states and jurisdictions of the US have websites that you can access to get specific information pertaining to initial license application and subsequent renewal of applications.

Some states have separate Allopathic and Osteopathic boards for licensure. Examples of States, which have separate Allopathic and Osteopathic Licensure boards include; Arizona, California, Michigan, Nevada, Pennsylvania, Tennessee, Utah, and Washington State.

Some states have a controlled substance license in addition to the medical license. Therefore, in order to be able to practice without limitations in prescribing controlled substances you will need to apply for and secure both licenses. We will discuss license requirements in individual states with emphasis on unique requirements for a particular state next.

**Alabama:**

The Alabama State Board of Medical Examiners is the state agency which has the exclusive power and authority to issue, revoke and reinstate all licenses to practice allopathic and osteopathic medicine in the state of Alabama. In addition, the board is responsible for issuing controlled substance certificates and to renew them annually.

The Board also investigates and reviews complaints against practitioners and pursues disciplinary actions when appropriate. It also establishes and reviews compliance with CME requirements for physicians. You may request an application package for a new license by mailing in a letter with the following information:

Full name and address, qualifying examination passed (USMLE, National Board of Medical Examiner, FLEX, etc.) and Board certification status (if you are already board certified in one of the specialties). If you are a current resident or a new graduate, this does not apply to you. You will need to send along a check or money order for $ 20.00 (as of September 2010) to the following address:

Alabama Board of Medical Examiner
PO Box 946
Montgomery, AL 36101

The web address is: www.albme.org and their phone number is: 334-242-4116

The general Licensure requirements for the State of Alabama are:

1.  A medical degree from a LCME accredited medical school or an ECFMGE-approved international medical school
2.  One year of allopathic or osteopathic graduate medical education in the US or Canada (3 years if you are an international medical graduate [IMG])
3.  No criminal records and adequate therapy for substance abuse problems.
4.  Fees: Application packet $20, Application fee $175, Criminal Background check fee of $65
5.  State of Alabama does accept your information gathered by the FCVS (see previous chapters on FCVS).
6.  3+ attempts at USMLE Step 3; 10 attempts at all USMLE Steps and you must complete all steps within 7 years; No limit on COMLEX (Comprehensive Medical License examination: levels 1,2, and 3) attempts or length of time to complete it.

**Alaska:**

You may download the application package from the state medical board at:

http://www.commerce.state.ak.us phone: (907) 269-8163

General Licensure requirements:

1.  A medical degree from an LCME or ECFMG accredited medical school
2.  On year (if you graduated from an LCME school prior to January 1, 1995) or two years of graduated medical education

(if you graduated after January 1, 1995). All international graduates (IMG) will be required to have completed at least 3 years of graduate medical education to eligible for licensure.

3. No criminal or substance abuse issues.
4. Application fee $250 (non-refundable), License fee $590
5. Accepts FCVS information
6. Must complete USMLE or COMLEX after only 2 attempts and must complete all steps of both examinations within 7 years (10 years for MD/PhD candidates.

**Arizona:**

Applications/information may be downloaded at: www.azmd.gov
Phone number: 480- 551-2700

General Licensure requirements:

1. A medical degree from an LCME or ECFMG accredited medical school
2. On year (if you graduated from an LCME school prior to January 1, 1995) or two years of graduate medical education (if you graduated after January 1, 1995). All international graduates (IMGs) will be required to have completed at least 2 years of graduate medical education to be eligible for licensure.
3. No criminal or substance abuse issues.
4. Arizona has no limits on the number of attempts at USMLE or COMLEX or the length of time to complete all components of either examinations.
5. Arizona does accept information submitted by FCVS

**Arkansas:**

Applications/information may be downloaded at: www.armedical-board.org phone: 501-296-1802

General License requirements:

1. A medical degree from an LCME or ECFMG accredited school
2. One year of graduate medical education in accredited residency program for LCME schools graduates (3 years for IMGs, unless actively enrolled in one of the University of Arkansas Healthy Sciences residency programs)
3. Must pass any component of USMLE after a maximum of 3 attempts and must successfully pass all USMLE components within 7 years (10 years for M/PhD candidates). No limits on the number of attempts at COMLEX or the number of years it takes to pass COMLEX.
4. Arkansas DOES NOT accept FCVS information. All information must be provided directly by the applicant to the board.
5. License application fee is $ 500.00

**California:**

The California board of medicine states that "California licensing board remains one of the most stringent in the nation" . This is probably true and it may take up to 9 month for a physician to receive a medical license. Therefore, it is imperative that you start early with the licensing process for California if you plan to practice medicine in California.

The state California licensing board also requires finger printing with your initial application process. If you reside in the state of California you will be able to complete this electronically by using the electronic finger printing form. However if you reside outside

California, you will have to request the hard copy form of the fingerprinting form from the board. Then you will have to go to your local police department for finger printing (there are fees for this process) and then mail the completed finger print forms along with all the demographic information to the board with the initial application form. The finger printing should be applied early because the security process is lengthy. The initial application processing fee is $ 442.00 and the finger printing fee is $ 51.00. You may be eligible for a reduced fee if you are a resident or a fellow in a graduate medical education program. In addition you may have to pay $ 25.00 towards the physician loan repayment program as part of your initial licensing application process fees.

California has two separate licensing application processes, one for allopathic physicians and another one for osteopathic physicians.

Allopathic Physicians License requirements:

www.medbd.ca.gov phone: 800 633-2322 or 916-633-2322

Application fee (non-refundable): $ 493.00

License fee: $ 805.00

The California board of Medicine has only limited acceptance of FCVS physician data. You can still request from the FCVS to submit your physician profile to the California board of medicine, however the board will review each application on an individual basis and will make a determination if your physician profile form the FCVS is acceptable to them. You may have to submit all your information directly to the California board of Medicine.

GME requirements: 1 year for US graduates, 2 years for IMGs.

The candidate must pass USMLE step 3 within 4 attempts. Passing scores on written examinations are valid for a period of 10 years from the month of examination.

California has specific and minimum requirements for courses in psychiatry.

California Osteopathic Board of Medicine:

The phone number for osteopathic board of medicine is: 916-928-8390

The application fee is $ 251.00. No limits on number of attempts at COMLEX or the length of time it takes to complete COMLEX.

**Colorado:**

You may obtain information and application forms at the Colorado State Medical Board website: www. Dora.state.co.us, phone number: 303-894-7690

The application fee is $ 522.00

The State Medical Board of Colorado does accept physician profile via the FCVS

GME requirements: 1 year of graduate medical education for LCME graduates and 3 years for IMGs.

The State of Colorado does not impose limits on the number of attempts at passing the USMLE examination or other previous examinations, however it does require that a candidate must successfully pass all components of USMLE within 7 years from first sitting for USMLE or COMLEX. This period is extended to 10 years for MD/PhD or DO/PhD candidates.

**Connecticut:**

General License requirements:

1. A medical degree from an LCME or ECFMG accredited school
2. Completion of two years of graduate medical education in accredited residency program for LCME schools graduates (3 years for IMGs)
3. Successfully completed one of the following examinations: USMLE step 1, 2, and 3 or National Board of Medical Examiners (NBME), the Federation Licensure Examination (FLEX), National Board of Osteopathic Examiners, or the Licentiate of the Medical Council of Canada (LMCC). The state does not impose any limits on the number of attempts, but does require the minimum passing score of 75 on most of these examinations. If you have completed FLEX component I in the past you will need to pass USMLE step 3 to qualify for a license.
4. CT does not accept FCVS information. All information must be provided directly by the applicant to the board including Medical school transcripts, residency programs completion and transcripts of examinations completed.
5. License application fee is $ 565.00 (as of 2010) payable to the treasurer, State of Connecticut, plus another check for $ 4.75 for National Practitioner Data Bank inquiry. *Do not combine* these fees in one check or money order.
6. An application form may be downloaded from the Board's website at: www.ct.gov. The completed and notarized application may be mailed to the board at the following address: Connecticut Department of Public Health, Physician Licensure, 410 Capitol Avenue, MS # 12 APP, PO Box 340308, Hartford, CT 06134. The Fax number is (860) 509-8457

**State of Delaware:**

General License requirements:

1.  A medical degree from an LCME or ECFMG accredited school
2.  Completion of one year of graduate medical education in accredited residency program for LCME schools graduates (3 years for IMGs)
3.  Successfully completed one of the following examinations: USMLE step 1, 2, and 3 or National Board of Medical Examiners (NBME), the Federation Licensure Examination (FLEX), National Board of Osteopathic Examiners, or the Licentiate of the Medical Council of Canada (LMCC). The state of Delaware does not impose any limits on the number of attempts, but does require the minimum passing score of 75 on most of these examinations. If you have completed FLEX component I in the past you will need to pass USMLE step 3 to qualify for a license.
4.  The state of Delaware does accept **FCVS** data submitted on your behalf. All information may be provided to the Board on your behalf by the FCVS.
5.  License application fee is $ 310.00 (as of 2010) payable to "State of Delaware"
6.  Request self-query from the National Practitioner Data Bank.
7.  Criminal background check is required.
8.  an interview is required with a member of the board.
9.  An application form may be downloaded from the Board's website at: www.dpr.delaware.gov. The completed and notarized application may be mailed to the board at the following address: Board of Medical Licensure and discipline. 861 Silver Lake Blvd, Suite 203, Dover, Delaware 19904. Phone: 302-744-4500, Fax 302-739-2711.

**District of Columbia (Washington, DC):**

There are five ways to become licensed in Washington, DC:

1. A medical degree from an LCME accredited school who passes USMLE step 3 after first attempt.
2. A medical degree from an LCME accredited school who passes USMLE step 3 after second or subsequent attempt. Candidates who have failed USMLE step 3, three times or more will be required to complete an additional year of post-graduate training in an ACGME accredited program before becoming eligible to apply for a medical license in Washington, DC
3. A medical degree from an LCME or ECFMG accredited school who passes one of the other examinations such as the NBME or FLEX 1,2 or FLEX 1,2, and 3 (prior to 1985).
4. A medical degree from an ECFMG accredited international medical school, ECFMG certificate, two years of postgraduate medical education in the US, and 10 years of experience outside the US.
5. A foreign-trained physician who has at least 10 years of experience in a specialty of medicine, is nominated by the Director of National Institute of Health or the Director of an accredited hospital in the District of Columbia and who meets other requirements for a license.

In addition the board conducts background checks and disciplinary actions that may have been taken against you. You may obtain the licensure application at the Board's website at: www.dchealth.dc.gov and their mailing address is:

Health Licensing Specialist, 717 14th Street, NW, Suite 600
Washington, DC 20005
Phone: (202) 724-4900 Fax: (877) 672-2174

**Florida (allopathic):**

General License requirements:

1. A medical degree from an LCME or ECFMG accredited school
2. Completion of three years of graduate medical education in accredited residency program.
3. Successfully completed one of the following examinations: USMLE step 1, 2, and 3 or National Board of Medical Examiners (NBME), the Federation Licensure Examination (FLEX) 1 and 2. FLEX 1,2 and 3 (if taken prior to 1985) or the Licentiate of the Medical Council of Canada (LMCC). The state does not impose any limits on the number of attempts, but does require the minimum passing score of 75 on most of these examinations. If you have completed FLEX component I in the past you will need to pass USMLE step 3 to qualify for a license.
4. The state of Florida does not accept FCVS information. All information must be provided directly by the applicant to the board including Medical school transcripts, residency programs completion and transcripts of examinations completed.
5. Pay the appropriate License application fee.
6. Background checks and Fingerprinting
7. An application form may be downloaded from the Board's website at: www.doh.state.fl.us

**Florida (Osteopathic):**

General License requirements:

1. A medical degree from an accredited Osteopathic Medical School
2. Completion of three years of graduate medical education in accredited residency program.

3. Successfully completed National Board of Osteopathic Examiners with a minimum passing score of 75 or higher.
4. The state of Florida does not accept FCVS information. All information must provided directly by the applicant to the board including Medical school transcripts, residency programs completion and transcripts of examinations completed.
5. Pay the appropriate License application fee.
6. Background checks and Fingerprinting
7. An application form may be downloaded from the Board's website at: www.doh.state.fl.us

**Georgia:**

The application for a medical license in the state of Georgia is completed on line. You will have to go the Georgia Composite Board of Medical Examiners, register (which requires you to enter your social security number) and then proceed from there.

General License requirements:

1. A medical degree from an LCME or ECFMG accredited school
2. Completion of one year of graduate medical education in an accredited residency program for LCME schools graduates (3 years for IMGs)
3. Successfully completed one of the following examinations: USMLE step 1, 2, and 3 or National Board of Medical Examiners (NBME), the Federation Licensure Examination (FLEX), National Board of Osteopathic Examiners, or the Licentiate of the Medical Council of Canada (LMCC). The state does require that USMLE step 3 be passed within 3 attempts, but makes exemption if you are board certified in a specialty. The Medical License Board of Georgia DOES NOT apply the ten year rule (see previous states), which means that

you do not need to take any additional examinations if they were passed over 10 years ago and you do not have to take the SPEX to get licensed.

4.  GA does accept FCVS information and has also recently contracted with Veridoc.org to streamline the application process. The Board will direct you to Veridoc.org website to register and it will help facilitate the licensure application process. Otherwise you may have to provide the transcripts, residency documentations to the board directly.

5.  Three reference letters directly sent to the Board by physicians familiar with your character and work.

6.  License application fee is $ 500.00 (as of 2010) payable to: State of Georgia, plus another check for $ 100.00 if you need a temporary license. There may be additional ancillary fess of up to $ 75.00

7.  The state of Georgia is considered one of the most efficient Licensing boards and there are reports of physician securing their license in as short as 29 days.

8.  If you need to start practicing and you meet all the requirements, the state will issue you a temporary license until the next scheduled Board meeting.

9.  An application form may be downloaded from the Board's website at: http://medicalboroard.gerogia.gov

**Hawaii:**

General License requirements:

1.  A medical degree from an LCME or ECFMG accredited school
2.  Completion of one year of graduate medical education in accredited residency program for LCME schools graduates (2 years for MGs and Canadian graduates).

3. Successfully completed one of the following examinations: USMLE step 1, 2, and 3 or National Board of Medical Examiners (NBME), the Federation Licensure Examination (FLEX), National Board of Osteopathic Examiners, or the Licentiate of the Medical Council of Canada (LMCC). The state of Hawaii does require all components of the USMLE to be successfully passed within 7 years.

4. The state of Hawaii does accept **FCVS** data submitted on your behalf, which includes your diploma, residency verification, and ECFMG (if applicable). However, you will have to submit the National Practitioner data bank (NPDB) verification, the American Medical Association (AMA) verification. *See below*

5. License application fee is $ 170.00 (as of February 2011) payable to "State of Hawaii"

6. Request self-query from the National Practitioner Data Bank.

7. AMA profile, which should be sent to the board directly. You will need to go the AMA website at: www.ama-assn.org to register and provide your profile if you do not have one established yet.

8. The state of Hawaii will NOT issue you a license if you are not a US citizen, a permanent resident (a green card holder) or have other documents that prove that you are legally allowed to work in the US or its territories.

An application form may be downloaded from the Board's website at: http://hawaii.gov/dcca/pvl/boards/medical The Board's address is :

Hawaii Medical Board
DCCA, PVL License Board
335 Merchant street, room 103
Honolulu, HI 96813
Phone: 808-586-3000

**Idaho:**

General License requirements:

1.  A medical degree from an LCME or ECFMG accredited school
2.  Completion of one year of graduate medical education in an accredited residency program.
3.  Successfully completed one of the following examinations: USMLE step 1, 2, and 3 or National Board of Medical Examiners (NBME), the Federation Licensure Examination (FLEX), National Board of Osteopathic Examiners, or the Licentiate of the Medical Council of Canada (LMCC). The state does specify that the applicant must pass any component of an examination after two attempts and the examination attempts must be completed within 7 years for MD and 10 years of MD/PhD candidates. If an applicant fails to pass an examination the second time she/he will not be eligible to take the same examination for one year.
4.  Two letter of recommendations from two physicians who have known the applicant for at least one year and who are familiar with the character and abilities of the physician.
5.  Fingerprinting and background checks are required for obtaining a license in Idaho.
6.  A passport-size photograph taken within the past year.
7.  License application fee is $ 400.00 (as of 2010) payable to: State of Idaho, plus a $ 10.00 application fee.
8.  The Board states that the applicant must be prepared to present for an interview if the Board determines that an interview is necessary.
9.  Idaho accepts FVCS data provided to the Board.

An application form may be downloaded from the Board's website at: http://bom.idaho.gov

Idaho of Medicine physical address is:

Idaho Board of Medicine
1755 N Westgate Drive, suite 140
Boise, Idaho 83704
Phone: 208-327-7000
Fax : 208-327-7005

You may email the board for any questions at: info@bom.idaho.gov

**Illinois:**

General License requirements:

1. A medical degree from an LCME or ECFMG accredited school
2. Completion of two years of graduate medical education in accredited residency program.
3. Successfully completed one of the following examinations: USMLE step 1, 2, and 3 or National Board of Medical Examiners (NBME), the Federation Licensure Examination (FLEX) 1 and 2. FLEX 1,2 and 3 (if taken prior to 1985) or the Licentiate of the Medical Council of Canada (LMCC). USMLE parts must be completed within 7 years and a total of 5 attempts for combined all components are allowed by the state of Illinois.
4. The state of Illinois does accept FCVS information.
5. The License fee is : $ 300.00

An application form may be downloaded from the Board's website at: **www.idfpr.com**

**The Board's phone number is: (217) 782-8556**

**Hopefully, by now you recognize that all Boards require graduation from an LCM or ECFMG medical school, we will discuss only those specific issues related to licensure application for the subsequent states.**

**Indiana:**

The state of Indiana requires one year of post-graduate training for US and Canadian graduates and two years for IMGs.

It allows three attempts at USMLE or other examinations such as the NBME or FLEX. All examinations must be completed within 10 years.

The license fee is $ 250.00

You may obtain further information and/or application forms at Indiana Board of Medicine website at: http://in.gov

The physical address for the board is:

Professional Licensing Agency
Medical Licensing Board of Indiana
402 W. Washington Street, Room W072
Indianapolis, Indiana 46204
Phone: 317-234-2060

**Iowa:**

The state of Iowa requires one year of post-graduate training for US and Canadian graduates and two years for IMGs.

The state of Iowa allows six attempts at USMLE steps I and II and three attempts at USMLE step 3. If the candidate exceeds these limits then she/he must complete three years of post-graduate medical education (residency) in order to qualify for a license. All components of USMLE or other examinations must be completed within 10 years in order to qualify for licensure.

The license fee is $ 505.00

Iowa does accepts credentials provided by FCVS

You may obtain further information and/or application forms at Indiana Board of Medicine website at: www.medicalbord.iowa.gov

The physical address for the board is:

Iowa Board of Medicine.
400 SW 8ᵗʰ street, Suite c,
Des Moines, IA 50309
Phone: 515-281-6641

**Kansas:**

The state of Kansas requires one year of post-graduate training for US and Canadian graduates and three years for IMGs.

The state of Kansas allows multiple attempts at USMLE steps I, II and III, but all components must be successfully passed within 10 years. Failure to pass all the three components within 10 years are handled on an individual basis.

Effective in 2009, Kansas State Board of Medicine requires criminal background check and fingerprinting as well as the National practitioner Data bank (NPDB) information

The license fee is $ 500.00 + NPDS fee of $9.50, and $ 50.00 for background check

Iowa does accepts credentials provided by FCVS

You may obtain further information and/or application forms at Indiana Board of Medicine website at: www.ksbha.org

The physical address for the board is:

Kansas State Board of Healing Arts
235 S. Topeka boulevard, Topeka, KS 66603-3068
Phone: 785-296-7413

**Kentucky:**

The state of Kentucky requires two years of post-graduate training for all candidates (US and Canadian graduates and IMGs).

The state of Kentucky allows 4 attempts at all USMLE steps and there is no limit on the time period during which these components are passed.

The state of Kentucky does require background checks which includes finger printing, the AMA profile as well as the National practitioner Data bank (NPDB) information

Kentucky also requires a 2-hour HIV/AIDS education from all applicants

The license fee is $300.00 + NPDS fee of $9.50, and $ 50.00 for background check, and any additional fees for the AMA profile that you may have to pay.

Kentucky does accepts credentials provided by FCVS

Because the Board meets quarterly, the application process may take 60-90 days, however, Kentucky does issue a temporary license that may use to practice until a full license is issued.

You may obtain further information and/or application forms at Indiana Board of Medicine website at:

The physical address for the board is:

Kentucky Board of Medical License
310 Whittington Pkwy, Suite 1B
Louisville, KY 40222
Phone: 502-429-7150

**Louisiana:**
Two years of post-graduate training for US and Canadian graduates and 3 years for IMGs.

The state of Louisiana has not limits on the number of attempts at USMLE step I, but Steps II and III must be passed within 4 attempts. All components must be passed within 10 years.

The state of Louisiana does require background checks which includes finger printing and the AMA profile.

Louisiana accepts credentials provided by FCVS

The Board also requires 2 letters of recommendation from physicians familiar with your work.

The license fee is $382.00 + any additional fees for background check, and the AMA profile that you may have to pay.

You may obtain further information and/or application forms at Board of Medicine website at: http://www.lsbme.la.gov

The physical address for the board is:

1515 Poydras Street, Suite 2700,
New Orleans, LA70112
Phone: 504-568-6820 email: lsbme@lsbme.la.gov

**State of Maine:**

*Allopathic physicians' license:*

Two years of post-graduate training for US and Canadian graduates for those who graduated prior to July 1, 2004 and 3 years for all other graduates including IMGs.

The state of Maine limits on the number of attempts at USMLE step III to only three attempts. All components must be passed within 7 years for all applicants. A waiver is required for applicants who have made > 3 attempts at USMLE III or have failed to pass all three components within 7 years. Other examinations such as NBME or FLEX are handled on an individual basis.

Maine requires credentials provided by FCVS.

There is a written that must be passed by all applicants. The material for the test may be found at the Board's website: http://www.docboard. org/me/me_home.htm

The state of Maine does require background checks which includes evaluation of your professional competence, ethics and character.

The license fee is $ 700.00 payable to: Main Board of Licensure in Medicine.

You may obtain further information and/or application forms at Board of Medicine website at: http://www.docboard.org/me/me_home.htm

The physical address for the Maine board of Medicine is:

Board of Licensure in Medicine
161 Capitol Street

137 State House Station
Augusta, Maine 04333-0137
Tel: (207) 287-3601
Fax: (207) 287-6590

**State of Maine:**

*Osteopathic License:*

A medical degree from an accredited Osteopathic Medical School

Completion of three years of graduate medical education in an accredited residency program.

Successful completion of the National Board of Osteopathic Examiners with a minimum passing score of 75 or higher.

The state of Maine does accept FCVS information. All information must be provided directly by the applicant to the board including Medical school transcripts, residency programs completion and transcripts of examinations completed.

Pay the appropriate License application fee.

Background checks for professional and ethical conducts.

An application form may be downloaded from the Board's website at: http://www.docboard.org/me/me_home.htm

**State of Maryland:**

The state of Maryland requires one year of post-graduate training for US and Canadian graduates and two years for IMGs.

The state of Maryland allows four attempts at USMLE steps I, II and III, but all components must be successfully passed within 10 years. Failure to pass all the three components of the qualifying examination within 10 years are handled on an individual basis.

A background check may be required.

The license fee is $ 816.00 for US graduates and $ 916.00 for IMGs.

Maryland does accepts credentials provided by FCVS

You may obtain further information and/or application forms at Maryland Board of Medicine website at: www.mbp.state.md.us

The physical address for the board is:

Maryland Board of Physicians
4201 Patterson Av.
Baltimore, MD 21215
Phone: 410-764-4777

**Commonwealth of Massachusetts:**

The Commonwealth of Massachusetts requires one year of post-graduate training for US and Canadian graduates and two years for IMGs.

The Commonwealth of Massachusetts allows six attempts at USMLE steps III, and all components must be successfully passed within 7 years. MD/PhD candidates are exceptions. Failure to pass all the three components of the qualifying examination within 10 years are handled on an individual basis.

The license fee is $ 600.00 for all candidates.

Massachusetts does accepts credentials provided by FCVS

You may obtain further information and/or application forms at Massachusetts board of registration in Medicine at: http://www.mass.gov

The physical address for the board is:

200 Harvard Mills square, Suite 300
Wakefield, MA 01880

The board may be reached by calling the main number 781-876-8200

**State of Michigan:**

**Allopathic:**

The State of Michigan requires two years of post-graduate training for all graduates (US and Canadian) and IMGs towards licensure application.

The State of Michigan does impose any limits at taking USMLE (or any of the previous qualifying examinations), however, USMLE step III must be passed within 5 years.

The state of Michigan has a medical license and a controlled substance license; however you apply for both of them together even though the states issues you two licenses.

The license fee is $ 225.00 ($ 150 for the medical license and $ 85.00 for the control substance license).

Michigan does accepts credentials provided by FCVS

You may obtain further information and/or application forms from Michigan Department of Community Health at: www.michigan.gov

The physical address for the Board is:

BHP, PO Box 30670, Lansing, MI 48909
Courier Mailing Address is: BHP, 611 Ottawa, 1st floor, Lansing, MI 48933
Phone: 517-335-0918

**Osteopathic:**

One year of post-graduate in an AOA-approved residency

No limits on COMLEX

The web address and the physical address are the same as the Allopathic information above.

**Minnesota:**

Minnesota requires one year of post-graduate training for US and Canadian graduates and two years for IMGs towards licensure application.

The State of Minnesota does impose limits at taking USMLE: 3 attempts at each USMLE step (or one of the previous qualifying examinations) and 4 if licensed in another state or board certified. USMLE step three must be passed within 5 years of step 2 or prior completion of a residency training program.

The license fee is $ 392.00

Minnesota does accepts credentials provided by FCVS

You may obtain further information and/or application forms from Minnesota Board of Medicine at : www.state.mn.us

The physical address for the Board is:

Minnesota Board of Medical Practice
University Park Plaza, 2829 University Avenue, SE, Suite 500
Minneapolis, MN 55414
Phone: 612-617-2130

**Mississippi:**

Mississippi requires one year of post-graduate training for US and Canadian graduates and 1-3 years for IMGs (individualized) towards licensure application.

The State of Mississippi does impose limits at taking USMLE: 3 attempts at USMLE step 3 and all components must be passed within 7 years. No limits on COMLEX.

The license fee is $ 600.00

Mississippi does accepts credentials provided by FCVS

Mississippi no longer accepts paper applications.

You may obtain further information and/or application forms from Mississippi State Board of Medical License at: www.msbml.state.ms.us

The physical address is:

Mississippi Board of Medical License
Crane Ridge Drive, Suite 200-B
Jackson, Mississippi 39216
Phone: 601-987-3097

**Missouri:**

Missouri requires one year of post-graduate training for US and Canadian graduates and 3 years for IMGs towards licensure application.

The State of Missouri does impose limits at taking USMLE: 3 attempts at USMLE 3, all steps of USMLE or one of previous examinations (FLEX, NBME) must be successfully completed within 7 years. No limits on COMLEX.

A notarized copy of a birth certificate or passport is required

The license fee is $ 300.00

Missouri does accepts credentials provided by FCVS

You may obtain further information and/or application forms from Missouri State Board of professional license: www.po.mo.gov

The physical address is:

Missouri Board of Medical License:
3605 Missouri Boulevard
P.O. Box 4
Jefferson City, MO 65102
Phone: 573-751.0098
Fax: 573-751.3166

**State of Montana:**

Montana requires two years of post-graduate training for US and Canadian graduates and 3 years for IMGs towards licensure application.

The State of Montana does impose limits at taking USMLE: 3 attempts at USMLE 3, all steps of USMLE or one of previous examinations (FLEX, NBME) must be successfully completed within 7 years. Exceptions can be offered to MD/PhD candidates. No limits on COMLEX.

The license fee is $ 325.00

Montana accepts credentials provided by FCVS

You may obtain further information and/or application forms from Montana Board of Medical examiners at: www.bsd.dli.mt.gov

The physical address is:

Board of Medical Examiners
301 South Park, 4th floor
PO Box 200513
Helena, MT 59620-0513
Phone: 406-841-2360
Fax: 406-841-2305

**Nebraska:**

Nebraska requires one year of post-graduate training for US and Canadian graduates and 3 years for IMGs towards licensure application.

The State of Montana does impose limits at taking USMLE: 4 attempts at USMLE 3, all steps of USMLE or one of previous examinations (FLEX, NBME) must be successfully completed within 10 years. Exceptions can be offered to MD/PhD candidates. Same limits on COMLEX.

The license fee is $ 300.00

Nebraska DOES NOT accept credentials provided by FCVS

If you have never been licensed in another state, the State of Nebraska requires that a certified copy of your Medical School Diploma be sent directly to the Board as proof of graduation from a Medical school. IMGs will also need to submit a copy of their permanent ECFMG certificate.

Criminal background check and fingerprinting is required for initial licensing.

The state of Nebraska does accept reciprocity if you have been licensed in another state for at least one year.

Nebraska DOES issue temporary licenses for locum tenens for physicians who have a full and unrestricted license in another state.

You may obtain further information and/or application forms from Montana Board of Medical examiners at **their** website

The physical address is:

Licensure Unit
PO Box 94986, Lincoln, NE 68509-4986
Phone: 402-471-2118

**Nevada:**

Nevada requires 3 years of post-graduate training for all graduates. For Osteopathic physicians: 3 years or 2 if the resident commits to practice in the state of Nevada.

The State of Nevada does impose limits at taking USMLE: 3 attempts at USMLE 3, and all steps must be passed with a total of 9 attempts. All components must be passed within 7 years. The same would apply for one of the former examinations such as FLEX or NBME. No limits on COMLEX.

A notarized copy of a birth certificate or passport is required

The license fee is $ 650.00

Nevada does accepts credentials provided by FCVS

Nevada does accept licensing by endorsement provided that the applicant has an active license to practice in another state and has passed one of the recognized examinations by the board.

You may obtain further information and/or application forms from Missouri State Board of professional license: www.medboard.nv.gov

The physical address is:

Nevada Board of Medical License:
1105 Terminal way, Suite 301
Reno, NV 89502
Phone: 775-688-2559

**New Hampshire:**

New Hampshire requires 2 years of post-graduate training for all graduates.

New Hampshire does impose limits at taking USMLE: 3 attempts at each component of USMLE. All components must be passed within 7 years. The same would apply for one of the former examinations such as FLEX or NBME. No limits on COMLEX.

The license fee is $ 250.00

New Hampshire does accepts credentials provided by FCVS

New Hampshire does accept licensing by endorsement provided that the applicant has an active license to practice in another state and has passed one of the recognized examinations by the board.

You may obtain further information and/or application forms from New Hampshire State Board of professional license: www.ng.gov./ medicine

The physical address is:

New Hampshire State Board of Medicine
2 Industrial Park Drive # 8
Concord, NH 03301
Phone: 603-271-1203

**New Jersey:**

Graduation prior to 7/1/2003: one year for US/Canadian graduates; 3 years of IMGs.

Graduation after 7/1/2003: All graduates (US/Canadians and IMGs) must have completed 2 years of graduate medical education in the same field and must have a contract for a third year of graduate medical education in order to be eligible for a license.

New Jersey: Hampshire does impose limits at taking USMLE: 5 attempts at USMLE III or COMLEX. All components must be passed within 7 years. The same would apply for one of the former examinations such as FLEX or NBME. No limits on COMLEX.

The license fee is $ 250.00

New Jersey does accepts credentials provided by FCVS

Criminal Background check form must be completed and submitted with your application

Child support form must be filled out and submitted with your application (even if you do not have children!)

You may obtain further information and/or application forms from Missouri State Board of professional license: www.nj.gov./medicine

The physical address is:

New Jersey State Board of Medical Examiners
140 East Front Street, 3rd Floor
Trenton, NJ 08608
Phone: 609-826-7100

**New Mexico:**

*Allopathic Medicine:*

New Mexico requires 2 years of post-graduate training for all graduates.

New Mexico does impose limits at taking USMLE: 6 attempts at each component of USMLE. All components must be passed within 7 years (10 years of MD/PhD candidates). The same would apply for one of the former examinations such as FLEX or NBME. No limits on COMLEX.

Criminal background checks including fingerprinting are required by the State of New Mexico medical board.

The license fee is $ 436.00 payable to: New Mexico Medical Board. (unless you are a resident in training and you are applying for a public service license (fee $50.00). Your program Director will have to submit a letter in your support for a public service license.

New Mexico accepts (and highly recommends) credentials provided by FCVS

New Mexico does accept licensing by endorsement provided that the applicant has an active license to practice in another state, has passed one of the recognized examinations by the board and is certified by an American Board of Medical Specialty.

You may obtain further information and/or application forms from New Mexico Medical Board: http://www.nmmb.state.nm.us

The physician address for the Board is:

New Mexico Medical Board
2055 S Pacheco St., bldg. 400
Sent Fe, NM 87505
Phone: 505-476-7220

**New Mexico:**

*Osteopathic Medicine:*

New Mexico requires 1 years of post-graduate training for osteopathic graduates.

New Mexico does NOT impose limits COMLEX.

Criminal background checks including fingerprinting are required by the State of New Mexico medical board.

The license fee is $ 436.00 payable to: New Mexico Medical Board. (unless you are a resident in training and you are applying for a public service license (fee $50.00). Your program Director will have to submit a letter in your support for a public service license.

New Mexico accepts (and highly recommends) credentials provided by FCVS

New Mexico does accept licensing by endorsement provided that the applicant has an active license to practice in another state, has passed one of the recognized examinations by the board and is certified by an American Board of Medical Specialty.

You may obtain further information and/or application forms from New Mexico Medical Board: http://www.rld.state.nm.us/osteopathy

The physical address for Board of Osteopathic Medical Examiners is:

2550 Cerrillos Road, Second Floor, Santa Fe, NM 87505
Phone: 505-476-4950
Fax: 505-476-4645

**New York:**

New York requires 1 year of post-graduate training for US graduates and 3 years for IMGs.

New York does NOT impose limits at taking USMLE or COMLEX.

Criminal background checks including fingerprinting are required by the State of New Mexico medical board.

The license fee is $ 735.00 payable to: New York State Medical Board.

New Mexico encourages US graduates to use FCVS. For IMGs credentials provided by FCVS is a requirement.

New Mexico does accept licensing by endorsement provided that the applicant has an active license to practice in another state, has passed one of the recognized examinations by the board and is certified by an American Board of Medical Specialty.

You may obtain further information and/or application forms at: http://www.op.nysed.gov

The mailing address for the Board is:

New York State Education Dept.
Office of Professions
PO Box 22063
Albany, NY 12201
Phone: 518-474-3817 (extension 560)

**North Carolina:**

North Carolina requires 1 year of post-graduate training for US/Canadian graduates and 3 years for IMGs.

North Carolina does impose limits at taking USMLE: 3 attempts at each component of USMLE or COMLEX. All components must be passed within 7 years (10 years for MD/PhD candidates). The same would apply for one of the former examinations such as FLEX or NBME. No limits on COMLEX.

The license fee is $ 350.00

North Carolina does accept credentials provided by FCVS. If you submit your credentials via the FCVS, then the board will process your application by endorsement. In this case you may fill out your application at the Board's website listed below.

Criminal background checks including fingerprinting are required by the State of North Carolina medical board.

You may obtain further information and/or application forms from New Hampshire State Board of professional license: www. ncmedboard.org

The physical address is:

NC Medical Board
PO Box 20007, Raleigh, NC 27619 or 1203 Front Street, Raleigh, NC 27609 (Use this address for express/overnight deliveries)

**North Dakota:**

North Dakota requires 1 year of post-graduate training for US/ Canadian graduates and 3 years for IMGs.

North Dakota does impose limits at taking USMLE: 3 attempts at each component of USMLE or COMLEX. All components must be passed within 7 years (10 years for MD/PhD candidates). The same would apply for one of the former examinations such as FLEX or NBME. No limits on COMLEX.

The license fee is $ 200.00

North Dakota does accept credentials provided by FCVS.

Criminal background checks including fingerprinting are required by the State of North Dakota medical board.

You may obtain further information and/or application forms from North Dakota State Board of professional license: www.ndbomex.com

The physical address is: 418 E Broadway Avenue, Suite 12, Bismarck, ND 58501
Phone: 701-328-6500, Fax: 701-328-6505

**State of Ohio:**

The State of Ohio requires 1 year of post-graduate training for US/Canadian graduates and 2 years for IMGs.

Ohio does impose limits at taking USMLE: 4 attempts at each component of USMLE or COMLEX. All components must be passed within 10 years. The same would apply for one of the former examinations such as FLEX or NBME. No limits on COMLEX.

The license fee is $ 300.00

Ohio does accept credentials provided by FCVS.

Criminal background checks including finger printing are required by the State of Ohio. This includes background evaluation by the Federal Bureau of Investigation (FBI).

Ohio may also require passing an English test for International Medical Graduates and/or an interview.

You may obtain further information and/or application forms from The Ohio State Board of Medicine: www.med.ohio.gov

The physical address is:

State Medical Board of Ohio, 30 E. Broad street, 3$^{rd}$ floor
Columbus, OH 43215
Phone: 614-466-3934

**State of Oklahoma:**

*Allopathic Medicine:*

The State of Oklahoma requires 1 year of post-graduate training for US/Canadian graduates and 2 years for IMGs.

Oklahoma does impose limits at taking USMLE: 3 attempts at each component of USMLE or COMLEX. All components must be passed within 10 years. The same would apply for one of the former examinations such as FLEX or NBME. No limits on COMLEX.

The license fee is $ 500.00

Oklahoma does accept credentials provided by FCVS.

Criminal background check: This can be accomplished by completing an application form at the Board's website. The cost for this procedure is currently (as of 2011) $ 21.99 and may be paid using a credit or debit card.

You may obtain further information and/or application forms from The Ohio State Board of Medicine: www.oakmedicalborad.org

Or you may request an application for a medical license by contacting the Oklahoma Board of Medicine at the following address:

OSBMLS, PO Box 18256, Oklahoma City, OK 73154

Fax: 405-962-1440
Email: licensing@okmedicalboard.org

**Oklahoma State:**

*Osteopathic Medicine:*

The State of Oklahoma requires 1 year of post-graduate training for Osteopathic physicians.

Oklahoma Board of Osteopathic Medicine does NOT impose limits at taking the COMLEX.

The license fee is $ 575.00

Oklahoma does accept credentials provided by FCVS.

Criminal background check: This can be accomplished by completing an application form at the Board's website. The cost for this procedure is currently (as of 2011) $ 21.99 and may be paid using a credit or debit card.

You may obtain further information and/or application forms from The Ohio State Board of Medicine: www.ok.gov

You may contact the Oklahoma Board of Osteopathic Examiners at the following address: 4848 North Lincoln Boulevard, Suite 100, Oklahoma City, OK 73105

Phone: 405-528-8625, Fax: 405-557-0653

**Oregon:**

The State of Oregon requires 1 year of post-graduate training for US/Canadian graduates and 2 years for IMGs.

Oregon does impose limits at attempts at passing USMLE: 3 attempts at component III of USMLE or COMLEX plus one year of graduate medical education. All components must be passed within 7 years. A waiver may be granted for MD/PhD candidates or if the candidate had a serious illness. The same would apply for one of the former examinations such as FLEX or NBME. No limits on COMLEX.

The license fee is $ 375.00

Oregon does accept credentials provided by FCVS, but this is not a requirement by the board.

Criminal background check and fingerprinting: This can be accomplished by completing an application form at the Board's website and pay the appropriate fee (which varies from time to time).

Medical Practice Act and DEA Laws test: an open book tests that is usually attached to your License application.

Competency Examination: A one-day computerized examination on general medical knowledge (not your specialty) for new applicants.

You may obtain further information and/or application forms from The Ohio State Board of Medicine: www.oregon.gov/OMB

Or you may request an application for a medical license by contacting the Oregon Board of Medicine at the following address:

Licensing Services Department
1500 SW 1st, Suite 620
Portland, OR 97201-5847

**Pennsylvania:**

*Allopathic:*

The State of Pennsylvania requires 1 year of post-graduate training for US/Canadian graduates and 3 years for IMGs.

Pennsylvania does NOT impose limits attempts at taking USMLE

The license fee is $ 35.00 for Accredited US medical schools and $ 85.00 for graduates of other medical schools

Pennsylvania does accept credentials provided by FCVS, but this is not a requirement by the board.

A certificate of good moral character provided by two physicians licensed in the US or Canada

You may obtain further information and/or application forms from The Pennsylvania State Board of Medicine: www.dos.state.pa.us

Or you may contact the board by mail on the following address;

Pennsylvania State Board of Medicine
PO Box 2694
Harrisburg, PA 17105-2649
Phone:717-783-1400, Fax: 717-787-7769

**Pennsylvania:**

*Osteopathic:*

The State of Pennsylvania requires 1 year of post-graduate training for graduates of an Osteopathic Medical School

Pennsylvania does NOT impose limits attempts at COMLEX

The license application fee is $ 45.00

Pennsylvania Osteopathic Board of Medicine does NOT accept credentials provided by FCVS.

A certificate of good moral character provided by two physicians licensed in the US or Canada

You may obtain further information and/or application forms from The Pennsylvania State Board of Medicine: www.dos.state.pa.us

Or you may contact the board by mail on the following address;

Pennsylvania State Board of Medicine
PO Box 2694
Harrisburg, PA 17105-2649
Phone:717-783-1400, Fax: 717-787-7769

**Rhode Island:**

Rhode Island requires 1 year of post-graduate training for US/Canadian graduates and 2 years for IMGs.

Rhode Island does impose limits at taking USMLE: 3 attempts at each component of USMLE or COMLEX. All components must be passed within 7 years. The same would apply for one of the former examinations such as FLEX or NBME. No limits on COMLEX.

The license fee is $ 570.00. There is an additional fee of $ 140.00 for controlled substance registration.

Rhode Island requires submission of credentials provided by FCVS.

You may obtain further information and/or application forms from The Rhode Island State Board of Medicine: www.health.ri.gov/licensing

The physical address for the Rhode Island Board of Medicine is:

3 Capitol Hill, Providence, RI 02908

**South Carolina:**

South Carolina requires 1 year of post-graduate training for US/Canadian graduates and 3 years for IMGs.

South Carolina does impose limits at taking USMLE: 4 attempts at each component of USMLE or COMLEX. All components must be passed within 10 years. The same would apply for one of the former examinations such as FLEX or NBME. No limits on COMLEX.

The license fee is $ 600.00.

South Carolina requires submission of credentials provided by FCVS.

You may obtain further information and/or application forms from The South Carolina Board of Medicine:www.llr.state.sc.us

The physical address for the Board is:

Synergy Business Park
Suite 202
110 Center view Drive
Columbia, SC 29210
Phone: 803- 896-4500
Fax: 803-896-4515

**South Dakota:**

South Dakota requires successful completion of a residency program as a pre-requisite for Licensure to all applicants.

South Dakota does impose limits at taking USMLE: 3 attempts at each component of USMLE or COMLEX. All components must be passed within 7 years. The same would apply for one of the former examinations such as FLEX or NBME. No limits on COMLEX. MD/PhD candidates will be allowed up to 10 years.

The license fee is $ 200.00.

South Dakota highly recommends submission of credentials provided by FCVS.

Criminal background check is required. You will to complete this procedure on your own based on what is available in your community.

You may obtain further information and/or application forms from The South Dakota Board of Medicine: http://www.sdbmoe.com

The physical address for the Board is:

101 N. Main avenue, Suite 301, Sioux Falls, SD 57104
Phone: 605-367-7781

**Tennessee:**

*Allopathic:*

The State of Tennessee requires 1 year of post-graduate training for US/Canadian graduates and 3 years for IMGs.

Tennessee does NOT impose limits attempts at taking USMLE, but all components must be passed within 7 years unless licensed in three other states.

The license fee is $ 410.00

Tennessee does accept credentials provided by FCVS.

A certificate of good moral character provided by two physicians licensed in the US or Canada

You may obtain further information and/or application forms from The Tennessee State Board of Medicine: www.health.state.tn.us

Or you may contact the board by mail on the following address:

Tennessee State Board of Medicine
425 5th Avenue North
Nashville, TN 37242
Phone: 615-741-3111

**Tennessee:**

*Osteopathic:*

The State of Tennessee Osteopathic Board of Medicine requires 1 year of post-graduate training for graduates of an Osteopathic Medical School

Tennessee does NOT impose limits attempts at COMLEX

The license application fee is $ 410.00

FCVS credentials are accepted.

You may obtain further information and/or application forms from The Pennsylvania State Board of Medicine: www.health.state.tn.org

Or you may contact the board by mail on the following address;

Tennessee State Board of Osteopathic Medicine
425 5th Avenue North
Nashville, TN 37242
Phone: 615-741-3111

**Texas:**

The State of Texas requires 1 year of post-graduate training for US/ Canadian graduates and 2 years for IMGs.

Texas does impose limits at attempts at passing USMLE: 3 attempts at each component of USMLE or COMLEX. All components must be passed within 7 years. The same would apply for one of the former examinations such as FLEX or NBME.

The license fee is $ 885.00

Texas does accept credentials provided by FCVS.

Criminal background check and fingerprinting: This can be accomplished by completing an application form at the Board's website and pay the appropriate fee (which varies from time to time).

Jurisprudence test must be passed as part of the licensure process.

A personal interview is often required.

You may obtain further information and/or application forms from The Texas State Board of Medicine: http://tmb.state.tx.us

The first step in obtaining a license in the State of Texas is to access the above website and fill out your information for the so called "Pre-License screening". After you pass this process (which involves submitting more documentations), then you become "eligible" to apply for a license in Texas. You should be able to complete most of your application process online or via email. If you do need to contact the Board here is the Board's address is:

333 Guadalupe, Tower 3, Suite 610
Austin, TX 78701
Phone: 512-305-710

**Utah:**

Utah requires 2 years of post-graduate training for all graduates.

3 attempts at passing component III of USMLE or COMLEX. All components must be passed within 7 years. A waiver may be granted for MD/PhD candidates for up to 10 years to pass all components.

The license fee is $ 200.00

Utah requires credentials provided by FCVS.

You may obtain further information and/or application forms from The Utah State Board of Medicine: www.dopl.utah.gov

Or by contacting the Board at the following address:

Po Box 146741, Salt Lake City, Utah 84114
Phone: 801-530-6628

**Vermont:**

*Allopathic:*

The State of Vermont requires 1 year of post-graduate training for US/ Canadian graduates and 3 years for IMGs.

Vermont does impose limits on attempts at taking USMLE: 3 attempts at passing component III of USMLE and all components must be passed sequentially within 7 years.

The license fee is $ 500.00

Vermont does accept credentials provided by FCVS.

You may obtain further information and/or application forms from The Vermont State Board of Medicine: www.healthvermont.gov

Or you may contact the board by mail on the following address:

Vermont Department of Health
108 cherry street
Burlington, VT 05402
Phone:802-863-7200 Fax: 802-865-7754

**Vermont:**

*Osteopathic:*

The State of Vermont Osteopathic Board of Medicine requires successful completion of one year of post-graduate training in an accredited Osteopathic program or 3 years in an allopathic ACGME accredited program.

Vermont does impose limits attempts at COMLEX: All components must be completed sequentially within 7 years.

The license application fee is $ 500.00

FCVS credentials are accepted.

You may obtain further information and/or application forms from The Vermont Osteopathic Board of Medicine: www.healthvermont.gov

Or you may contact the board by mail on the following address;

Vermont Department of Health
108 cherry street
Burlington, VT 05402
Phone:802-863-7200 Fax: 802-865-7754

**Virginia:**

The State of Virginia requires 1 year of post-graduate training for US/Canadian graduates and 2 years for IMGs.

Virginia does NOT impose limits on attempts at taking USMLE, however all components must be passed within 10 years unless the candidate is Board certified in one field.

The license fee is $ 302.00

Virginia does accept credentials provided by FCVS.

You may obtain further information and/or application forms from The Virginia State Board of Medicine: www.dhp.state.va.us

Or you may contact the board by mail at the following address:

9960 Maryland Drive, Suite 300
Henrico, Virginia 23233-1463
Phone: 804-367-4400

**Washington:**

*Allopathic:*

The State of Washington requires 2 years of post-graduate training for all applicants regardless of country of medical school.

Washington does impose limits on attempts at taking USMLE: 3 attempts at passing component III of USMLE and all components must be passed sequentially within 7 years.

The license fee is $ 500.00

Washington does accept credentials provided by FCVS.

You may obtain further information and/or application forms from The Washington State Board of Medicine: www.doh.wa.gov

Or you may contact the board by mail on the following address:

Washington State Department of Health
243 Israel Road SE
Po Box47866
Olympia, Washington 98504-7866

**Washington:**

*Osteopathic:*

The State of Washington Osteopathic Board of Medicine requires successful completion of one year of post-graduate training in an accredited Osteopathic program.

Washington does NOT impose limits attempts at passing the COMLEX.

The license application fee is $ 825.00

FCVS credentials are accepted.

You may obtain further information and/or application forms from The Washington Board of Medicine: www.doh.wa.gov

Or you may contact the board by mail on the same address above in the allopathic section.

**West Virginia:**

*Allopathic:*

The State of West Virginia requires 1 year of post-graduate training for US/Canadian graduates and 3 years for IMGs.

West Virginia does impose limits on attempts at taking USMLE: 3 attempts at passing component III of USMLE and all components must be passed sequentially within 7 years.

The license fee is $ 400.00

West Virginia does accept credentials provided by FCVS.

You may obtain further information and/or application forms from The Washington State Board of Medicine: www.wvbom.wv.gov

**West Virginia:**

*Osteopathic:*

The State of West Virginia Osteopathic Board of Medicine requires successful completion of one year of post-graduate training in an accredited Osteopathic program.

Washington does NOT impose limits attempts at passing the COMLEX.

The license application fee is $ 200.00

FCVS credentials are accepted.

You may obtain further information and/or application forms from The Washington Board of Medicine: www.wvbom.wv.gov

**Wisconsin:**

Wisconsin requires 1 year of post-graduate training from all applicants regardless of their country of Medical School.

Wisconsin does impose limits at taking any component of USMLE: 3 attempts per component and all components must be passed within 10 years. No limits on COMLEX. The same would apply for one of the former examinations such as FLEX or NBME. No limits on COMLEX.

The license fees are as follows: Initial fee:$ 165.00, which includes $ 75 for credentialing, $ 75.00 for State Law examination and $ 15.00 for contract examination fee.

Wisconsin accepts submission of credentials provided by FCVS.

You may obtain further information and/or application forms from The Wisconsin Board of Medicine:www.drl.state.wi.us

**Wyoming:**

Wyoming requires 1 year of post-graduate training from all applicants regardless of their country of Medical School.

Wyoming allows 7 attempts at each component of USMLE, however all components must be passed within 7 years. No limits on COMLEX. The same would apply for one of the former examinations such as FLEX or NBME. No limits on COMLEX.

The license fees is: $ 400.00

Wyoming requires submission of credentials by the FCVS.

You may obtain further information and/or application forms from The Wyoming Board of Medicine at: www.wyomedboard.state.wy.us

## Other tools you will need to practice medicine:

### Hospital privileges:

When you join a residency program, the institution will automatically grant you hospital privileges to work as a resident physician. You will practice medicine under the supervision of staff physicians, but you will not be allowed to admit patients under your own name and perform procedures on patients independently. This arrangement is fine during your residency training where you are gradually learning medicine and there are always fully qualified attending physicians to guide you and answer questions you may have with patient care. However, if you decided to "moon light" at another facility, then you will need to obtain hospital privileges in order to practice as an independent physician. Different hospitals have different procedures for this and some are more stringent than others and for some hospitals it may take up to three months to get your privileges approved, however there are some general guidelines that all hospitals in the US will follow and can be summarized as following:

- You must have an unrestricted license to practice medicine in that state
- The hospital will conduct primary source verification, which includes your Medical School and residency training program
- The hospital will need letters of recommendations from at least two physicians familiar with your work
- The hospital will specifically ask you if you have felony or criminal charges against you (past and present).
- You will also need your personal Drug Enforcement Agency Identification (DEA) number. You can obtain a DEA number after you get your unrestricted medical license by applying to the DEA at EDA.gov. As long as you are fully licensed and you pay the fees and you have no criminal records, there are usually no issues with securing a DEA number. You will also need to obtain a National Practitioner identification number (NPID #). If you are a new graduate and still do not have an NPID #, your employer should help you obtain one.
- The hospital will want you to fill out specific forms that have to do with what specific procedures you will be granted privileges to perform at that particular hospital such as tracheal intubation, central venous catheter insertion, lumbar puncture, chest tube insertion, etc. This is where your residency procedure log book comes in handy. Some hospitals may require

that you demonstrate that you are competent at performing some of these procedures and that you have performed enough of them in order for you to perform these procedures independently.

The same procedures will apply for securing Hospital privileges following your graduation from your residency program and when you start applying for full-time positions (jobs) as an independent physician.

**Background Checks:**

Most hospitals and prospective employers conduct background checks on physicians who are applying for hospital privileges or applying for a position as an employed physician. Therefore, following your graduation from a residency training program/and or a fellowship you should expect that hospitals and employers will conduct a background check on you if you are applying for a job or seeking hospital privileges. The motivation for conducting a background check on you as a physician is patient safety and to ensure a safe practice environment for other healthcare provider, but there is also the liability issue for hospital and employers. A business can be held liable for injuries to patients, accidental or intentional, that may be the result of inadequate screening of employees prior to employment. When a background check is conducted, it shows that the organization did its due diligence is assessing the safety and competencies of physicians applying to practice medicine at that particular institution.

What is involved in background checks? The process involves three areas 1.credential verification 2.reference checking and 3. additional background investigation

*Credential verification*: includes a review of the physician's complete education, training, residency, licenses, and any certification (such as board certification), and often involves the physician's previous hospital privileges, malpractice claims history, and peer reviews.

*Reference checking:* involves verifying dates of previous employment (if any), titles at previous positions, and contact references to speak with them about the qualifications of a physician.

*Background investigation:* is often done by a third party agency. The extent of this investigation varies from one organization to another, but generally involves evaluation of the following:

- Criminal and Civil court records for convictions, arrests, and lawsuits
- The National Practitioner Data Bank for malpractice cases and medical board sanctions.
- Medicare sanction list of the Office of Inspector General in the US Department of Health and Human Services
- Sex offender and terrorist data base
- Social Security number; and
- Motor Vehicle records and driving record status.

Some investigations include credit checks, which can cover credit payment history, bankruptcies, tax liens, and referral to collection agencies for no payments. However it is illegal during a background check of a physician to search for information related to a candidate's age, religion, race, sexual orientation, or any other protected category under the Federal Civil Rights Act. It is also illegal under the federal fair credit reporting act for a third party consumer reporting agency to perform an employment background check in secret. The applicant, in this case the physician, must authorize this process by signing a standalone disclosure form.

*Disclose, Disclose, Disclose:*

Physicians should do whatever they can to ensure that individuals in charge of hiring them are not surprised by what turns up in a background check. The most important issue, a physician who is applying for a job, to recognize is that if there is something negative in their background that could be professionally damaging if discovered, she/he should bring it up to the people who will be hiring her/him early in the process of contract negotiation. If you don't bring up an issue or deny it, it implies that you are dishonest or perhaps you have not come to terms with what happened. Physicians are generally willing to give their colleagues a second chance in credentialing or employment if they are forthright. However, the opposite is an automatic exclusion.

Another issue is that physicians should inform the references they list on their applications or CV that they could be contacted to verify information. This is will alert them and will allow time for them to organize their thoughts about the applicant in order to provide the best possible answer. With regard to this issue, choose your references carefully. This applies not only for employment, but also with regard to residencies and fellowships. It is not uncommon for a reference not to know that a physician (who listed them as a reference) is looking for a job or someone that they do not like listed them as a reference.

## Medical Malpractice/Law suites

As you begin to practice medicine as an independent physician following graduation from your residency program and/or fellowship, medical malpractice and the possibility of being sued by a patient or her/his family is a reality that you will have to recognize and understand. In a report which collected data on malpractice by the American Medical Association in 2007-2008 and made public in august of 2010, close to 6000 physicians were surveyed regarding this issue. The AMA survey showed that 42% of physicians surveyed were sued at least once during their career and that 25% of surveyed physicians stated that they have been sued two or more times. 5% of these physicians stated that they have been the subject of a medical malpractice law suit in the preceding 12 months. Overall, there were 95 medical liability claims filed for every 100 physicians. The good news for physicians is the information that was gathered by the Physician Insurance Association of America, a consortium of medical malpractice insurers. This organization found that 65% of closed malpractice claims that were filed from 1985 – 2009 were either dropped or dismissed. Approximately 25% of cases were settled, 5% were decided by the so-called "alternative dispute resolution" and only 5% were resolved by trial. In cases that went to trial the physician prevailed in 90% of cases. So the message, for you as a physician (especially if you are in early parts of your career) is that: yes malpractice is a reality and that a significant number of physicians will be sued. However, only a small percentage of these cases actually do go to trial and if you do end up in a court the probabilities are very high that you will prevail. According to the data from the Physician Insurance Association of America the average payout was $ 212,722.00 across all specialties and the average expenses involved in defending a physician in a malpractice law suit was $ 47,937.00.

The table below shows the frequency of Medical Liability claims by physician specialty as reported by the American Medical Association for 2007-2008.

| Specialty | percentage sued | | last 12 mo | claims per 100 |
| --- | --- | --- | --- | --- |
| | Ever | ≥ 2 | | physicians |
| Family practice | 39% | 22 | 3 | 80 |
| Internal Medicine | 34 | 12 | 5 | 58 |
| Adult subspecialist | 40 | 21 | 4 | 86 |
| General surgery | 69 | 52 | 14 | 213 |
| Surgery subspecialist | 57 | 36 | 9 | 170 |
| OBGYN | 69 | 52 | 10 | 215 |
| Emergency Med. | 50 | 31 | 9 | 109 |
| Anesthesia | 42 | 15 | 2 | 67 |
| Radiology | 47 | 29 | 10 | 116 |
| Pathology | 35 | 9 | 3 | 55 |
| Pediatrics | 27 | 5 | 0 | 36 |
| Psychiatry | 22 | 8 | 2 | 39 |
| All others | 35 | 16 | 3 | 66 |

As you can see General surgery, OBGYN, surgical subspecialties, and emergency medicine have higher malpractice claims compared to pediatrics and psychiatry. Therefore, it is not surprising that Pediatric malpractice law suit is often described as " low-frequency", however, it is often of higher severity, which means that if you are a pediatrician you are statistically less likely to be involved in a law suit, however, if and when you are sued and the plaintiff prevails in the case the payout is much higher than law suits in other fields. This is partly because children have a much longer life span covered and the potential for a better quality of life and future earnings are much higher than say for a 90 year-old patient.

***Strategies to minimize the risk of being sued by patients or their families:***

If you did decide to "moon light" outside your home institution, remember that you are now at risk for a medical malpractice law suit. Here are few strategies you can use to minimize being sued:

- Documentation, Documentation, Documentation: if it is not documented it was not done.
- If you forgot to document an issue, you may go back to patient's record to document, but you have to add your documentation as an addendum with the new date and time and the reason why you did not document earlier.
- NEVER… NEVER attempt to alter medical records, even if you use the same pen and there is enough space for you to add more documentation and you think you are very good at doing that. If the case goes to court, plaintiff attorneys can call hand-writing experts to testify. They will show to the jury that you altered the patient's medical records. If you alter medical records your malpractice insurance is not responsible for defending you and paying the law suit verdict in some states. This issue will become less and less relevant with the advent of electronic health records (EHR) because with HER, every time you enter a note or any data, the system automatically introduces the date and the time of entry!
- "Prevention is better than cure": Controlling the course of events prior to the onset of mutual hostility between you and a patient or a patient's family is the key to avoiding a malpractice lawsuit. Explain procedures, interventions and prognoses in details and share as much information with patients or their families including any uncertainties. This is an excellent opportunity to establish a good Doctor-Patient relationship. Project a sense of realistic expectations while remaining reassuring and helping the patient or her/his family accept reality.

- Communicate effectively: First, assess patient's or patient's guardian (in case of children or elderly) level of understanding when a complicated medical treatment plan is about to be implemented. Include them as a team member and communicate with the importance of their involvement in the treatment plan. Speak in layperson's terms as much as possible and document that in the medical records. Use graphics if appropriate. Repeat information when necessary without showing impatience: e.g. get a chair and sit next to the patient's bed or take the family into a conference room and explain the situation or procedure to them. Allow time for questions.

- When dealing with a hostile, frightened or anxious patient or family members who often use anger to gain control of the situation, make your best effort to put aside natural feelings of disappointment, anxiety, defensiveness and hostility by listening well and remaining calm. For patients and their families who are upset and angry about the complications of a procedure or an outcome, it is best to remain silent until the outburst subsides and the patient or family members have calmed down. This technique of remaining attentive but being silent often diffuses angry people. Under no circumstances lose your temper. Showing anger is the best way to lose patient's trust and to guarantee a visit to the plaintiff's attorney. It has been clearly documented that lawsuits occur because patients or their families were angry at the physician and that there was not good rapport between them.

- Establish a two-way rapport with patients and their families: If it is not possible to establish rapport, suggest transferring the patient to another facility or in an office setting offer the patient to make arrangements to see another physician provider. It helps if you can reassure them that it will be done at no additional charge to patient or their families.

- Always remain accessible: If you are "moon lighting" and a complication or bad outcome occurs, make sure the hospital, patients or their families know how to get in touch with you. Do the same when you graduate and start practicing independently. One of the worst mistakes you can make in dealing with angry or dissatisfied patients or their families is to avoid them. This is likely to hasten their visit to an attorney. As difficult as it might seem the more you talk with and listen to angry patients or their families, the more likely you are to avoid converting an incident into a malpractice claim.

**Other preventive strategies for a malpractice law suit:**

*The most important factor is to be liked by patients, their families and later by the jury!*

You have heard the expression "you may not get a second chance to make the first impression" is very applicable to this situation. It may be too late to turn on the charm after the patient has already developed a complication or a bad outcome from a medical intervention or a procedure. Always show compassion and be genuine in whatever you say to patients and/or their families. There appears to be an unseen energy between human beings, which is sensed by all of us, the homosapiens. When you are honest, genuine, and sincere, people sense that and they appreciate it. Exhibiting compassion, empathy, and sympathy with every step in caring for your patients goes a long way in communicating with your patients and their families that you are putting in your best effort at helping them get better. Being positive, optimistic, but realistic about patients' condition will facilitate the building of trust between you and your patients and their families. When this confidence is established, people will recognize that best results were not possible despite our professional best efforts and medical malpractice law suits rarely occur under these circumstances. The Jury will look at you in the same way as the patients and their families. Even if a bad outcome was avoidable the verdict is likely to be less if the jury DOES NOT perceive you as arrogant, condescending and unrepentant.

The best preventive measure towards malpractice law suits is to critically evaluate yourself and ask yourself these questions: Do I care? Am I honest, caring, genuine, upbeat and encouraging when I speak to my patients and/or their families about their health? Do I express this to all my patients when I interacting with them on a daily basis. Try to incorporate these traits into your daily practice. You will gain the trust and admirations of your patients and then you may not have to "put on the charm" when you are sitting on the witness chair.

*Always make your best effort to follow a standard of care:*

For a plaintiff attorney to have a case, she/he must demonstrate that the standard of care was beached and that this breach resulted directly in an "injury" to the patient. When a standard of care is breached the physician or a hospital can be considered legally "negligent". The term "negligent" legally means that the physician failed to do what another physician of ordinary prudence would have done under similar circumstances. The jury will have to decide whether what you the physician (who is being sued) should have done in relation to what another physician of similar caliber and in a similar situation would/should have done. Juries have been heard to make statements such as "The Doctor should have known that a sick looking baby with high fever could have meningitis", or " He should have checked the results of the lab tests he requested". Many physicians believe that a standard of care should be determined by a panel of experts in that particular field of medicine, however the reality is that members of the jury are rarely experts in the medicine. In fact, physicians are often disqualified by the plaintiff attorneys during jury selection process and ordinary people will decide on the verdict of practically all malpractice cases.

Members of the jury want to see that at least you followed standard of care when you rendered a care to that patient.

Over the years physicians have lost a significant level of power over what is considered standard of care. Health care organizations and hospitals have adopted standards of care, presumably based on data from evidence-based medicine, the private accreditation arm of healthcare facilities such the joint Commission for Accreditation of hospitals and the reimbursement services of the federal government such as the Center for Medicaid and Medicaid. In adopting these approaches testimonies from experts in a particular field have become merely a popularity contest between "expert witnesses" who may be perceived by the jury as "hired guns". So, what is a physician to do in order to do her/his best to avoid a law suit? Make sure you are familiar with and follow the guidelines put forth by these organizations with regard to a specific entity that you are treating. There are numerous examples, and citing all of them is beyond the scope of this book, however here are some examples of clinical guidelines for certain diseases (as of 2010):

Asthma:

Use of systemic corticosteroids during hospitalization for acute exacerbation of asthma and a prescription for systemic steroids at the time of discharge from the hospital. Providing the patient with written instructions on asthma management and instructions on what to do for maintenance therapy for asthma as well as during flaring up of symptoms. Follow up instructions at the time of discharge from the hospital. No following these guidelines would be considered breach of standard of care if the patient leaves the hospital and then several days later dies of a severe attack of asthma before reaching the hospital.

Myocardial infarction:

Use of Aspirin and a beta-blocker upon arrival to the hospital and percutaneous coronary angioplasty within 90 minutes of arrival (if indicated). Providing the patient with a prescription for beta-blocker and aspirin at the time of discharge as well an ACE inhibitor or angiotensin-receptor blocker at the time discharge for patients who have left ventricular systolic dysfunction. Documentation of education on smoking cessation for the patient.

The judge who is presiding over the case will have the power to admit "evidence-based clinical guidelines" based upon their proven integrity, as scored using level-of-evidence and class-of-recommendation parameters. In this case the court may have to hear "evidence of these guidelines" to determine if conflicts in clinical guidelines actually identify the proper standard of care. To achieve this, your attorney may have to present to the court the classification of the levels of evidence from the medical literature as follows:

*Level A:* recommendation based upon evidence from multiple randomized controlled trials or meta-analyses of controlled trials

*Level B:* recommendation based upon evidence from a single randomized trial or nonrandomized trials.

*Level C:* recommendation based upon expert opinion or case reports.

After the court evaluates levels of evidence, it may have to quantify the relative strength of the recommendations and conduct a risk/benefit analysis, which may include an evaluation of the conflicting findings that may be present in different studies. In this process a class of recommendations is established as follows:

**Classes of recommendation**

*Class I:* conditions showing evidence and/or general agreement that a given treatment or a medical procedure is useful and effective for the patient.

*Class II:* conditions exhibiting divergence of opinion about the usefulness/efficacy of a procedure or treatment;

*Class IIa:* weight of evidence is in favor of usefulness/efficacy

*Class IIb:* usefulness/efficacy is less well established by evidence

*Class III:* exhibiting evidence and/or general agreement that the procedure is not useful or effective, and in some cases, may be harmful to the patient.

To put these evidence-based data scoring systems into a clinical example, Let us use the statistics compiled by the American College of Cardiology and the American Heart Association. A closer look at these data show that there are currently over 1900 recommendations from 16 active guidelines. Of the Class I recommendations, only 19% are based on Level A evidence. Most of the recommendations are Class II, and they are most commonly supported by Level C evidence.

It has been demonstrated that practitioners do not limit their medical decisions only on evidence derived from Level A or Class I, and in fact the majority of them do not follow that path. You need to bring these facts to the attention of your attorneys and instruct them to argue that in front of the judge in charge of the the case in the event that your medical liability law suit goes to trial.

**Additional Factors relevant to Medical Malpractice:**

**Informed Consent, A very valuable tool to prevent and defend A law suit!**

Every time you render a treatment or you plan to perform a procedure, you should secure an informed consent from the patient or her/his legal guardian. The legal guardian could be a parent or another individual who has the authority to sign for medical treatment. Occasionally a patient such as a child may be the ward of the state, in which case you have to secure a consent from the appropriate authorities in the specific department in that state, otherwise your treatment may be considered a battery. When patients are admitted to a hospital, the patient or the legal guardian signs a consent for general treatment, but you should still consider securing consent for specific treatments or procedure, particularly invasive procedures. Hospitals have a risk management department which in conjunction with other departments including the legal department formulate a comprehensive consent form, but if you are in a private practice setting where you perform procedures you should make sure that your consent form is a comprehensive one. Here are some important elements of consent:

**Names:** make sure that the consent form bears the name (and any medical record numbers) of the patient. It should also include the names of the primary physician who will be performing the procedure as well as the names physicians who are assisting the primary physician.

**Detailed discussion:** about the procedure. This discussion should be conducted by and documented by the physicians who will be performing the procedure. It is inappropriate to have a nurse or an inexperienced resident physician obtain the consent. You should document that this discussion was in "layperson's terms" as much as possible.

Also, document the procedure in simple English as much as possible. e.g. putting in a breathing tube into the wind pipe for respiratory failure instead of " tracheal intubation" or "removal of the uterus" instead of hysterectomy. If the patient does not speak English, secure the help of a translator officially appointed by the hospital or if your hospital does not have this service, there are various sources for translation via telephone. If appropriate use a staff member who speaks patient's language. In either case document that a translation took place and have the staff member sign in the chart or document other the source of translation.

DO NOT USE a family member to translate. Often due to the stress and with the passage of time the family member may forget what was discussed or he/she may alter what was discussed.

**Signatures and Dates:** The physician who will be performing a procedure should sign and date the consent form and state that he/she was present during the consent process. Only an adult with capacity can sign consent. Incapacitated adults and minors must have their consent signed by a legal guardian. In either case the person who is signing the consent should legibly write their full name (so that the name is easily readable). Also, add how the person who is signing the consent is related to the patient. e.g. Mother. Most comprehensive consent forms have all these elements.

**Variations in the consent form and how frequently you should consent?** A general consent with a space for a specific procedure is sufficient. For example, your hospital may have a general consent form with a space to write the specific procedure e.g. Insertion of a catheter into the subclavian vein/internal jugular vein. Or "red blood cell transfusion". It is preferable to have a patient or a legal guardian sign a new consent every time you discuss a new procedure or treatment. For certain procedures e.g. deep sedation for radiotherapy in a child, one consent is often considered valid for one month in many institutions. Make sure a copy of the consent is saved in the patient's medical record.

**How should you list risks of a treatment or a procedure?**

You should document in the consent that "risks that are relevant to the procedure were discussed with the patient or the legal guardian and that they agreed to proceed". The problem with attempting to list all the possible complications is that they may be too many and that the patient may develop that one complication that you did not list on the consent. If you decide to list some of the risks associated with a procedure or a therapy, make sure you qualify with a statement that these risks are not all-inclusive.

*How powerful is an informed consent?* A consent form is so powerful that some Law firms will not accept a " medical malpractice case" if they see a valid and informed consent as part of the evidence. This is partly because your (defense) attorney can use your informed consent forms along with procedure notes or other notes to build a defense in medical malpractice cases which allege lack of informed consent.

**Secure a witness for the consent:** the best witness is a staff member such as nurse, a respiratory therapist or one of your assistances. The witness does NOT have to be present while you are discussing a procedure with a patient or her/his legal guardian. What the witness will attest to; is that the patient or the legal guardian "appears" competent, that they indicate that they had a conversation with the physician who will be performing the procedure and that she/he witnessed the person sign the consent the form.

*Rashed Hasan, MD, FAAP*

**Should you settle if you are sued? Who should make this decision? You, or your insurance company?**

The first question that you will have to answer is whether to settle out of court or not. Obviously, if you strongly and objectively believe that you have rendered a medical care that is within the standard of care and you and your lawyers believe that the law suit is frivolous, then you may decide that you do not wish to pay the patient or her/his family since a liability does not exist. However, consider other factors such as the time it takes to go through the process until the case gets to trial, your reputation in the community that you practice in, the effects of a potentially large verdict on your insurance policy and even your insurability in the future and the emotional distress you and your family will have to go through. However, it is critical to remember that If you settle and you decide to pay for any damages, your name will automatically be added to the national practitioner data bank regardless of the amount of money you pay. Even if you pay $ 1000.00, your name WILL BE LISTED IN THE NATIONAL PRACTITIONER DATA BANK!!

To make a final decision about settling or not, is a process that involves consideration of a number factors. Here are some factors to consider when making such a decision:

*Detailed evaluation of the case:*

Objectively evaluate the case with the following questions in mind; Will I be able to support the fact that I actually followed standard of care in this case with the records that are available to me, the plaintiff attorneys and the jury? ;and will these medical decisions be defensible, and believable by the jury, when the plaintiff attorneys will attempt to make a circus out of the case in the court of law and in this process they will attempt to point out every possible breach of the standard of care using the most glaring language?

Secure copies of any existing review of the case by "experts". One of the procedures that are typical for insurance companies to do is to obtain an impartial review of the case by an independent reviewer as part of their initial effort to thoroughly evaluate the case. If review of the case by an expert outside reviewer has not been conducted, please ask for one, and in the meantime ask for any internal review (in writing or verbal) that may have been conducted by your medical liability insurance company.

*Evaluate your medical liability policy thoroughly:*

One of the major elements of your medical liability policy that you should know (if you don't know, you need to find out now) is whether it has a clause called "consent-to-settle". If your policy does contain this clause, then the insurance company must secure your consent before settling. On the other, if your medical liability insurance policy does not contain this clause, which may be the case because insurance companies often sell a policy at a lower cost if it does not contain this clause, then it can settle the case without your permission if it will expedite the process of closing the case and as long as the settlement is within the limit of your liability insurance coverage: e.g. $300,000.00 per incident, total annual coverage of $ 600,000.00 per annum.

*Have detailed discussion with your medical liability insurance companies regarding other factors that may affect the case:*

You need to discuss with your medical liability insurance company and the attorneys that have been appointed to defend you (either by your insurers and/or by the hospital that you work for) if there are other factors that may impact the outcome of the case. If the attorneys have been appointed by the insurance company, you have to take into consideration the "bias" of the attorneys towards the decisions of the insurer, even though attorneys are obligated to represent you in the best possible manner according the code of ethics of the American Bar Association. Therefore, it may not be a bad idea to consult another attorney in the field of medical liability at your own expense or the expense of the entity that is your employer. If the opinion of this attorney is that the jury most likely would render a verdict in favor of plaintiff, you may want to insist on settling the case out of court. Alternatively, if your personal attorney believes that the case is weak in favor of the plaintiff you may want to insist on proceeding to a trial. Other factors to consider are: the role of the local media on the case; the caliber of the law firm representing the plaintiff; the jury pool, the judge, and the effects of sympathy on the case by the jury and the local community. Your insurer and your attorneys should be able to give you some idea about these issues.

Your insurance company has some of the interests that you have and that is to settle the case and get it over with as soon as possible, however, there may be few disagreements in which case your personal attorney may be able to help you in this regard.

One important factor is the potential of the verdict to exceed the limits of your liability, in which case your personal asset may be at risk. Some insurance companies offer excess assurance in case they insist on going to trial and you and your personal attorney insist on settling the case out of court. If the insurance company agrees on excess assurance in writing and the case does go to trial, the insurance company will be obligated to pay the verdict and any amounts in excess of the limits of your liability insurance. Again, your personal attorney may be able to help you with this regard.

*What happens if you settle the case?*

Even if you do agree to settle the case, your name and the amount of settlement will be recorded in the National Practitioner Data Bank

(NBDB). Then every time you apply for hospital privileges, a state license, or enrollment with an insurance company or a managed care organization, this information will appear on your data. Although the risks are not very high, this information may adversely affect your applications for any of these entities.

*What if you decided to go to court for a trial?*

Going to trial is a lengthy process. It will definitely take months if not few years. You will have to fill out forms that involve your personal and financial information, you will have to appear for depositions once or few times. It can be emotionally draining if you are not used to dealing with attorneys and the court system. Attorneys are used to it and usually not bothered by harassing and intimidating you; in fact they probably enjoy it. Attorneys will attempt to test your character during a deposition; their goal is make you appear condescending, arrogant, nervous, or not confident of your answers. During a deposition provide concise and accurate answers to the plaintiff attorneys' questions. Do not provide them with any additional information that is not part of the question. Your attorney should be with you during a deposition and she/he will object at the appropriate time if a question is inappropriate (in the same manner that she/he would object during an actual trial in the court). If you don't recall certain information say so. I am sorry, I do not recall. Plaintiffs' attorneys may show medical records to refresh your memory; if this happens, read the information as it appears in the patient's medical record without adding or deleting any information. You may ask to refer to medical records if you do not recall certain information. Be consistent with your answers.

If and when you do go to trial, Plaintiff attorneys will attempt to take the same approach in court in front of the jury. They will make every effort to discredit you and your medial decisions. Therefore, if you do go to trial, dress modestly, appear calm, be respectful of the court, the attorneys, and the jury. Make eye contact with the jury often and make sure that,you are also addressing members of the jury with your answers and not only the attorneys.

Whether you decide to go to court or not is also a business decision. Therefore, weigh the costs of settlement against the costs and time involved with going to court and the potential damaging effects of the verdict on your finance health (the verdict may exceed the limits of your liability), your reputation in the community and with NPDB as well as your insurance policy in the future.

### What is it like to be sued for malpractice? The after-reaction

Sixty percent of physicians are sued by the time they reach age 55, according to a report by the American Medical Association in 2010. The average cost of resolving a medical liability case in 2009 was approximately $325,000.00, which was up by 14% from a prior report from 2000. Defense payments in 2009 averaged $48,000.00, an increase of more than 65% compared to a similar report from 2000.

In addition to the financial burden, physicians who have been sued at any point in their career must note the lawsuit when applying for medical liability insurance and when applying for hospital privileges. Often they have to provide details of the law suit to these insurance companies, hospitals and health care organizations, which may trigger bad memories.

physician's acceptance by managed care organizations panels may be adversely affected and referrals can go down. Experts have stated that the stress associated with a medical malpractice lawsuit manifests in different ways, in different physicians, but it often affects all aspects of a physician's life. From the time that the physician becomes aware of the prospects of a lawsuit until the end of the trial and beyond, the physician is impacted emotionally, mentally, physically and financially. How long a case weighs on a physician depends on the individual physician, the emotional support she or he receives and the outcome of the case, experts say. Therefore, it has been reported that some physicians get nightmares of the events leading to the lawsuit, the trial and events beyond the trial. Some physicians go through a phase where they question everything including questioning their worth as a doctor. For some it may take years to accept that there is a process going on outside of their control, and that the jury and others might come to a conclusion that is different from the perception they have of themselves. Talking about feelings associated with a lawsuit is especially difficult, because legal troubles are perceived as private issues. Complicating matters is the fact that physicians are usually advised by their attorneys not to talk about case details to anyone. This may make the physician feel like keeping it to herself/himself and the physician may feel that she/he is alone, and there's not a lot of help out there for him/her. Therefore, having a strong social support network is essential when enduring litigation. The physician must have an outlet to talk about her/his, anger or symptoms of depression. "There is suffering, and then there's suffering *alone*.", said one expert in the field. If your spouse is also a physicians, you may be one of the lucky ones, because they understand the field of medicine and what it is like to be sued for malpractice, particularly when you believe that "you did nothing wrong".

*How to prepare yourself for a lawsuit?*

You need to prepare yourself for the lawsuit and the trial both psychologically and refreshing on the medical knowledge relevant to the case. Prepare yourself psychologically, because sometimes the damage to you may not come before or during the trial, it may come after the trial is over. During the trial, be prepared to accept the fact that you may not be allowed to tell your story the way you would like to tell it. This happens because of the tactics of the plaintiff attorneys. When getting grilled by the plaintiff's attorney on the witness stand, some physicians have reported that "little voice inside their head saying: maybe you are guilty". If these feelings intensify, you may lose your conviction! Other physicians have reported that surviving a lawsuit is akin to overcoming death. Some physicians go through phases of denial, grief and acceptance. The psychological impact of a lawsuit varies from individual to individual, but it could last a lifetime. So prepare yourself for the lawsuit. Experts recommend that if you are sued you should seek mental and emotional assistance during and after legal battles. Here are starting places where physicians can turn for resources:

**Your local medical society:** Many medical societies have assistance programs for physicians going through medical liability lawsuits. Some offer mentor-type programs that match defendant physicians with physicians who have been through similar experiences.

**Seek help from your liability insurer:** Insurers such as The Doctor's Company offer programs to help physicians manage the stress of lawsuits (here is their website:http://www.thedoctors.com). Each year across the US, the insurers conducts several Litigation Education Retreats, which include lectures from attorneys on what to expect from the legal process and tips on how to be an effective witness.

**Consider counseling:** Experts say counseling and psychiatric assistance enable physicians to recover more quickly after lawsuits. The Center for Professional Well-Being, for example, offers services for management of litigation stress (and here is their website: http://www.cpwb.org).

You need move on with your life:

Your perception of patients may change after a lawsuit and you may notice that you practice more cautiously. You may notice that your document issues in a more obsessive-compulsive manner and that you write down even minor conversations with patients for fear that the information might be necessary someday in a legal setting. You may be far less likely to take on more challenging cases.

A year after a verdict, some physicians still feels as if they are still recovering, but for most of physicians their zest for life and family activities would have returned to normal by this time. You may want to continue to seek the guidance of medical professionals who have been through similar experiences.

### Should you apply for a Fellowship during or after your residency?

Most fellowships involve 3 additional years of training in a specific area within the general specialty. For example, following completion of your residency in Internal Medicine, you could do a fellowship in Adult gastroenterology or Adult Hematology/Oncology both of which will require 3 additional years of training. Fellowship is different from residency in that you spend all of your time in one specific sub-specialty. You will learn about that particular area in depth and become an expert in it. You will also become competent in procedures related to that field so that by the time you complete your fellowship you should be able to practice and perform procedures independently. Fellowship training also involves research and scholastic activities, which include writing abstracts, presenting abstracts at Medical conferences and writing scientific papers for publication in medical journals. Because Fellowships are much smaller than residencies and you train in one narrow field, you tend to be under a closer scrutiny at all times. During your residency you spend one month in each one of the sub-specialties and when you are done you may never go back to that particular subdivision for the rest of your residency training years and if you are in a big program you may not see the attending physicians in that field (at least not often). In contrast, during your fellowship you will face your attending physicians on a daily basis for 3 consecutive years. This has the advantage of developing some sort bonding with them, they will get to know you better, know your strengths and weaknesses, but it will also put a higher level of pressure on you as a trainee. It is this extra pressure that is character building and it is this pressure that will help make you an expert in that particular field once you have successfully completed the fellowship.

Additionally, it involves 3 additional years of training during which you are still considered a trainee, albeit you get a little bit more respect than being a resident. You will still be receiving a stipend during your fellowship which usually starts at the salary of PG Y 4 with benefits. So, unless you get an opportunity to "moon light", your income will still be limited and you will have to consider the potential financial losses during these additional 3 years training.

With some fellowships you can recuperate some the financial losses following graduation, but this is by no means guaranteed for all sub-specialties. So, it is worth exploring whether you should do a fellowship or not as you approach the end of the second year of your residency training program from all aspect: financial, social, personal etc.

Although the choice of physicians to enter fellowship is based on many factors, economic considerations are important. In a recent study published in Pediatrics (the official journal of the American Academy of Pediatrics) in 2011, the authors analyzed the financial returns of fellowship training in pediatrics and compared them with those generated from a career in general pediatrics. Specifically, the authors used standardized financial techniques to estimate the financial returns that a graduating pediatric resident might anticipate from additional fellowship training followed by a career as a pediatric sub-specialist and compared them with the returns that might be expected from starting a career as a general pediatrician immediately following residency. The authors also evaluated the effects of including the newly enacted federal loan-repayment program and of the changes that have occurred in the length of fellowship training.

The results of this study showed that the financial returns of pediatric fellowship training varied greatly depending on which subspecialty fellowship was chosen. Pursuing a fellowship in most pediatric subspecialties was associated with a negative financial decision when compared with pursuing no fellowship at all and practicing as a general pediatrician. The authors suggested that incorporating the federal loan-repayment program targeted toward pediatric subspecialists and decreasing the length of fellowship training from 3 to 2 years would substantially increase the financial returns of the pediatric subspecialties.

Other studies conducted in the past have produced conflicting results. For instance in late 1990s there was a push towards rewarding primary care physicians with higher compensation and benefits in order to encourage new graduates to choose primary care as their field of practice, but studies conducted in early 2000 did not show any significant benefit to practicing primary care compared to specialists.

The bottom line is that continuing into a fellowship training following your residency will depend on the field that you choose if you look at it purely from an economic standpoint. For examples certain subspecialties such as Adult Cardiology may be more financially rewarding compared to Adult Infectious diseases.

*I am a graduate of an International Medical School, may I apply for a fellowship without having any residency training in the US?*

You may find programs that will accept you as a fellow in their fellowship program if you have significant experience in that field. However, your training will not be acceptable by the American Board of Medical Specialties if you plan to set for your board in that sub-specialty. In order to become board-eligible you have to complete a residency in an accredited program in the US in the general field of that particular subspecialty. e.g. Internal Medicine for Cardiology, Pediatrics for Pediatric Critical Care, etc. Occasionally, some physicians have succeeded in securing a position in a residency program following completion of a fellowship program, but these circumstances are rare and are not guaranteed.

**Board Certification:**

The majority of physicians choose to become board certified in their field. Following completion of your residency program you will become board-eligible if you are also licensed to practice medicine in one of the 50 states of the US, the District of Columbia, or one the territories such as Porto Rico or Guam. If you train in a combined residency you will be board-eligible for both boards e.g. Internal Medicine and Pediatric Boards if you finish a combined Internal Medicine/Pediatric residency. If you plan on working in an academic center then you are more likely to need to be board certified because you will be teaching residents and medical students and board certification indicates that you have been tested to assess your knowledge, skills, and experience in a specialty and that you are deemed qualified to provide quality patient care in that specialty. Most hospitals also require board certification in order for them to grant you privileges to practice medicine in the hospital caring for hospitalized patients. Some hospitals will grant you privileges when you are board eligible if you are a new graduate, but will demand that you become board certified within 5 years, otherwise the hospital may not renew your privileges. Board certification requires preparation. There are preparatory courses offered through various organizations and agencies such the AMA, the American Academy of Pediatrics and the American College of Surgeons. There are two levels of board certification through the 24 medical specialty boards. A physician can be board certified in 36 general medical specialty boards. If you completed a fellowship in a particular sub-specialty you may become board certified in 88 subspecialty fields. For example you could be board certified in Internal Medicine (general board), and also become board certified in Adult Gastroenterology. Today, virtually all board certifications require recertification within 7-10 years. Some prospective employers will pay for the expenses involved in board preparations and the costs, application fees, and travel expenses for board certification. Yet, others will pay a bonus if you pass your boards and become board certified. So, there is room for negotiation with matters related to these issues and so do not forget to bring it up during the contract negotiation with prospective employer (see the section on contract negotiation).

**Continuous Medical Education (CME):**

We live to learn! It is very true for physicians. Learning does not stop when you complete your residency or Fellowship training programs. As a physician you will have to continue to learn on a constant basis and to receive credits for what is called CME credits. Most states require a minimum number of CME per year in order for you to be able to renew your license. CME credits are divided into category I and category II. You can receive CME credit by attending a medical conference in person in your hospital, at a local society, or by traveling to attend a medical conference in another local. You can also receive CME by listening to CDs and then answering a quiz or by reading certain review articles which are followed by a quiz. Most employers or prospective employers will reimburse employed physicians who invest the time and efforts to receive CME credits. So do ask your prospective employer about the CME credit allowance, which ranges from $ 2000 – 6000 per year. If you are self-employed, or if you moonlight as a resident or fellow, you may be able to deduct expenses associated with CME (including travel expenses, lodging, conference fees, and meals) from your taxes.

## Financial and Economic Aspects of being a physician

Physicians are high earners compared to the average middle class (they often make 4-10 times more than the average middle class person). However, for physicians, living within their means is significantly different. However, it is important to recognize that physicians graduate later than those in other professions and when they are done they are left with significantly higher debt than the average profession. After graduation, they work longer hours than others and this may be a factor in burnout. Therefore, there are several reasons why physicians need to focus on their financial aspects early in their career.

Here are some general suggestions to help you get ahead and make up for the years lost in training.

**Have a saving plan early:**

Of course the ultimate goal of saving is for your retirement, however life may not proceed the way you have planned it. Make sure you have quality health insurance and perhaps catastrophic health insurance, a disability insurance and a term life insurance (read other sections of the book on these topics) and some savings for rainy days. Then the next questions you need to answer is: How much money you will need to for day-to-day living when you are healthy, in case you cannot work or for your retirement?

The general rule of thumb is that you should not withdraw greater than 4% of your total savings. For examples if you believe you will need to spend $ 100,000.00 a year during retirement, then you will need about $ 2.5 million of after tax assets! To get to this point, most experts recommend saving a minimum of 15-20% of your income throughout your career. The secret to doing this is making savings automatic. If money comes out of your pay-check each pay period, you are less likely to notice it and you never miss it. Do not bank on your retirement accounts alone, also do not get into the habit of saying "I will send a big check at the end the year", chances are you will spend the money and you will not save.

For example, even if you own your own practice, the most an individual can deposit into retirement accounts is $50,000 a year (as of 2013). Over 30 years, that would only net about $1.5 million. You need to think of other investments such as putting money into other accounts such as a joint taxable account, real estate, or purchasing a medical office building that you can use a portion of it and lease the additional space.

**Live as if you are still in training for few years!**

Following completion of residency/fellowship, physicians' salaries jump dramatically.

This is likely to lead to lead to "pent-up purchasing desires". Most physicians move from a low-paying residency/Fellowship positions, an old car, and an apartment; to quadrupling their income literally overnight. Instead of trying to catch up all at once and spend everything you earn, you might want to live like a resident for few years. It has been shown that physicians who are ultimately more successful are the ones who can still live on $50,000 a year and still be content.

Because of all of the years spends in education and training, physicians get a later start on savings than people in many other occupations. Early in your career, you need to make up for those lost years in training by saving, not spending. If you spend all of what you make you obviously will not be saving and you will be tied to your job longer than you wish.

**Your Debt**

Most physicians come out of school with a lot of debt, but look at the schooling debt as a speed bump on the road of your career rather than a roadblock to savings. Student loans typically come with competitive interest rates. Study your student loan often and if does not appear that you have a "good interest rate", work on consolidating your loans with better interest rates, which are usually available once you start practicing. It would be a mistake to pay off debts like student loans before starting to save for retirement. You will have more money when you retire if you begin investing what you can while still paying off loans (read individual sections on these issue elsewhere in the book).

**Building Financial Security:**

We always remind medical students who rotate with us by saying to them: "do you know you are the only people who are paying to be here?" their pupils dilate and they usually say "you are right". And so we always tell them to make it a habit to plan on learning few new things when they go through their rotations.

No one needs to remind you that by the time you graduate from Medical School you will have a substantial amount of debt to deal with. As you start your residency you will receive a stipend which will be enough for you to make a living. If you already have a family with children, it may be tough, but trust me you will make it through the residency. It will become more manageable compared to being a medical student and paying everyday just "to be there".

We present this aspect of your life at this stage in the book because we believe that financial literacy should start early in your career.

*Should you buy a house during your residency or rent?*

The answer depends on: Location, Location, Location!

In locations where the real estate market is always booming and there is constant housing demand, it might not be a bad idea to purchase a house (at the right prize) if you plan to live in it for at least five years. For instance if you think that you will stay in that area after your residency and you are certain that you will have a position, then it makes sense. However, if you plan to stay in the house for less than 5 years, then in general it is not a good idea to purchase a house, unless you believe that you can rent the house after you leave the area and/or you can afford to pay the mortgage in case you don't find a tenant to rent the house to.

From mid-1990 through 2007 the housing market in places such as San Francisco, Los Angeles, Boston, Las Vegas, and Miami were booming. It was not uncommon for the prize of a house in one of these locals to double within 5 years. But then came the economic crisis and housing market collapse in 2008 and the prizes plummeted and foreclosures were rampant. Home prices dropped by more than 50% in some areas. By August of 2010, there were indications that housing prizes were stabilizing and the markets which were hit the hardest began to show signs of stabilization.

While living in your own house gives you a high degree of satisfaction and independence as well as the potential for appreciation and equity building over time particularly during the housing boom, there important points to remember if you plan to buy a house:

- Can you afford to buy a house? You will need 20% of the purchase price in cash as down payment. Then you calculate your monthly mortgage payment based on the house price minus the down payment
- Don not forget to include the property taxes and insurance as additional monthly payments on top of the mortgage. If you purchase a house in an area where the property taxes are high, the monthly payment can be substantial. So always ask about property taxes and insurance.

- Whatever your monthly payment is (including the mortgage loan, the property taxes, and insurance) you will probably need an additional 30 – 40% for additional expenses related to repairs and maintenance of the house, higher utility bills and incidentals. Most calculators available on the internet that compare owning vs. renting don't take into consideration these variables!

- When you sell the house at a later date, you will have to pay a commission to the real estate agents, which is usually in the range of 4-7% depending on the location. So even if the price of the house appreciates by 5% over time, you will have to give that appreciation to the realtors. Additional costs would include registration, county and city fees, etc. That is why if you purchase a house and the value of the house appreciates by say 5% after 3 years, you may still lose money considering what you have to pay the realtors, county and city fees and whatever maintenance expenses you have throughout these three years.

However, there are advantages for buying a house if you plan to stay in the house for a significant period of time or if you think that you will be able to rent the house in case you relocate. Data from surveys of consumers' finances conducted by the federal reserve of the US, have consistently shown that there often a significant gap between the wealth accumulated by homeowners compared to that accumulated by renters. As a homeowner, you will build wealth in at least two ways: through appreciation of the value of the house if you are lucky to buy a house during a phase in the economic cycle when there are housing boom, and secondly through forced saving of paying down the mortgage. The younger you are when you get in the game the quicker you can get the appreciation to work for you.

*Buying a house gives you huge tax benefits, is that true?*

It is true that owning a house may give you tax benefits, but the benefits are often exaggerated! Everyone who files taxes gets a standard deduction. If you were married and you filed your taxes jointly with your spouse in 2010, you will get $ 11,400.00 in "free" deductions, even if you do not pay a penny in mortgage interest. If you buy a house and you are now a home owner with mortgage interest and other deductions totaling $ 12,400.00, the only advantage you would have over a renter who paid zero interest is an extra $ 1,000.00 in deductions. If you are in the 25% tax bracket, the $ 12,400.00 you spent gave you a tax break of just $ 250.00. Even if you get a decent deduction now, the tax "benefits" tend to shrink over time. Most mortgages are structured in such a way that you pay most of the interest in the early years. As the years go by, you will pay more principal and less interest. At the same time the standard deduction offered to all tax payers keeps adjusting upward, squeezing your tax break from both directions. Are you confused? You are not alone! Bottom line, the tax advantages of owning a home is exaggerated.

*So, Should I buy or rent?*

You are more likely to benefit from buying a home if you plan to do the following:

- You plan to stay in the house for 5 years or longer. Yes, it will take that long for any appreciation to offset costs associated with selling the house
- You find a nice quality house, which is not going to need any repairs and you have nice neighbors who are not going to make your family miserable. With renting you can call the landlord to come and fix things for you and if you don't like the neighbors you can move to another location, moving is not that easy with owning a house

- You have some extra savings just in case emergency repairs come up and then you will not have to borrow money to fix that house. Some people recommend that you have enough cash saved to cover at least two mortgage payments after you buy the house
- You manage money well and you are not going to borrow against the house (referred to as "Home equity line of credit") in order to spend it on other things in life such as vacations, repairs, a new care or a boat.

*Final words on buying a house:*

The housing collapse that started around 2007-2008 (after the peak in housing prizes of 2006) surprised many people who believed that the housing market will never collapse and that investing money in house is a secure bit. This housing slump affected the southwestern part of the US, Florida, Michigan and to some extent some parts of California the hardest. But very few cities and states were spared this housing collapse and this problem continues to linger and has affected parts of the country and communities once thought to be more or less immune to housing collapse because of the firm believe that these locals were economically diverse. Places like Seattle, WA and Minneapolis, MN have seen housing prizes drop more than the drop in cities like Las Vegas, NV and Atlanta, GA, which have seen (as of late 2010) prizes drop more than in Miami, FL and Phoenix, AZ. In Seattle, WA for instance, home prices fell by 30% from the peak prizes in 2007.

This significant drop in house prizes occurred when the questionable loans (often called "sub-prime" loans), which were issued to prospective home owners with questionable credits and ability to afford the houses they were purchasing started to deteriorate and people were defaulting on their mortgage. The resulting recession that began in 2008 with high unemployment, contributed further to the deterioration in the housing market. This housing slump in a place like Seattle, WA is reminiscent of the housing slump the city saw during the recession of 1982. Seattle, WA has not seen any housing slump since then, which would be over 25 years of prosperity in the housing market.

As of January 2014, uncertainty about the home prices continue and as long as the employment rate is high and the housing inventories in may places are high, home prices may not appreciate and in fact there a continued risk of further drop in houses prices. Therefore, before you buy a house, you need to do a risk-benefit analysis to see if buying a house in the area where you will be conducting your residency is a reasonable choice for you. The worst thing you can do with your limited income during a residency or a fellowship is to continue to lose the equity in your house over the next few years. If you did decide to proceed with purchasing a big ticket item for which you will need to borrow money, then you need to know: your credit score!

## Know your credit score!

Your credit score is an important financial number. We will discuss what is a credit score and how it is calculated in a short while, however, because credit score is critical when you decide to borrow money towards the purchase of expensive items such as a house or a car, you do need to become familiar with it and to take strategies that will enhance your credit score. The higher your credit score the lower will the interest rate that you will have to pay on a loan towards purchasing a home, a car, or financing a new or an existing practice.

Some of you might say that I am a physician and I am a high earner and do not need to worry about my credit score, but the reality is (and this may surprise some of you) income is often not included in the calculation of credit score!!

**How is a credit score calculated?**

A formula is used that predict risk associated with lending money or providing credit to individuals. Once the formula is solved it comes up with a number which is called the credit score. Also, an individual's credit file is reviewed and analyzed with respect to a number of factors including: Outstanding debts, credit in use, credit and payment histories, and new credit history.

There are different credit scores, however most corporations and institutions use the score developed by Fair, Isaac and Company, which is referred to in the US as the FICO score (FICO is a publicly-traded company, which means that you can buy a piece of this company as a stock under the symbol: FICO). To calculate the FICO score for you, your financial history is analyzed by reviewing your credit report (available with the credit report agencies) with focus on: your current outstanding debt, length of your credit history, new credit applications and current usage of whatever credit you have.

Here is a breakdown of the different components of credit report that are used towards calculation of your FICO score and the approximate contribution of each component to the score:

| | |
|---|---|
| Payment history | 35% |
| Outstanding debt | 30% |
| Credit history | 15% |
| Credit in use | 10% |
| New credit | 10% |

As you can see, *your income is not a factor,* therefore being a physicians and a high earner is not a positive influence on your credit score, but paying your bills that are due on time and keeping the level of your outstanding debt moderate (moderate use of the credit lines that are available to you) are major factors towards a good or high credit score.

The numerical expression based on a statistical analysis of an individual's credit files is called the CREDIT SCORE. Some form of credit scoring system is available in many western countries including the US, Canada, England, Germany, Sweden, Australia and some emerging market countries such as India.

Like we said, banks and lenders like to look at your credit score because that is how they evaluate your credit worthiness and the potential risk that you the borrower may default on paying back a loan. They use your credit score to decide whether you qualify for a loan, at what credit limit, and at what interest rate. They use the credit score to determine which borrowers are most likely to be associated with the most revenue for them. Use of credit score is not limited to banks and lenders. Other corporations such as your cell phone company, insurance companies, landlords, employers, and even some government departments use the credit score.

   In the US, FICO produces your credit score and this score is used by two of the major credits reporting companies, namely Transunion, and Equifax. The third credit reporting company, Experian uses its own scoring system called "PLUS system".

*So, What is your credit score ?*

Your credit score is a number that is a calculated from a combination of the above factors. The score ranges from 300 to 850, with a FICO score of 723 being the median score for Americans. An individual with a FICO score of less than 600 is considered a high-risk borrower. 620 is the dividing score between good and bad borrowers. A score of 640 or higher is considered "good" and 650 signifies average general credit-use behavior. A score of 720 or higher is considered excellent. One caveat is that there is another scoring system used by some credit reports called the Vantage Score and it ranges from 501-990 and has different classifications which can be confusing to creditors and consumers. So, do ask what scoring system was used to calculate your credit score.

Oh Canada.. How about Canada?

The system for reporting of credit scoring in Canada is similar to that in the US because the two system reporting agencies, namely the Equifax and Transunion are the same in both countries. There are some differences between the two countries however. One such major differences is that unlike the US when a person is allowed to have only one free credit score per years, in Canada a consumer may order her/his credit score as many a year as she/he wished as long as the request is in writing, is delivered in writing by mail, and is noted in the credit report. The documentation in the credit report does not have a negative effect on the credit score of the individual. Data from Equifax Score, show that FICO score in Canada ranges from 300 – 900. The Canadian government published a free handbook called "Understanding your credit report and credit score". It provides samples of credit reports and credit scores with explanations of codes and any notations that are used in these reports. It is available at the Financial consumer agency of Canada website. Alternatively, consumers may purchase their credit score for a fee from one of the credit bureaus or directly from Fair Isaac. Credit scores can also be made available for free through subscription to one of the credit report monitoring services.

*Do not damage your credit score!*

Most individuals know the importance of avoiding late payments of bills, making the minimum payments on credit cards, not maximizing your credit limits and avoiding major events such as filing for bankruptcy or defaulting on a mortgage, so that a house is not subjected to foreclosure. However, many people probably are not aware of other issues that can adversely affect your credit score. Here are several issues that you should try and avoid:

A. Do not settle past-due debts with creditors in order to pay less than what you owe: if you take this route and "get rid of your debt", it will stay on your records as "settled" rather than "paid off" and updated on your credit report as such. Because your credit report is more heavily weighted towards recent events rather the time when you originally secured these loans, it works against you and it adversely affects your credit score.

B. Do not close old credit card accounts: If you have old credit cards that you have not used for a while, it is not in favor of you from a credit score standpoint to close these accounts. Remember the longer is your credit history, the better is your credit score (at least this is one factor). So if you close old accounts it may shorten your credit history. Another factor is, that creditors like to see in your credit report that you have several credit lines that are available, unused and that you have not had any problems with these accounts. There is a small probability that these accounts misused through fraud, but if you check your credit score and your credit report periodically you should be able to identify any irregularities and take care of them.

C. Avoid the temptation of transferring from a high-interest rate account to a new low-interest rate account: When you open a new account it works against you. It involves credit reporting (every time somebody inquires about your credit report or score; it negatively affects your score) and if you consolidate all your debts into one credit card it translates to less credit utilization (see B). Remember creditors want to see that you have credits available from multiple sources. If you believe that you can save significant amount of money by consolidating, remember that it may adversely affect your credit score.

D. Do not pay off your mortgage: Creditors like to see different types of revolving loans and installments in your credit report and 10% of your credit score is dependent on what the industry calls "credit mix". If you pay off your mortgage, you have less credit mix and one less revolving line of credit.

E. Do not pay off your car loan: the same issues that apply to a mortgage apply to a car loan.

F. Do not stay debt free!!: your credit score is based on how well you handle your credit. If you have no history of having lines of credit and how you have handled them, your score will be low even though you may not have any debts! In the future, if you need to borrow money to open a practice, expand your practice, or buy a home or a car, if you have never been in debt with a line of credit, you have not history of how you can handle a line of credit and accordingly your credit score may be low and your borrowing cost may be higher!

Based on what we have discussed in this section on credit scores, here are some factors the industry looks at when evaluating your credit worthiness:

1. The ideal number of credit inquiries is 0-3 in the preceding 6 months. Individuals who have more than 6 credit inquiries are likely to have lower credit scores and may have difficulty securing a loan

2. 6-12 lines of credits with a mixture of mortgage, auto loan, credit cards, store credit cards, home equity line of credit… etc. as you can see it is difficult to imagine that you would be penalized for having too many credit accounts as long as you are managing them well. Therefore, DO NOT close old credit card accounts (unless you are paying high annual fees) even if you are not using them. They tell a story about the length

of your credit. The longer you have had a credit the better it is for your credit score.

3.  You need to have a credit history that is 5 years or longer. This ties in with the item in F above. It is difficult to assess your credit worthiness if you have never borrowed. So have credit lines and make your minimum payment for many many years in order to get a good credit score.

4.  If the utilization of your credit lines are somewhere between 5-85% that is considered good.

## Protect yourself from identity theft and scams

Identity theft:

One of the major concerns when it comes to identity theft is your social security number. The social security number is used by those involved in identity theft because it is intertwined with so many other issues of your identity in your life. It is required by financial institutions which issue you credit cards, lines of credits mortgages, and bank accounts. These institutions treat the social security number as an authenticator, even though the social security card (which bears your social security number) is basically a piece of a cardboard (as of 2014) and does not contain any biometrics that identify the person. This makes it impossible to ascertain whether a person using a certain social security number is truly the person it was issued for, but most people assume that only you know your social security number. To protect you, the Internal Revenue Services (IRS) suggests that if you are asked for your social security number, you should first ask which law requires its use. Congress has also proposed laws that restricts use of a social security number and bans its application for certain commercial transactions such as rental applications.

We probably do not need to tell you about the common sense approach that you should take to this issue such as not giving your social security number, your credit card number or your bank account number to any sources that you are not familiar with or that are not an essential part of your career, finances, or daily life, but there are also other ways that people that do not wish you well can get a hold of your social security number. The social networking web sites are one source for criminals to try and find out your social security number and here is one approach to finding out your social security number and then use it to their benefits and to your detriment.

Your social security number consists of 9 digits and at least recently (2010) the numbers were not randomly selected. The first 3 digits were based on the location where you applied for your social security number, which is to some extent dependent on the zip code. So, if you live in the new England area, where the zip codes start low such as 01 or 02, your social security number also is likely to start with low digits such as 01, 02. For example the zip code for Boston, MA is in the range of 02115 or 02118 and so if your social security number was issued in Boston, then it is likely to start with 01 or 02.

On the other in California the zip codes are higher and are in the 900 range such as 94199 for some areas of San Francisco. Therefore, if your social security number was issued there, it is likely to start with numbers in the 9 depending on the exact city where it was issued. As a result people who applied for their social security number in the east coast have social security numbers that are low and the number increases as you move westward.

Once they know your locations, your hometown or your city (provided you have not moved), criminals can probably guess the first 3 digits of your social security number if they work hard enough at it. The second two digits are also not issued at random, they are also based on when and where you applied for your social security number.

Again your local is important. The last 4 digits are supposed to be random, but to a certain extent are based on your date of birth. Therefore, if you make your date of birth public at one of those social network sites, it is likely to help thieves figure out your social security number. Researchers at Carnegie Mellon University established a computer program that was able to construct the correct social security number of close to 10% of Americans by knowing the above information.

The lesson here is to be careful where you put and how much of your personal information on line.

Just as trivia information for your own knowledge base, here are additional information about social security numbers that you may find interesting:

1. As of 2010, the first three digits of a social security number cannot be between 734 to 749 or above 772

2. Any of the components of the social security numbers (first 4, middle two, or last 4) cannot be all zero e.g. 000- or -00- or -0000

**Beware of Scams!**

**Financial scams that you should be aware of !**

Here is a list of financial scams published by the better business bureau that you or your spouse should be aware of, because you may actually lose money getting involved in them rather than making money. And remember, as a physician, you are a high-earner and you are likely to be a target for these scams.

**Reselling your time share condo:** According to data from the better business bureau in 2010, complaints against this type of business increased by 40% during this period. As a physician you are likely to have a time share condo or apartment. Scammers target people who are desperate to sell their time share because it may be too expensive for their budget. They will approach you and tell you that they have a buyer waiting to buy your time share. However, you will have to pay thousands of dollars as transaction fees. The process is simple, you agree and pay the fees, but then you never hear from the prospective "buyer" and you end up losing your money.

**Free trial offers:**

This may be an offer for a free trial for a variety of things such as membership in auctions, clubs, internet services, diet and vitamin supplements and money making schemes. The free trial may seem to be a no-risk trial, but once they get a hold of your credit card you may have to go through many loopholes to cancel your services and by then they would have charged your card for few months before cancelling your service.

**Work from home and make a lot of money!**

This may be a trap for your spouse (if he or she does not work and stays home). The work from home scammers post adds on the internet and on street corners. They claim that they will help you establish a home-based business that will make you a lot of money, but you will have to pay fees to set up your business. In the process these scammers may steal some of your most valuable information such as your social security number, your credit card number or your bank account number. Some people have found that "doing business from home" involved marketing and selling stolen goods. The bottom line is that you may lose thousands of dollars if you get involved in these scams.

**Home Repairs:**

Be careful hiring individuals who knock on your door and offer to do repairs on your house including renovations of a bathroom, finishing a basement or repairing your roof or replacing it. The individual may ask for a "down payment" for doing some work on your home, then take your money and never show up to complete the work. Often it is very difficult to track these individuals down to recover your money. Instead, seek work from a company that is well known in your area and which is bonded and insured to finish the job for you. Occasionally one does come across a handyman who has a track record of doing repair jobs on homes. Make sure you get references from reliable sources.

**Debt Relief and Settlement services:**

Whenever the economy goes sour and peoples' debt skyrockets, so does the number of "companies" that claim that they will assist consumers wipe out their debt. These companies post adds on the internet and media avenues. They often ask for fees up front, which may amount to hundreds or even thousands of dollars. These additional fees may leave you in more debt and without any resolution to your original debt.

**Lottery Scams:** Scammers in this scheme may claim that they are a nationally or internationally known company. They may send you a letter in the mail or an email claiming you have won a large sum of money from a lottery drawing. Then, they will proceed to ask you that in order for you to receive the millions of dollars that you have won you must wire money for the fees involved in delivering your money to you or foreign taxes on the wining amount. You wire the money but "your millions" that they claim you have won is never delivered.

**Loan Scams:** You as a physician who owns a practice may be the perfect victim for this scam. They target businesses such as a medical practice that they perceive as having financial problems or in need of extra cash. They promise that because you are a physician with a successful practice, you have qualified for a large loan to rebuild or expand your practice and we are here to lend you that money. They may state that you have qualified for $ 100,000.00 in business loan at a low interest rate as part of "a government reinvestment act". However, you must pay upfront fees, which often amounts to thousands of dollars and that you should wire those fees to a certain account before you receive the loan. The naïve physician wires the money (fees), but never receives the loan.

**We overpaid you!**

In this scam, which targets small businesses such as a medical practice, the scammers overpay with a check. Then they will contact you and ask you to wire the overpayment to a certain account or send a check to a fraudulent entity. You send the money, but their original payment turns out to be a forged check and you never receive any money in the first place.

**Top Ten Financial Tips that are conducive to a healthy financial future:**

**Before we proceed further into other financial issues we would like to discuss these important points that are likely to be lead to a healthier financial future:**

1. Never cosign for anyone: If a family member or a friend approaches you to co-sign a loan, it is probably better to say " I am sorry I cannot do that for you" because more often than not the borrower has financial issues and she/he is likely to default at some time in the future or make late payments. In this case you risk lowering your credit score (see section on credit score) or losing money. You, the co-signer are ultimately responsible for the loan and so if the person you are co-signing for defaults it appears as if you have defaulted. If you really

have to help this person, it is probably better to offer a loan to that person with specific terms and interest rates in a promissory note. Also, make sure that the person has a collateral that is worth the amount of the loan or more.

2. Save money for yourself FIRST! Think about yourself first. Your retirement should come before college funds for your children. You will help your children more if you are financially secure. If you save money for college, but you do not have enough money saved for your own retirement, then you could potentially be a burden on your children during retirement if you cannot work for whatever reason e.g. illness or disability. There are plenty of college loans that your children can apply to when the time comes, but we are not aware of any loans for retirement!!

3. Be involved in your finances: Do not hand over your finances to your spouse, your partner or a "financial advisor": Be an active participant by getting involved in family and business expenses and your (your family) investments. It will require additional work and time, but it is worth it. You work hard for your money and therefore, you need to be informed at every step along the way with your expenses and investments. Some experts suggest that getting involved may actually improve your relationship. There is an old French proverb that goes like "good accounts makes good friends" suggesting that when people have a good understanding of their mutual finances, that strengthens the relationship.

4. Protect your assets: You as the physician are a high-earner. If your prospective spouse does not work or has an income that is significantly less than yours, then think of a prenuptial agreement! What is a prenuptial agreement? It is an agreement that usually states that anything you bring into the marriage is not automatically shared, but it is yours. However, assets that are accumulated during the marriage are entitled to both

of you. Of course, a pre-nuptial agreement can be written (usually by an attorney) in any fashion that both of you agree on and can include items that is accumulated during the marriage. Because this is a sensitive issue, you may want to discuss it at the appropriate time with your prospective spouse.

5. "Blames be gone": Do not blame your financial illiteracy on others (your parents did not teach you enough about money, The society does not teach us enough about finances, I feel that we should learn more about finances in the Medical School). You need to go and find out for yourself about personal finances. Allocate 1-2 hours a week to learn about finances by reading, talking to someone who is more literate in this subject than you, or watch some of the financial channels such as CNBC.

6. After you make it, take care of it (it is your money): In the same manner that you take care of your spouse, your children, or your parents, your car etc. Try and learn to cherish money in the same way that you cherish other things in your life. You can do this by finding good investments for your money, monitor your investments often and see in which direction it is going. If you are invested in mutual funds, you should get quarterly statements. The same thing would apply to your retirement accounts. When you get your statements, carefully review them and make sure you understand them. If you do not understand certain issues or items, direct questions to the appropriate individuals.

7. Control your own destiny: have a goal for your finances. e.g. to accumulate a million dollar in assets by age 50 or to have 2.5 million by the time I retire (see the section "the idea of becoming a millionaire). Then keep your eyes on the ball and sprint forward no matter what others tell you and how much they will try to deter you from achieving your goal. You are a high-earner and you should be able to accomplish this goal. Take the steps that are the right steps and not the easy ones.

8. Do not make your minors the beneficiary of a life insurance. You should have life insurance, but remember that in the unexpected case that you die, insurance companies DO NOT pay your life insurance payout to children under the age of 18. What you should do is to establish a trust account and name the trust as the beneficiary of your life insurance policy. Your children can the beneficiaries of the trust.

## Money saving strategies for physicians

Pay Cash Instead of using a credit card:

As a high-earner, you should be able to pay for some of your purchases in cash. Studies have shown that having a credit card entices you to spend more compared to if you had you pay in cash. This is logical because when you use the plastic card it does not feel that you are actually paying for an item. You only feel it when the bill arrives at the end of the month.

While it has been difficult to demonstrate how much you actually save by paying in cash, what is certain is that you will avoid paying high interest rates on a purchase, you avoid paying any overdraft fees and other fees that may be associated with a credit card.

Let us take a simple example of gasoline for your vehicle. If you pay attention you will notice that prize at most gas stations is approximately 10 cents lower if you pay in cash. If you drive a large vehicle such as an SUV, which takes about 20 gallons, you save $ 2.00 every time you fill up the tank if you pay in cash. Have the same strategies when you go to the mall alone or with your spouse, you will notice that you will spend less money at the mall if you pay in cash.

The worse situation is probably when you and/or your spouse have department store credit cards. You will spend a lot more and not feel it until the bills arrive at the end of the month. The only exception to this rule is, if you consistently promise to pay all the credit card bills at the end of each month so that you do not have any balances that you will have to pay interest on. If you follow this strategy, you may be able to make money off your credit card if your credit card pays you rewards, let us say 1% cash reward. In that case use the credit and pay for items using your credit card up to the maximum allowable monthly or annual credit. If your credit card company pays you 1% up to a maximum of $ 500.00 per month, then use your credit card for purchases up to $ 50,000.00 a year, in which case you should get $ 500.00 reward at the end of the year. Be careful though, because like we said earlier spending can easily get out hand when using the plastic card. If you do decide to put up to $ 50,000.00 on your credit card, remember that you will be able to spend up to $ 4200 a month using your credit, but then you will have to make sure that you pay that balance (of $4200.00) every single month in order to avoid paying hefty interests to your credit card company.

Maximize contribution to your retirement account(s):

If you are an employed physician, contribution to your 401k (for private for-profit corporations) or 403b (for non-for-profit institutions) is your only option to contribute to your retirement. As of 2012, you can contribute up to a maximum of $ 17,000.00 per year. If you are 50 years or older you may contribute an additional $ 5500.00 for a total of $ 22,500.00 a year. Contributing maximally to your retirement account is a great way to save money for physicians because physicians are high-earners and are therefore in the highest tax bracket usually in the 30-35% range. So, if contribute $ 1000.00 to your retirement account you will skip paying $ 350.00 in taxes on that money and it will stay in your retirement account and grow tax free until you decide to withdraw it when you retire. Of course when you retire your income will be significantly less and you will be in a lower tax bracket and therefore you will pay fewer taxes on that money.

If you are self-employed such as having your own practice or if you are employed, but have a side income from moonlighting activities you can even contribute more to other types of retirement accounts such as a the self-employed personal IRA. (see section of this book on retirement for more details).

Save regularly:

Establish a saving account at your bank and instruct your bank to transfer a small amount into that saving account every month. Even if you save $ 100.00 every month, you will save $ 1200.00 at the end the year, multiply that mount by 30, that is $ 36,000.00. If you add to the compounding interest rate over the years, your money may multiply to a significant amount. Albert Einstein once said "there is nothing more powerful than the power of compounding". Remember that you can withdraw the money at any time if you need it for an emergency.

Shop for auto insurance and raise your deductible:

One of the expensive monthly payments you make is your auto insurance and it adds up if you have more than one car and let us face it, which physician has only one car. The reason you need to shop arround for auto insurance is that auto insurance companies premiums change from year to year depending on what they have to pay for claims. If you thoroughly research it you will find that the lowest premiums rotate among different companies. An auto insurance which has the lowest premiums this year may not have the same lowest premium rate next year. If you know an auto insurance agent who is honest with you and who happened to be a friend, she or he would be the person to tell you which auto insurance company has the lowest premium for that particular year.

Another way to decrease your expenses for auto insurance is to increase your comprehensive and collision deductible on your auto insurance. Just like any deductible, this is the predetermined amount of money that you will have to pay in case you are involved in an accident before your insurance company starts paying the claim.

How does this work?

Let us say that you were involved in an accident and the costs to repair the damages are $ 2250.00 and your deductible is $ 250.00. You will pay the first $ 250.00 out of your pocket and the insurance company will then pay the balance of $ 2000.00. If you can afford to raise your deductible to $ 1200.00, you may be able to save up to 25% on your monthly premium, which when added over a 12 months period and over many years could be a substantial amount of saving.

Buy in bulk if you have a big family

This is particularly true for nonperishable items such as paper towels, toilet paper, vitamins and some alcoholic beverages. For toilet papers for instance you may save up to 50% buying in bulk and for vitamins you may save up to $ 1.00 on a bottle if you buy it in bulk. Costco and Sam's club are examples of places where you can buy items in bulk.

*How to really save when you buy in bulk?*

Buying in bulk is cheaper on most things (about 85% of the stuff we buy), but you can save even more if you know some of dos and don'ts of shopping at bulk stores.

*1. Should you purchase a membership?*

Most bulk stores e.g. Sam's club and Costco require membership in order for you to enter the store and shop. Their annual membership fees range from $ 50.00 to $ 100.00. Because each store carries and has different products you may be tempted to get two or more memberships. This will cost you money, which adds up to your overall cost. One way to get around this cost is to share membership with a friend or not buy a membership at all. Most of these stores allow you to bring a friend along while you are shopping, which means that you go shopping at one these stores for free.

*2. Always think of the price as price per unit*

That means if you pick up an item e.g. canned fruit that contains let us say 12 cans, translate the price into the price per can. Even though most of the items are cheaper when bought in bulk, about 15% of items are not cheaper when translated into price per unit and it might be cheaper to buy such items at a grocery store. This leads us to the next issue

*3. Do not always assume you or your kids will like that item:*

This is very important to recognize for perishable items. If you buy perishable items in bulk, but you do not eat them, you will lose money. One way to get around this issue is to share perishable items such as fruits and vegetables with a friend. In that way you are more certain that your family or your friend's family will actually consume what you purchase. This issue is more important during your residency and fellowship if you have a family and you live on a budget.

*4. Buy the store brand*

Many of the bulk stores carry their own brands of products such as paper towels, toilet papers, cleaning products, detergent, pet food, and some nonperishable foods. And the store brand usually costs less.

*6. Freeze perishable food before it goes bad*

Instead of wasting countless perishable items because you just did not eat them in time, learn to start checking expiration dates and freezing whatever is left before it goes bad.

*7. Don't plan too far ahead*

If you don't have a large household, it can take weeks or even months to use up a bulk size. And if you get sick of it—or no longer need it—you've wasted money. You're better off sticking to staples like flour, sugar, or rice and avoiding the giant-sized frozen barbecue shrimp altogether.

*8. Make use of store perks and discount offers*

Some bulk-food stores such as Costco, come with extras such as a gas station, a tire and car-care center, a cafeteria in order to make the most of your membership. So use all of the perks the store offers. And most extras have a discount (like tires, which are dirt-cheap at Sam's Club), so you'll save even more.

Other money saving strategies

If you have a habit that seems to be costing you money such as going to a bar every day after work and buying a drink for $ 10.00 or going to eat out every day, which again can get very expensive, try and change your habit and exercise these activities less frequently. You will save money and you may enjoy it more and appreciate it more.

So, the bottom, you need to shop smartly! Shopping can be a lot of fun, but it can also cost you a lot of money and even put you into a lot of debt.

## The stock Markets

You notice that we said markets and not market. Yes, there are several stock markets that you can invest in ranging from the US stock market (The new York stock exchanges, the NASDAQ, and the American stock exchange), to the European stock markets (London's FTSE, Paris's CAC 40, and Germany's DAX), and the stock markets in other countries such as Brazil, Russia, India, China (BRIC) or other countries, which are collectively called "the emergent markets". We suggest you stay close to home, but if you would like to have exposure to other stock markets, you can do it in a much safer way by investing in the American depository receipts of foreign companies (which are priced and traded in US dollars), exchange traded funds or mutual funds.

We suggest that you set your priorities straight. Before you put your money in the stock market, allocate your resources to other more important areas of investment and wealth building. These include:

- Buying a home (if that is appropriate for your circumstances) that will be your primary resident and that you and your family will enjoy in a nice neighborhood with good school systems and other amenities of daily living that are important to you and your family. Like we said earlier, if you plan to stay in one local for longer than 5 years, then it is probably a good idea to purchase a house.
- Maximally contribute towards your retirement accounts:
    These may include a 401 K or a 403b or other retirement accounts. As of 2013, the maximal annual contribution is $ 17,500.00 and if you are over the age of 50, you can add an additional $ 5500 per year (referred as catch up contribution). This amount is determined by the Federal government and it increases periodically. You can have your employer deduct certain amounts from your paycheck e.g. $ 634.00 per pay check every two weeks. It comes out of your paycheck

and is deposited into a retirement account. Because you don't see it, it is surprising that you don't feel that you are losing certain amounts from your pay check every two weeks. The contribution can be invested in stocks, bonds or even money markets and it grows tax free until the age of retirement. Your employer will usually have a contract with one of the financial institutions to invest your money. Usually they are invested in mutual funds.

— *What are mutual funds anyway?* Since a significant percentage of physicians are employed in one form or another and because all of the contributions towards 401 K or 403b are invested in mutual funds it is a good time to discuss what mutual funds are?

The financial institution which has a contract with your employer to manage employee's retirement accounts will give you a list of mutual funds that you can invest in for your retirement account. If you have no background about this area it can a daunting task and confusing, therefore, it is important to educate yourself about what mutual funds are?

— A *mutual fund:* is a company that pools all investors' money into one pot and then invests them in stocks, bonds, or money market. In terms of the legal structure, a mutual fund is a corporation that receives preferential tax treatment by the Internal Revenue Services (IRS). The assets of a mutual fund consist of stocks, bonds, and cash that it holds. Unfortunately, with your retirement contribution towards your retirement account you have to select a number of mutual funds that are on the list that is provided to you by the financial institution that manages the employee's retirement account. You will not be able to invest that money on your own, even if you are experienced in buying and selling stocks and bonds. Your only choices to purchase a select numbers of mutual funds from a list of the mutual funds that the financial institution (that your employer has contracted with) gives you.

– *What are some of the theoretical advantages of investing in mutual funds?* Under ideal circumstances if the mutual fund you are investing in is very large and has money managers (those financial guys who take your money and turn around and invest it for you) who have experience in buying and selling stocks and bonds it may provide you (the investor) with the advantage of efficiency, diversification (selection of stocks and bonds from a diverse groups of industries), low cost, and convenience. However, in the real world it does always turn out that way. Money managers may not do well in buying and/ or selling stocks and bonds at the proper time, as a result your portfolio of stocks and bonds may lose value, which translates into an overall lowering of the total value of your retirement account. This is particularly true when the stock markets go through bad periods when markets around the world crash and lose over half of their values. This is exactly what happened in March of 2000 when the NASDAQ (the stock market which has stocks of companies in the field of technology) crashed from 5000 to 1200 in a matter of months (it lost 75% of its value). Now if you bought mutual funds that invest primarily in technology stocks, you would have lost 75% or more of your retirement money during that period. A lot of people lost more than that. A similar event happened in the market crash of 2008 when both the Dow Jones industrial average and the NASDAQ lost more than 50% of their values.

– *How does buying a mutual fund work?* A mutual fund issues shares to investors like you in exchange for cash. So every two weeks or every month your employer take certain amount of money e.g. $634.00 out of your pay check and sends the money to as a mutual fund that you (the investor) decided to invest in. The mutual fund company takes that money, deposits it into its account, and then the money managers who work in the mutual fund company use the money to purchase stocks and bonds or keep a portion on the money in a money market account (which will collect interest). You as the investor become part-owner in the mutual fund.

—   *How is a mutual fund valued and prized?* Each day, the appropriate staff at a particular mutual fund add the value of all the stocks, bonds, and cash that the mutual fund owns, deduct all liabilities the fund has, and come up with a net overall value for the mutual fund. They then divide the net assets by the number of shares outstanding. This gives them a number called the *net asset value* (NAV), which is the price of a share that investors buy and sell from the mutual fund. The NAV for a particular mutual fund is published in may newspapers on a daily basis, which is a requirement by federal regulations. You can use the NAV to assess how that mutual fund you bought is doing.

Let us look at an example to clarify how mutual funds work. You invest $ 1000.00 of your retirement money in a new mutual fund (let us say it is named: xyz) and you purchase 100 shares at $ 10.00. The mutual fund company takes that money and turns around and buys 50 shares of General Electric (GE) stocks at $ 20.00 each for a total of $ 1000.00. One year later GE stock has appreciated from $ 20.00 to $30.00 per share. Now those 100 shares are worth $1500.00. When the accountants at the xyz mutual fund calculate the NAV, they will take the total assets for that mutual fund (which is now $1500.00) minus any liabilities and expenses (office rent and utilities, money manager fees, accountant fees, etc.) which are $ 100.00 and come up with the net value for the fund: 1500 – 100 = 1400 divided by the total number of shares (50) = 28. So, the NAV for the mutual fund that you purchased at $ 20 has appreciated to $ 28.00.

—   *Load and no-Load funds, what does that mean?* When you purchase a mutual fund you hear about the terms "Load funds" and "No-Load funds".

A no-load-fund, is a fund that has no charges associated with purchasing that fund. If you would like to invest $ 1000.00 in that fund, you will be able to use that entire $ 1000.00 to purchase shares of that mutual fund. This will lower your cost and it will allow your investment to appreciate faster. "Load funds" on the other had charge fees for purchasing their shares. The charges ranges from 0.1% to 2%. What does that mean? If you decided to purchase a "load fund" with your $ 1000.00 and the fund charges you 2% to purchase shares, you will have only $ 980.00 (2% of 1000 is $20) to purchase shares. Obviously this will add to your cost and will dampen appreciation in your investment. Some mutual funds have front load and back load, which means that the fund will charge you a fee when you purchase its shares and will also charge you fees when you decide to sell the mutual fund shares. *You should always try to purchase "no-load" funds for your investments. Often, a broker is supposed to help select and purchase a "load fund", but with little effort and knowledge you should be able to purchase "no load funds", which you will have to select and purchase on your own.*

Mutual fund companies are well regulated, but you should still make a good effort to invest in mutual funds of companies that have established reputations for themselves over time. Some of the larger mutual funds have such a large number of mutual funds across a diverse spectrum of companies and industries and have becomes very large. e.g. are Vanguard group of mutual funds, Fidelity group of mutual funds.. etc.

— *Buying and selling mutual fund share, how do I do that?* For your retirement account it is not an issue, because the financial institution that manages the retirement accounts for your employer will do that for you. All you have to do is to make an informed decision and select a number of funds (usually 5-10) from a list of fund that they will offer to you as an investor. However, if you decided to make additional investments in stocks and bonds then you need to learn about how to purchase mutual funds. Now we are talking about the processes involved when an investor buys or sells shares in a mutual fund. The first and most convenient way would be for you to open a brokerage account with one of the financial institutions. Examples include: TD Waterhouse, Scottrade, Schwab etc. After you open an account and your account is approved you can start trading stocks, bond, and mutual funds. Mutual funds like stocks have symbols which you should be able to find at your brokerage website after you log in. You identify a mutual fund that you would like to invest in, find the symbols, then you go to your account and place 'an order",akin to a physician order for a patient, to purchase certain number of shares of a particular mutual fund.

If you do not wish to open a brokerage account, but still would like to invest in mutual funds. you can still purchase mutual funds, but the process is a little bit different. In case of "load-funds" you may get more help from the mutual fund company (because they are charging you a fee). However, with "no-load funds) you deal directly with the mutual fund in question and the process is easy. The mutual fund representatives are usually available to help you through a toll-free telephone number. If you do not have any knowledge about the mutual fund you would like to invest in the first step you should do is to call the toll-free number for the fund and request a prospectus. A prospectus is a booklet of information that is issued annually and that describes the investment philosophy of that particular mutual funds and it will also include all the financial numbers for the fund and how the fund has performed compared to peers and the financial market over the previous several years. The most important aspect of a mutual fund is the investment objective of the fund. This tells the investors the goals the fund seeks to achieve and how the fund intends to achieve them. Often the name of the fund gives you an idea of the objectives of the mutual fund. For example a balanced mutual fund will generally buy and hold stocks and bond. A fund seeking growth will utilize primarily stocks of companies which are growing fast and therefore their stocks are expected to appreciate faster than the rest of the market. On the other hand a mutual fund with the main objective of "income" will invest primarily in bonds with little or no concern for growth and appreciation of the capital. Other types of mutual funds include: growth funds, fixed income fund, international funds (invest in international or multinational companies including American multinational companies), and money market funds. This should give you a good idea of what that mutual fund is about and how the money managers in that fund have performed compared to the market in general and other mutual funds in the same sector in particular. So, before you invest in a mutual fund ask yourself the question of what are my objectives with this investment. Do I want growth and appreciation of my money, but I am willing to take the risk that I may lose capital, or I would like to have an income and preserve my capital and I am not concerned about any growth?

Then if you are satisfied with a particular mutual fund and would like to invest in it, you may ask for an application. The application will arrive in the mail; you fill it out and mail it back with a check for the specific amount that you would like to invest. Most mutual funds have a minimum investment amount that ranges from $ 500.00 - $ 5000.00. Once the cash is received, the mutual fund will allocate certain number of shares based on the NAV for that mutual fund and the amount of money you plan to invest in that mutual fund. Then periodically the mutual fund will send you statement describing how the fund has performed since you have purchased the shares and also the details of all transactions, including purchases, sales and any dividends. Selling a mutual fund is even easier. All it takes is a telephone call to the mutual fund company or your broker. You instruct a broker at the mutual to sell a portion or the entire shares of the mutual funds. The shares are sold usually within one business day and the cash proceeds are deposited into your account.

—   Here are some of the investment objectives in mutual funds:

Growth: of your capital is achieved by investing in stocks of companies which are known to be growing fast and their stocks are also appreciating fast in the stock markets around the world. With potentially higher rate of return comes risks too. If a company's earnings disappoint in a quarter or two the stock price my plummet, if the mutual fund has purchased shares of many growth companies whose earnings disappoint, then NAV of that mutual fund can drop and you can lose substantial amounts of money!

If you would like to preserve capital and have liquidity: invest in short-term bonds (both US and international bonds can accomplish this objective for you)

If you need to supplement your income: invest in bonds

If you do not need income, but would like to see your money appreciate at a lower risk, then you may consider balanced mutual funds which invest in both stocks and bonds in a balanced fashion.

Mutual funds are rated by various companies, the most prominent of which is Morningstar. It provides information on most mutual funds and rates them on a scale. You can find the rating of a particular fund in the prospectus, at Morningstar website and at most financial websites most notably CNBC.com.

*What are some of the advantages and disadvantages of mutual funds:*

These are some of the advantages of mutual funds as often quoted by financial literatures: "convenience with professional management, and diversification".

Convenience: Buying mutual funds is convenient because others will do the work for you. You make few phone calls, set up your investment objectives and the brokerage or in some cases the mutual fund company will match you with a list of mutual funds that meet your objectives. You may also purchase mutual funds on line using a brokerage account.

Cost: Another advantage of investing in mutual funds is lower costs by virtue of their size, the magnitude of trading (stocks and bonds), spreading of the costs (internal and external) over a large number of shareholders.

Diversification is another major advantage of owning mutual funds. For a low dollar amount of investment, you can own hundreds of individual securities in a single fund, thus spreading your risk. Even if some of companies that are in the mutual that you have purchased go bankrupt and their stocks become worthless, the impact on the mutual fund that you own, (which in turn owns hundreds of securities) may be tempered.

In addition there are different types of mutual funds that will allow the investor to participate in many types of securities, e.g. small companies (small cap mutual funds), technology stocks, financial stocks, foreign stocks (European, Asian, Latin American etc.), foreign bonds etc. Therefore, you could assemble a portfolio of mutual funds that invest in different asset classes and have the maximum diversification.

*What are disadvantages of mutual funds?*

Investing in mutual funds make tax planning more difficult. Mutual funds buy and sell securities. In that process the mutual fund may make profits and you the investor are responsible for the taxes on those profits/gains. Because the timing of taxable distribution is uncertain, **it may be difficult to make tax planning, if you are invested in non-retirement (taxable accounts).** If you invest in mutual funds for your retirement accounts (where taxation is deferred) it should not be an issue. Mutual funds are managed by 'money managers". These managers trade frequently in stocks, bonds and other investment vehicles, which are part of that particular mutual fund. However, these transactions are not disclosed to the public or the investor (until after the fact; for competitive reasons) and therefore, it is difficult to track what your money is actually invested in. However, if you invest in a technology mutual fund, you are almost certain that, this particular mutual fund will not trade in financial companies for instance. Additionally, changes in management of the fund such as the fund manager may not be disclosed to the investor in a timely manner. And finally, some mutual funds have expenses that you have to pay when you purchase the fund and additional expenses that you have to pay when you exit the fund. These are called loaded fund. One way to overcome these expenses is to invest in no-load funds. e.g. "indexed funds", which are mutual funds that track the performance of a particular index such as the S&P 500 and are not actively managed and thus have lower fees.

*Can you invest in mutual funds and still be tax efficient?*

Like we discussed earlier, one of the issues with buying and selling mutual funds in an investment account that is not part of your tax-sheltered accounts (retirement plans) is taxation, that you as an investor will have to deal with. When you purchase a mutual fund as an investor, the money managers in that particular mutual fund are constantly buying and selling stocks (or less commonly bonds), in some cases almost on a daily basis. If a stock is sold at a profit, which is good and means that your investment has done well and has appreciate. However, the profits are capital gains and the mutual fund must pay taxes on them. Because you, the investor made money (capital gains), they will pass the taxes on to you the investor. Mutual funds usually send investors (shareholder in that particular mutual fund) the tax bill in December of each year. If you are still holding the mutual fund in your account and have not sold it, you are still responsible for paying the taxes. So you have to come up with extra money at the end of the year to pay taxes on any gains you have made on those mutual funds.

In order to avoid the issue of taxes with mutual funds, one option is to invest in the so called tax-managed mutual funds. These mutual funds attempt to limit the tax liability by using a number of strategies including limiting income from dividend that is taxed at higher than 15%, selling stocks at lower long-term capital gains taxes, and harvesting losses to offset gains in stocks.

Morningstar, the agency that tracks mutual funds and rates them has accumulated data on most tax-managed mutual funds in the US and has reported a tax ratio of 0.46% of their assets compared to 0.85% for all US stock mutual funds. However, some experts believe that there are no major advantages between tax-managed mutual funds and other funds and that past tax efficiency is no guarantee to future tax efficiency.

Another strategy to deal with taxes when investing in mutual funds is to invest in the so called "index-funds". These mutual funds are indexed to one of the major indices such as the Standard and Poor 500 (S&P 500). Because these funds hold stocks that are part of that particular index and accumulate these stocks over time, there is less turnover in buying and selling stocks and consequently less tax issues. And finally always look at the pre-tax and post-tax return for a mutual fund you plan to invest in to evaluate the tax-efficiency of that particular mutual fund.

*Buying and selling individual stocks in the stock market:*

In this type of investment you actually purchase stocks of individual companies. You may purchase one stock e.g. General Electric (symbol: GE). Each stock (like mutual funds) has a symbol, which ranges from 1 to up to 4 or 5 letters.

Buying and selling stocks as an individual investor has undergone significant changes over the past 5 decades. Here is how buying and selling has evolved over the years:

In the 1960s, there were no online accounts such as Scottrade.com, TD Waterhouse.com. If you wanted to buy a stock, you would call your broker, who then entered the order in the system of the brokerage that he/she works for. The order (e.g. 100 shares of GE stock) would be called onto the floor of the NYSE, where your order to buy 100 shares of GE was matched with an order to sell 100 shares of GE by a seller.

If the stock you wanted to buy was an over-the-counter (OTC) stock, that is, it was not listed on the NYSE or Amex, but still traded, the broker called around by phone to market makers who quoted different prices to buy or sell the stock.

Things have change gradually over time. In 1969, the first crack in the wall was that the first Electronic Communication Network (ECN), which was called "Instinet" was founded. It was created to allow brokers to post offers to buy and sell stocks after regular market hours.

In the 1970s, The National Association of Securities Dealers, an association of over-the counter (OTC) market makers created the first electronic stock market: the National Association of Securities Dealers Automated Quotations (NASDAQ) market.

NASDAQ was different from the NYSE in two ways:

- There was no physical floor
- Instead of one market maker (the specialist at the NYSE), there were multiple market makers, often up to a dozen securities dealers who posted offers to buy (called "bids") or sell (called "ask") stocks over computers. These terminologies are still in use today and often a broker will talk to you with something like this " the ask for that stock is $ 30.50 and the bid is $ 29.45", translation: if you want to buy this stock you will bay $ 30.50 per share and if you want to sell it, you will get paid $ 29.45 per share. The selling prize is usually lower than the buying prize for all stocks.

Subsequent to that there another change that led to erosion of NYSE specialists and rise of Internet trading. But this wasn't "electronic trading" in the way we understand it today. Initially, it was just a computerized bulletin board which merely posted bids and offers. However prices were updated only once a day! Orders were not matched by computers, they were still taken over the phone well into the mid-1980s. Still, it did serve to bring down the bid-ask spread and thus help lower the cost of trading.

1975: Fixed commission was abolished by the Securities and Exchange Committee (SEC). This allowed for the rise of discounted commissions and facilitated the growth of internet brokerages.

1976: NYSE introduced its Designated Order Turnaround (DOT) system, which allowed brokers to route 100-share order directly to specialists on the floor. These were not true electronic executions because the specialist still matched the orders, but it did bypass floor brokers.

The 1980s: The rise of electronic trading and the emergence of broker-ages such as Ameritrade, Scottrade and others.

1984: NYSE adopted a more sophisticated Super DOT system that allowed orders of up to 100,000 shares to be routed directly to the floor and thus more floor brokers on the NYSE floor were cut out.

Soon thereafter, Electronic trading took another leap forward as NASDAQ expanded the Small Order Execution System (SOES), which allowed dealers with small trades to enter their orders electronically rather than over the phone. This was done because during the 1987 stock market crash many broker-dealers simply stopped answering their phones.

Market makers were now required to accept SOES orders, within certain volume and price limitations; this greatly improved the liquidity in many smaller stocks, but was flawed because some traders found ways to game the system. Still, it was another towards abolishing of order executing by phone.

The 1990s: Further erosion of the NYSE specialist business and the rise of online trading with the expansion of online trading brokers.

1996-1999: Online trading begins to explode as Internet traffic dramatically increases. Small traders suddenly had the same access to real-time pricing as professional brokers. The word "day trader" enters the vocabulary.

"Day trading" became possible because of more powerful personal computers and high-speed internet combined with higher volume and faster access to bids and offers, which was provided by electronic communication networks. This led to a dramatic drop in commissions which made online trading more profitable. Now individual investor could buy and sell stocks with commissions as low as $ 25 -30 per trade or less. The bull market (when the stock market was going only in one direction: UP) of the 1990s generated more interest from individual investors in trading stocks on line from their personal computers and from the comfort of their home. This fueled day-trading further.

In 1997, stock trading was allowed in increments of one-sixteenth of a dollar, down from one-eighth of a dollar. e.g. prior to this year the lowest fraction a stock could trade at was 1/8, but now the fraction was as low as 1/16 e.g. from $ 16 $^1/_8$ 16 $^1/_{16.}$

2001: Stock trading in pennies begins instead of fractions. e.g. instead of $ 16 $^1/_8$ it was changed to $ 16.05. This combination of faster technology and going to pennies created big changes:

It practically abolished the potential profitability of the old system. Once trading went to a penny, it became difficult for a specialist and a market maker to make money even when committing large amounts of capital. Now you couldn't make a sixteenth of a dollar off a trade, you could only make a penny, so it had to be a big scale business for a specialist on the floor of the NYSE to make a profit on a transaction. However faster computers (and faster trading) also allowed the creation of more sophisticated algorithms that permitted computers to decide the timing, pricing, and quantity of orders based on rules developed by a programmer in a particular brokerage firm. Traders could now slice up big orders into hundreds of tiny orders. This paved the way to the so called "high-frequency trading", a type of trading which employs algorithms but uses those algorithms to make millions of trades a day at very high speeds.

Instead of big money on a few trades, they make pennies (or fractions of a penny) on millions of trades. It's been estimated that 60 percent of the volume is now done by high-frequency traders."

In the early to mid-2000's, these developments were given a further push by the SEC, which was actively seeking to foster competition. They encouraged electronic trading over traditional, floor-based trading and created a new regulatory structure to foster that goal.

In 2001, the NYSE introduced the so called "Direct+" trading, which provided immediate automatic execution of limit orders (which means, the buyer states that she/he would like to buy a stock at a very specific prize e.g. $ 15.55) up to 1,000 shares. This was a real electronic trading (automated matching of buy and sell orders) and was the beginning of the end of the old floor specialist system. In 2008, the NYSE eliminated floor specialists and renamed them Designated Market Makers, though still in charge of maintaining a fair and orderly market in their stocks.

Today an individual can open a brokerage account with any of the online brokerages and start trading stocks, bonds, mutual funds, exchange traded funds, and even commodities using a personal computer and with modest commissions. That is very tempting to physicians who are high earners and tend to have high disposablel incomes. So, you need to be cautions and not get carried away. Otherwise you could lose substantial amounts of your hard-earned money.

Whenever you are investing in a stock market (whether you do the trading by yourself or through a broker = the guy who manages your money at a financial institution) always have one thing in mind: Position yourself to protect your portfolio (the bunch of stocks, bonds, and cash that you own) from another downturn in the market. Always take a cautious, sensible, defensive stance so that you have the resources to take advantage of opportunities when the stock market takes a beating and drops significantly.

Many people will tell you that it is difficult to time the market and you should dollar-cost average, which means that every month you put certain amount of money into the stock market. With this approach you can still lose money. For examples, we all remember the jubilation when the Dow Jones Industrial average (which is an index that contain 30 stocks of 30 companies in different industries of the US) crossed the 10,000 mark. That was in 1998. The Dow did go up from that milestone and reached a little bit over 14,000 in 2008. Then came the financial crisis of 2008 and the Dow dropped from 14,300 to around 6500 and fluctuated between 9000 and 10,000 for the a while. Now, people who used the dollar cost average and continued to invest regularly bought stocks when Dow was at 10,000, but also bought stocks when Dow was at 14,300. This means that their average cost for buying stocks was high and overall their portfolio did not actually appreciate over the preceding 10 years. When you speak to some of these physicians, their portfolio did not return to where it was following the market crash of 2008/2009 until sometimes late in 2013!

Another strategy that you can follow, is not to invest in the stock market every month and perhaps not even, every year. With this strategy you keep your money in cash or short-term bonds and not invest in the stock market *during the years when the market has appreciated significantly.* For example, after the Bush tax cut of 2002, the Dow Jones Industrial Average appreciated from around 7500 and reached a peak of 14,400 in 2008. When the stock market (in this case the Dow) doubles over a period of time, chances are that it will pull back. Indeed this is exactly what happened in 2008 when the Dow plummeted from 14,400 to 6,500. A lot of people lost substantial amounts of money when the market plummeted.

If you have money in the stock market that is managed by so called "Financial Advisors" at different financial institutions, you may want to meet with them regularly and ask them: "what are your strategy in dealing with my money during times of crises, when the market crashes"?. You may be amazed to see that they have little or no plans in protecting your assets even though the stock market may have doubled over the preceding years. Be your own advocate, if the stock market has appreciated significantly and your portfolio has appreciated you may want to consider scaling back on certain stocks that have appreciated substantially. One rule of thumb that you can use is that if a stock had doubled in value you may consider selling half of the stocks and hold on to the other half. Some financial experts (Jim Cramer of CNBS's program Mad Money is one of them) call this strategy "playing with the houses' money". With this approach if the stock continues to appreciate you will continue to make more money. On the other hand if the stock plummets you have preserved your assets and may still keep some of the gains in the stock.

When the stock market crashes, like the situation in 2008, when the Dow dropped from 14,400 to 6,500, that may be the time to slowly get into the market. It is true that no one can time the market, and no one can predict the absolute bottom, but when the market drops significantly you can buy your favorites stocks in smaller amounts at a time, dollar cost average and build up a profitable portfolio. You probably agree that buying stocks when the stock market has plummeted to 7,500 is better than buying stocks when the stock market has doubled to 14,400. Of course, you will only be able to buy if you have been hoarding cash prior to the cash.

What is dollar cost-averaging? You probably have heard that expression before. However, what most people mean by that is to buy stocks every month (with your retirement contribution for example) and hoping that you will buy a stock or a mutual fund at different prices throughout the year, but the overall cost will average out over the course of the year. However, there are reasons why this strategy does NOT always work. During the week that followed 4th of July weekend in 2010 the stock market jumped 5% in a matter of few days. When your money is in a mutual fund or being managed by a "Financial Advisor" you never know when they actually buy stocks for you. If they bought stocks for you after the 5% jump you obviously bought stocks after they have had a huge run upward. Considering that the expectations for stocks is to appreciate approximately 10% per year, then it might be too late to buy at a time when the stock market has made half of its expected annual gain. And so even though your

"Financial advisor" may tell you that we are dollar cost averaging, in reality that may not be happening if you are investing into the market on a monthly basis.

We suggest that you dollar cost-average when the stock market has crashed and not when the market is at its peak. The strategy is not very different from shopping. You like an item in a particular store, but you don't want to pay the full prize for it. You can go window shopping as often as you like, but you wait and when that item goes on sale then you buy it. That item may not go on sale every month, but may go on sale once a year or sometimes less often than that. Let us use an example of a stock that may be purchased at a cheap prize.

General electric (GE) is a very reputable American company. It is a multi-industrial (from airline engines to media) and multi-national (has businesses in many countries). It has been around for a long time and probably will be around for many decades to come. GE stock (symbol: GE) was trading at around $ 60.00 in 2000, it dropped to $ 30.00 during the economic downturn of 2002, then increased gradually over the course of several year to reach $ 40.00 in 2008. During the financial crisis of 2008/2009 it dropped to a miserly $ 6.00 in March 2009. Now it is true that you could not have timed the market, but had you kept your money liquid and slowly accumulated shares of GE at let us say $ 9.00, $ 8.00, $ 7.00 and $ 6.00, you would end up with an average cost of $ 7.50. Isn't that better than paying $ 50.00 or $ 40.00 per share in 2007. Since the generational low of $ 6.00, GE stock has creased in price $ 25.00 as of January 2014. That is an more than four-fold increase in the value of the stock.

People who supposedly "manage" your money would like you to be invested all the time. Because that is how they have a job with a nice salary and get a nice bonus at the end of each. That is why they want you to dollar-cost average. Of course you can be smarter than them. No matter how much they pressure you, tell them I would like to stay in cash for now. Until the stock corrects or crashes, which means that the market drops by at least 10% or more often 20% or more. Then you can slowly get into the market and dollar cost average over a period of weeks to months. But always, always keep some of your money (10-20% in cash) no matter how tempted you are to invest it in stocks.

If you decide to invest in the stock, you need to be informed. You need to watch the market on a daily basis. The best resource in the US is CNBC, the financial channel that follows the markets around the globe minute by minute. Bloomberg is another financial channel that you may access is via television or at their website.

Also, during uncertain times, which means the economy is in a bad situation (recession) take the following steps to protect yourself:

*Before you start investing your money, always make sure that you have a plan. If you think you will need the money within a few years, for instance you are planning to buy a house, then keep that money in a saving's account or a certificate of deposit (with the time-limit that is consistent with your plan; let us say a 12-month CD), both of which will preserve your capital but also gave some interest over time.

*Another option if you want to take some risk (although minimal) is Treasury notes. Treasury notes are backed by the US government; you can safely maintain your capital, while receiving interest during the specified period, e.g. 3-year treasury notes, or 5-year treasury notes.

Few things to remember about US treasury bills/notes are:

- The longer the period of holding, the higher the interest rate you get paid. For instance the 2-years treasury notes gives you less interest than the 5-year note and so on.
- If for some reason the economy recovers and the interest goes up, then the treasury notes decrease in value a little bit, and so you may lose some of your principal, but usually it is in the low single digit range and nothing stocks, where you could easily lose half of your assets.

Don't forget to dollar cost-average as the stock market is recovering. Remember we said earlier always have some of your money in cash. So if you bought GE stock at $ 9,8,7, and $6.00 and your average cost is $ 7.50, but the stock market recovers and GE stock is now $ 12.00, you can still buy some more shares at let us say $ 12.50. As the stock market continues to go up and the GE stock increases in value you will still make money and your portfolio appreciates because your dollar cost average is still lower than the current stock price.

If you don't like all this complicated way of investing, there are mutual funds in various sectors of the economy (national and international) that you can invest in. However, remember that when the market drops, these mutual funds drop in value too. There is one way to hedge against this with mutual funds. There is a category of mutual funds called "long-short funds". When the stock market appreciates, your portfolio increases in value too, but when the market drops, the hedging in these mutual funds helps ameliorate the precipitous drops in your portfolio. You may want to ask you financial (Brokerage) institution about this category of mutual funds.

**Consider buying stocks that pay dividends!**

Stocks of certain companies pay you dividends, which are like interests that you get if you were to keep your money in a savings account or in a certificate of deposit. But the payment you receive from these companies for purchasing and owning their stocks are called dividends instead of interests and there are significant tax ramifications.

Unlike interests which are taxed at your ordinary income tax rate, dividends are taxed at a much lower rate. As of 2010, the tax rate for dividends earned on pre-taxed accounts (these accounts that are not part of your retirement accounts is set at only 15%. In 2002, then, President George W. Bush, cut taxes on dividends down to 15% (from 40%), in 2010, president Obama tried to abolish the so-called Bush-taxes, but after heated debate in congress and opposition by republicans, he decided to keep the rate at 15%. If you buy stocks that pay dividends for your retirement accounts, there are no tax implications.

The dividends are paid usually every quarter into your account and you have the option of taking them as cash deposited into your account or reinvestment them by buying more of the stocks of the same company.

### How do you know which stocks pay dividends?

If you go to any financial website e.g. CNBC.com, and type in the symbol of a stock let us say "Merk" symbol (MRK), which is a pharmaceutical company, it will provide you with a quote for that particular moment, but among other things it will also indicate if MRK pays dividends. You will find this information listed as follows: dividend + yield 1.52 (4.3%) to indicate that if you purchase and own the stock of Merk (MRK), you will get paid $1.52 per share, which translates to a yield of 4.3% on your money.

So, let us say that you buy and own 100 shares of MRK and the stock is trading at $ 35.25 per share and you pay $ 3525.00 to buy these shares (plus the commission, which is between $ 5 -12.00 one-time fee to purchase the stocks). Every quarter, MRK will pay you $ 1.52 per share = $152.00 (152/3535 = 4.3% on your money). MRK will pay you this amount every quarter as long as you hold the stocks. If the prize of the stock goes up, you will still receive $ 1.52 per share, but the percentage will change. So if the stock appreciates to $ 45.00 after say one year, you will still receive $ 1.52 per share, but now it is a lower percentage (1.52/45 = 3.37%). On the other hand if the stock price drops to $ 25.00, you will still receive $ 1.52 per share, but that is a now a much higher percentage of the stock prize (1.52/25 = 6% of your investment). Good companies tend to increase their dividend over time, which means that you will be able to make more money over time.

**How powerful is dividend as part of your investment?**

The simple answer: Huge!

*The bulk of growth in investments over the past century has been due to dividend and dividend growth!*

As companies increase their dividend over time, you get paid more for purchasing and owning a stock, you invest those dividends into more stocks, you get more dividends and so on and so forth.

How can companies afford to pay you dividends?

Companies, which are publicly traded, which means that you can buy a piece of those companies as stocks, make profits every quarter. They have expenses that they will have to pay, but once these expenses are paid they are left with profits. A portion of these profits are paid to their shareholders (people who have purchased and own the stocks of that particular company) as dividends. Companies which pay dividends are in general considered strong companies because that means that they have a good business, they are generating profits and are able to reward their shareholders with dividends.

However, always check the fundamentals of a company and make sure the company is solid from all other business and financial aspects and DO NOT INVEST in a company simply because they pay you dividends.

Good companies which are publicly traded have a track record of being able to not only pay dividends over time, but also to demonstrate dividend growth i.e. able to increase their dividend over time, over many years and often decades. MRK and GE are such examples.

Be aware of companies which pay very high dividends yield though: A dividend yield in the 3-5% is understandable. For instance in

December of 2010, the dividend yield for major cell phone carriers in the US and around the world was approximately 6%. Examples include AT& T, Verizon, and Vodafone. Most of these companies were doing reasonable well and it was clear that people will continue to carry cell phones and the younger generation will continue to purchase more cell phone. However, if you see a company that offers 15% dividend yield and the business model or the business cycle for that company is suspect, then you should be careful in buying the stock of that company, because they may either not be able to pay that high dividend down the road or the company may run into major financial problems and you may lose your entire investment. In 2008 – 2010 during the financial crisis some of the financial stocks and mortgage-related stocks were in this category.

How do I find high dividend paying stocks?

Nowadays you can simply go to google.com and type in "high dividend stocks" and it will come up with a list of websites that can give you a long list of companies with high dividend paying stocks. Then do your research and select companies with strong financial record, good products, and a track record of dividend growth. Avoid the temptation of buying stocks of bad companies, which pay very high dividend yield.

**Words of Wisdom: Before you invest in the stock market you consider doing the following:**

- **Pay off all your credit card debts**
- **Make sure you have adequate insurance coverage: health, dental, catastrophic medical coverage, disability, and life insurance for you and your family members.**
- **Without these essentials, you and/or your family could get wiped out financially if you are hit with a catastrophic**

**health problem or a disability. The credit card interests you pay every month will wipe out all the income that you may have from trading in the stock market. So, be wise, and have your priorities straight!.**

## The Idea of becoming a millionaire!

According to a poll conducted by the financial channel CNB and the Associated Press (CNBC-AP poll) in 2010-2011, most Americans doubt they save enough for retirement in order to live comfortably during the "golden years".

The idea of becoming a millionaire is even more remote for most Americans. Approximately 30% of US residents (US citizens and others) believe that they need between $ 100,000.00 and $ 500,000.00 in order to live comfortably during retirement years. However, 22% believe that you need at least one million US dollars in order to retire comfortably during retirement.

The survey also shows that only 1 in 5 U.S. respondents think it is likely that their net worth will total at least one million dollars in the next 10 years, while 62 percent said that is very unlikely The consensus from the majority of respondents (61 percent): It is "extremely" or "very difficult" to become a millionaire in the United States today. However, many American residents are still trying to hit that million-dollar mark and luckily millions of them have already attained that goal. The number of millionaires in the US is growing. The U.S. has more than 10 million of them. Despite the European debt crisis and worries about the U.S. economy, a May 2011 report from the Deloitte Center for Financial Services projected that the number of millionaire households in the U.S. will more than double to 20.5 million by 2020, with combined wealth of $87 trillion, up from $39 trillion in 2011.

Money makes money, but it has been tough to make that money grow during the rocky financial markets (of 2008 through 2011). The

CNBC- AP poll reported that roughly 60% of U.S. residents stated that their confidence in investing in the stock market has been shaken by recent volatility in the stock market. That sentiment had increased over the preceding 12 months.

Respondents in this poll stated that they are making saving and investing their top priority. The reality is that investors who stayed the course (despite volatility in the stock market) and did not pull their money out of the market in the last few months (as of 2011) may actually have fared better. Despite an almost 8 percent decline since mid-July of 2011, the broader stock market, represented by the S&P 500 Index, was up nearly 8 percent over the preceding 12 months. Certainly it's been a rough few years with the S&P 500, down 8 percent in five years. But over the preceding decade, the broader stock market has appreciated up by more than 10 percent, a fact that speaks favorably in favor of investing in the stock market. The key to learn from this experience, is when markets crash, unless you absolutely need the money, then do not sell because once you sell, you have locked in your losses. You may want to wait it out, just like millions of American who did following the market crash of 2000 and 2009.

*The road to becoming a millionaire:*

You as a physician are a high-earner and you have an opportunity to becoming a millionaire sooner than others, however, in most cases, the road to financial security in retirement comes with steady savings, strategic investing, and probably a later retirement date than you may have envisioned at the start of your career. In order to achieve the goal of becoming a millionaire you need to keep the following rules in your mind:

1. Live within your means. Even though you are a high-earner, you still need to spend money wisely and try to spend within your means. The financial news is replete with high-earners

such as professional athletes who have lost their homes and claimed bankruptcy even though they had astronomically high incomes.

2.  Commit to saving a certain amount every month at an early age (perhaps starting during your residency/fellowship) and be disciplined with this strategy (read the chapter on retirement).
3.  Keep your investment in a diversified portfolio: that means a mix of stocks, bonds, cash and alternative investments (commodities and real estate) and rebalance that mix to attain your goals for growth.

*So how long will it take until you're a millionaire?*

Assuming that you start with an initial $10,000 investment and your portfolio grows by 5 percent every year, here's how much you need to save each month to reach your $1 million goal by age 70, according to the calculator available at Bankrate.com

25-year-olds have to save $500 a month. That's just about $17 a day for the rest of your working years.

35-year-olds have to save $900 a month, which is just $ 30.00 a day for the rest of your working years assuming that you will retire at the age of 70 years.

45-year-olds have to save $1,700 a month.

55-year-olds have to save $4,000 a month.

However, one has to remember Inflation. Inflation increases over time, which means that the value of money decreases over time. Assuming an average inflation of 3%, a $1,000,000 nest egg will only be worth $642,000 in today's dollars. Therefore, you will likely need to save more. However, because you are a high-earner, you should be able to save more each month, but the key is to start early in your career and have a disciplined approach and you are likely to become a millionaire sooner than many other people.


**How to protect your assets that you have worked hard for?**
You as a physician are a high-earner, but you really work hard for every penny you earn. All the assets you have accumulated can be lost instantly if they are not protected and you are involved in a law suit.

Getting sued is part of the life of a physician, however understanding that certain assets should be protected from being lost in case you are sued or in case you have to file for bankruptcy (see the section of this book titled "Bankruptcy for physicians") is critical to your financial success and your livelihood.

We live in a litigious society, and therefore, planning to protect your assets should be a priority. Do NOT put yourself at risk for a disaster you can mitigate with proper planning. By choosing the asset-protection structure or structures that best suit your situation, you should be able to safeguard your finances for yourself and your family.

Who is at risk?

Any physician is at risk. You are at risk not only during the course of your practice as a physician, but also in your personal life: There are a number of circumstances under which your assets can be attacked or garnished; these include getting divorced, filing for bankruptcy, or if you are on the defensive end of a law suit. Here are some examples for the last situation. If someone slips and falls while walking into your office or in your driveway and she/he breaks her hip, you are liable for the consequences and you could be sued. If your teenager is involved in a bad car accident and someone is seriously injured or killed, you are liable for your child's actions and you could be sued.

Here are the steps that you should take to protect your assets:

The first level of protection is to have enough insurance:

Of course you should have your home owner's insurance and insurance for you and your family members. After that is done you should consider getting an umbrella policy that limits liability. This umbrella policy is offered by most insurance companies that offer you your home and auto insurance, however, insurance companies usually do not volunteer to offer it to you as an option. Accidents are statistically the most common incidents that we as physicians face; often it is out of our control but we have to prepare for it. Examples are when you or one of your family members get involved in an auto accident or when someone is hurt on your property (your office or your home). Other examples are boat, jet skis and rental property accidents. When you think about it the cost (premium) is not that much when you consider the amount of coverage you get. For example, for a two- million dollar umbrella coverage, your premiums may not exceed$ 1500.00 a year. Some physicians purchase expensive umbrellas. For instance for $ 10 million dollar umbrella the cost is in the range of $ 2000- 3000. You may also request that the policy be written in such a way that it includes separate coverage for legal fees in case of lawsuit.

Another easy step is to see what is automatically protected by the states where you reside (discussed below). Some states have homestead laws that allow primary residences to be excluded from lawsuits. Illinois and Pennsylvania have laws that protect the equity in a home when it is owned jointly if one spouse is sued. Assets in retirement accounts, and some types of insurance policies also have some protection from creditors. Assets transferred into trusts for the benefits of heirs is another way to shield assets. If they are worded to give plenty of discretion to a trustee in making distributions, trusts can also serve double duty and protect children from lawsuits or divorce settlements.

If you are really rich you have the option of setting up asset protection trusts in states like Alaska or Delaware that have laws allowing these shelters, or can go to offshore jurisdictions, like the Cayman Islands. For the very wealthy the local onshore versions are relatively new, with most dating back to the 1990s. Because of this, these plans have not yet been legally tested and so if you are very wealthy you need to keep that in mind when establishing a trust. The other thing to remember is that if you establish a trust and you frequently dip into it and use the cash for various expenses, it would be difficult to make the case that the money was beyond the reach of creditors.

Some experts recommend that if you have accumulated at least 3 million dollars in cash then it is better to put it in an asset protection trust offshore to make sure the assets are beyond the reach of United States creditors because the bottom line is, if the assets and the trustees, all the components are here in the United States, they're going to be less protected. However, it can cost up to $25,000, to set up one of these trusts. One point to remember also is that on rare occasions, courts had jailed people for contempt when they refused to bring offshore assets back to the United States to satisfy creditors. The bottom line is that if you are very wealthy you need to talk to an asset protection attorney and a financial advisor who is also an expert in asset protection, but it does not hurt to educate yourself on these issues so that you are better prepared to ask appropriate questions.

What assets are protected by law?

Federal and State laws determine what assets are protected from creditors and judgments. Here are some examples of assets that are protected under the law:

*Traditional retirement accounts and Roth Individual Retirement Accounts (Roth-IRA):*

Contributions and earnings in your traditional IRA and Roth IRAs have an inflation-adjusted protection cap of one million dollars from bankruptcy proceedings. The court has the discretion to increase this cap in the interest of justice. In addition any money that rolled over from qualified plans such as 403 b and 547 b plans have unlimited protection in case of bankruptcy. However, these plans may not be protected from other judgments awarded in courts other than bankruptcy.

*Qualified Retirement plans:*

If you are an employed physician, employee-sponsored plan assets have unlimited creditor protection from bankruptcy, regardless of whether the plan is subject to so called "Employee Retirement Income Security Act or ERISA". Included under this umbrella are: self-employed IRA (SEP-IRA), SIMPLE-IRA, defined benefits, defined contribution, 403 b, 457 plans and government and church plans under the law (code section 414).

*Your primary residence:*

Your home that you live in is protected from creditors. In some states, it has to be jointly owned and occupied with your spouse in order for it to be protected. The value of the home that is protected varies from state to state, with some offering unlimited protection as long as it is jointly owned (you and your spouse) and jointly occupied, while others offer limited protection, and few states offer no protection. Since the law changes periodically, please do check your state laws on a regular basis if you own an expensive house in a prime location and you have substantial equity in the house.

*Annuities and Life Insurance:*

Like the protection that you get on your primary resident, state laws determine the amount of protection you receive on these assets. Some states fully protect the cash surrender value of a life insurance and the proceeds from an annuity contracts from attachment or garnishment by creditors. Other states protect beneficiary's interest to the extent that it is reasonably necessary for support of beneficiaries. Please check your state laws.

## How to protect your other assets?

There are legitimate strategies available to protect your assets that you have and continue to work very hard for. The principle here is to put as many road blocks as you can in front of the creditors before they can get to your assets. The creditors will at some point find this information about you and then they are more likely to reach a settlement with you or your insurance instead of getting themselves involved in another long and expensive litigation process in their attempt to garnish your assets. Here are some common and legitimate methods that may be used to protect your assets:

Asset protection trusts:

Some wealthy individuals have and perhaps continue to use trusts overseas to protect their assets from creditors. Examples include accounts in Cayman islands or Switzerland. These trusts can be expensive to establish and maintain. Currently (as of 2011), several states including Alaska, Delaware, Nevada, Rhode Island and South Dakota allow asset-protection trusts. You do not necessarily need to be living in one of these states to establish these trusts, but a portion of your assets must be in your state of residence. Asset protection trusts offer a way to transfer a portion of your assets into a trust run by an independent trustee and you can receive occasional distribution from the trust and the assets may be shielded from creditors in favor of your children. However, asset protection trusts have the following requirements:

1. It must have an independent trustee located in the state; this could be a bank or a trust company licensed in that particular state.
2. It must be irrevocable
3. Distribution is made at the discretion of the trustee
4. It must have a spendthrift clause
5. A portion of the trust's assets must be located in the trust's home state
6. The trust documents and administration must be in the state where the asset-protection trust is established.

Account-Receivable Financing:

If you own your own practice or another business you could borrow money against your accounts receivable. Then take that money and deposit it into a non-business account. This would make the debt-encumbered assets less attractive to the creditors in case of a law suit and it may even not be reachable to creditors.

Strip Out Your equity in a business

Let us say that you own a house that you rent out and you get a monthly cash flow from it. You bought the house for $ 200,000.00 and you put down 20% of the purchase price for a total of $ 40,000.00. You could take a loan against the equity in that house and deposit the cash in a protected asset account (see above) provided your state does provide protection for these accounts from creditors.

Family Limited Partnership:

Family Limited Partnership (FLP) is a limited partnership established by an agreement between family members. It is often used as a business and financial planning entity that has the power of combining business operations with financial planning, estate planning and asset protection. FLP is typically established with one general partner (which could be you) and several limited partners (which could be your spouse and your children). The general partner (in this case you) is entitled to the so-called *pro-rata* share of the partnership's profits and losses, and enjoys all the rights of management and control of the partnership (i.e. you are the general manager of this partnership and you control the operations). The limited partners have some pro rata rights to the profits, losses and distributions, but they have no rights of management or control of the partnership. The general partner (the general manager) can be you (the parent), but it can also be another entity such as a corporation or a limited liability company controlled by the you the parent. Initially when the children are still young you, the parent can be the general partner and a limited partner.

FLP is an asset-protection plan because it offers protection for the assets you (intend to) transfer to the partnership (and thus to your children) while at the same time it allows you to have total control over the management of the assets. You are in total control of the assets and you can buy or sell assets in the partnership, retain proceeds from those sales or distribute the proceeds to general (you) and limited partners (your children and your spouse). Because the FLP owns the assets, they are protected from creditors under the Uniform Limited partnership Act. There is not market for the shares you receive and therefore, the value of the shares is significantly lower than the value of assets exchanged.

How does FLP protects your assets?

Let us say that your teenage son is involved in automobile collision and the other driver and a passenger are seriously injured. They sue your son and you and the court judgment is for $ 500,000.00 against you. The automobile insurance limit of coverage is $ 100,000.00, but the plaintiff would like to satisfy judgment from assets you own and so their attorney has decided to come after your personal assets. However, the attorney soon finds out that you no longer own bank accounts, investments or property as an individual. Instead, most of these assets are held by the FLP in which you have controlling interest. Generally, the plaintiff will not be able to seize partnership assets to satisfy the judgment against you, nor can a judgment creditor reach into the partnership and take specific partnership assets to satisfy a partner's debt or judgment. Since title to the assets is in the name of the partnership, the assets in it may NOT be taken to satisfy the judgment.

How can the creditors recover some of the money?

You do not have an interest in the FLP, the creditor can attempt to satisfy its judgment through use of something called "a charging order", which gives it the right to any distributions from the FLP to the debtor/partner. This order remains in effect until the creditor has been paid in full or until the expiration of a statutory time limit. In other words, money paid to you out of the partnership can be seized by the creditor until the amount of the judgment is satisfied. To avoid this issue, the general partner and controlling member of the FLP can direct that the partnership retain rather than distribute distributions.

In addition to the charging-order remedy, some states allow a creditor to foreclose on the debtor/partner's interest. An order of foreclosure means that the creditor can seize and sell the debtor/partner's interest in the partnership. This action entitles the creditor to the debtor/partner's share of the FLP, even to an amount exceeding the value of the judgment. A creditor with foreclosure rights is in a better position to satisfy his claim from partnership assets if you are, in fact, a partner.

Another option to prevent creditors from having access to your assets is to establish the FLP in such a way that neither you nor your spouse is a partner of the FLP, you have no direct partnership interest to seize. One way to accomplish this is to set up the FLP interest to be owned by a trust specifically created for this purpose.

Since we have introduced the concept of trust, let us go over some common types of trusts.

Revocable Living Trust:

This is the standard trust for transferring assets to beneficiaries at the time death. Assets such as properties in such a trust may be transferred without the involvement of a court. If there is not a trust, the properties will have to pass through the probate court, which is a lengthy process and involves costs in the form of fess. However, with a revocable trust the property may be transferred as soon as the terms of the trust dictate.

Irrevocable Life Insurance Trust:

This type of revocable trust is used to own life insurance for the benefits of your spouse and your children. Why would you want a trust to own your life insurance? Because when the trust owns your life insurance policy, the value of the policy will not be included as part of your estate and therefore, you will avoid estate taxation on the life insurance payout, which in case of physicians may amount to a million dollar. *If you leave your life insurance in your estate, the federal government and tax laws state that it will be included as part of your total taxable estate.* However, if you go this route you cannot be the trustee of the trust and you will no longer have control over the trust or its assets. But, that should not be an issue, because the assets are distributed to your loved ones after you die!

Quality Personal residence Trust:

Your home is not only your castle, but is often the most expensive asset you own. Its loss could have emotional and financial consequences that are disastrous. Therefore, it behooves you to protect this valuable asset of yours with a qualified personal residence trust. This type of trust can protect your home and transfer its ownership to your children over time.

Can you establish a Personal residence Trust and still live in it?

Yes, After transferring your interest in the home to the trust, you retain the right to live there for a specified number of years. At the end of the term or at your death, whichever occurs first, the home passes to the trust beneficiaries (usually your children). Again the advantage of having this trust is that the house will NOT be included in the value of your estate, and thus will escape estate taxation, if you outlive the term of the trust. However, if you die prior to the end of the term, then the entire value of the home is included in your estate.

**What is Fraudulent Conveyances?**

While protecting assets from potential claims is both practical and necessary, deliberately hiding assets from a creditor whose claim has already been realized (which means usually after a judgment has been rendered) may be considered in legal terms as "a fraudulent conveyance" punishable by fine, imprisonment or both.

If you deliberately shelter assets to defraud or delay creditors, your liability may extend beyond the assets you are trying to protect. Check with your attorney about the fraudulent-conveyance laws in your state to be sure your asset-protection plan stays clear of violating any of these issues if you are that situation.

**What are some of the less Complex Ways to Protect your assets?**

There are some inexpensive, simple ways to protect assets that anyone can implement:

- You could transfer assets to your spouse's name. However, if you get divorce, the end results could be different from what you intended them to be.
- Put more money into your employer-sponsored retirement plans because it might have unlimited protection from creditors in case you are sued.
- Buy an umbrella policy that protects you from personal-injury claims above the standard coverage offered in your home and auto policies. Ask your auto or home-owner insurance company. Often you can buy an umbrella policy for up to two million dollars for 20-30% higher premiums.
- Make the most of your state's laws regarding homesteads, annuities and life insurance. For instance, paying down your mortgage could protect cash that is otherwise vulnerable.
- Do NOT mix business assets with personal assets. That way, if your company runs into a problem, your personal assets might not be at risk and vice versa.

**Some Final Words of Caution**

Often you come across adds on infomercials and on the internet from some self-proclaimed asset-protection "experts" advertising their seminars. Make sure you do extensive research, including checking with your local Better Business Bureau before deciding to use any of these services. And before you take any of the steps discussed in this section of this book. Hire an attorney who is familiar with the laws of your state and an expert in the asset protection field. Most importantly, do NOT wait until you have a judgment against you. By then it may be too late, and the courts could declare that you made a "fraudulent transfer" to get out of meeting your obligations.

## Interesting tax issues for you, your parents, your children and other family members

*What should you do with stocks or mutual funds that have made substantial gains towards the end of a year? Should you sell and take profits or stay the course?*

We are discussing this issue in this section purely from a tax-point of view and for investment accounts that are pre-tax accounts and are not part of your retirement accounts (in which the taxes are deferred and are not an issue).

For example in 2010, the capital gain tax rate was 15% and there were intense discussions about raising the capital gains tax rate from 15% to 20%. Under those circumstances, one option would be to sell a portion of your stocks that have appreciated and pay only 15% in taxes on the gains as opposed to waiting until the next year, when you may have to pay 20% in capital gains taxes. So, it is worth keeping in touch with the financial news and with your accountant towards the end of the years to keep abreast of these important issues. We are not suggesting that you sell your stocks or mutual funds based purely on tax issues. You should look at the overall picture of your investment and taxes one important factor to consider when you are contemplating selling stocks or mutual funds

*What about stocks or mutual funds which have gone down and you have lost money on them?*

If you have stocks which have appreciated and you plan to sell them, but also have stocks which have gone down and you have lost money on them, what you can do is to sell the loser and claim capital losses against capital gains. For examples if you own 1000 shares of GE stocks that you purchased at $ 7.00 each for a total of $ 7000.00, but you also purchases 1000 shares of China mobile at $ 20.00 per share for a total of $ 20,000.00 during the same year and the GE stock appreciated to $ 17.00 per share, while the shares of china mobile dropped from 20 to $10 per share, you have gained $ 10,000.00 from GE, while you have lost $ 10,000.00 from China mobile. If you sell both stocks your net gain is zero and you do not owe any capital gain taxes.

*What is the "wash-sale" rule?*

This is a tax rule, which prohibits an investor from claiming loss on the sale of an investment such as stocks or mutual funds and repurchasing the same investment (stocks or mutual funds) within 30 days. As the name implies, this rule applies only to stocks or mutual funds sold at a loss. If you sell stocks or mutual funds at a gain and for one reason or another those stocks or mutual funds go down and you would like to purchase them at the lower prize you can do that and the rule does not apply to this situation. You can still keep the profits you made from the sale without incurring a penalty. So if you are holding a stock or mutual fund you have made gains on and you believe that the capital gain taxes may go up next year (let us say from 15 to 20%) you can sell these investments in the last week of December, pay only 15% on the gains and repurchase the same investment in the first week of January if that stock or mutual fund goes down. We recognize, that this may be a complicated issue for those of you who are not familiar with buying and selling stocks or new to this issue, but it help to become familiar with this issue if you plan to buy and sell individual stocks in the future.

*Paying taxes on dividends:*

As of 2010, the taxes on dividends earned from holding stocks or mutual funds is 15%. However, tax laws change and there are periods when the gains on your investments from dividends are taxed as ordinary income, which means that you will be taxed at your tax bracket on any gains in your portfolio from dividends. So, if you are in the 35% tax bracket (and most physicians are) and your investments makes $ 2000.00 from dividends you will owe $700.00 in taxes instead of $ 300.00 if the earnings from dividends (capital gains) was taxed at 15% and no considered ordinary income. Like we discussed earlier, in 2012, when the so called Bush tax cuts expired, they were amended so that capital gain taxes remain at around 15%.

*What about the Estate Tax?*

In the past the estate taxes were high; 55% of estates are valued at more than one million for individuals and two millions for couples. In 2002, then President Bush introduced a new tax provision which abolished these estate taxes. At some point in the future these estate taxes may return to where they were. So, if your assets are in that range you may want to discuss this issue with your accountant and come up with strategies that will minimize paying a hefty estate tax in case the unexpected happens and you suddenly die.

As of 2010, there is a proposal for two year extension of the so called "Bush tax" in which taxpayers will receive an exemption for estate tax for up to $ 5 million. This proposal, if passed, will also allow survivors combine their exemption with that of a deceased spouse for a total of $ 10 million. This means that people who have a estate that is worth up to $ 10 million dollars are almost guaranteed that they will not have to pay any estate taxes. If you are not rich yourself yet, but have a parent who is rich and who may have a estate which is worth that much you may want to advise her/him on these issues. You never know it may benefit you. You may get some of that money instead of Uncle Sam.

Overall, estate taxes are a small percentage of the total taxes collected by the treasury department, however with this tax law exemption an estimated 40,000 of the estates will escape estate taxes, which amount to an estimated $ 300 billion dollars over ten years as estimated by Brookings Institute. As of 2010, congress is debating this issue, and if this tax law passes and the "Bush Tax" stays, which means that there are no estate taxes for up to $10 million, the law will more than likely will be for only two years and no one knows what happens in the future, which makes it even more critical for individuals who are high earners and have significant assets to keep an eye on this issue for any future changes in the law.

*How about some gifts for family members?*

As a taxpayer who is a high-earner and a high-net worth individual you can reduce the size of taxable estate every year and over the years by taking advantage of the *annual gift tax exclusion*. Here are some guidelines on how to approach this issue:

1. The Internal Revenue Service (IRS) allows any taxpayer to make an annual tax-free gift of up to $14,000.00 (as of 2014) per recipient. You can give this gift to as many individuals in your family as you wish. A married couple can give up to $28,000.00 per recipient annually. You can give these cash gifts to your parents, your children, your cousins, or anyone you would like to give to.
2. Instead of cash, you can use stocks that have appreciated in value considerably and give them to your children or your parents as a gift.

*What is the advantage of doing that?* Instead of you paying capital gains at your higher tax brackets, your children can pay taxes on these asset at their tax brackets, which is usually considerably lower than yours. One caveat is that the child has to be 24 years of age in order for you to avoid paying taxes at your tax bracket. Therefore, this strategy works best for your parents who may be living only on social security benefits and have limited income or if you have older children (older than 24 years) who are not employed or have limited income and are in one of the lower tax brackets.

3.  Another way to reduce your taxable estate is to contribute towards a 529 college plan for your children or grandchildren. You can contribute up to 14,000.00 per year or you and your spouse can contribute up to $ 28,000.00 per child per year.

4.  If you would like to reduce the size of taxable estate further you can elect the 5-year plan towards a 529 college fund. This provision allows you ($ 65,000.00) or you and your spouse ($ 130,000.00) to contribute the corresponding amounts towards a 529 plan for a child or a grandchild in one single year instead of annual contribution over five years. You may also receive state tax deductions for these contributions.

5.  529 college plans for grandchildren (or children) have some advantages which include tax-free growth (no federal taxes and often no state taxes on any appreciation) and the ability to transfer the plan to another sibling (if it is not used by the child), a cousin, and even parents or in-laws as long as the fund will be used towards a college education.

*"I really need extra money right now, can I tap into one of my retirement accounts?"*

The financial crisis of 2008 brought with it a number of issues for Americans including tapping into their retirements as a source of emergency funds. Can you do that? Can you withdraw money from retirement accounts?

Yes, you can. But there are tax consequences for withdrawing money from these accounts. Remember, the money in your retirement account is pre-tax money; money that was not taxed when you made the contribution to these accounts. Therefore, if you withdraw any portion of it out, you will have to pay taxes on that money at your current tax bracket. In addition, there is a 10% penalty for early (before your retirement age; 59.5 as of 2010) withdrawal and you will also have to pay state taxes according to state of residence. Most physicians are at the highest tax bracket of 35-39%, which means that when you withdraw from any of retirement accounts, you will have to pay close to half it to taxes. But there are ways to minimize taxes on early withdrawal from a retirement account. Here are some examples:

A.  Borrow money from an IRA account: You can take money out of any retirement account (that is not Roth-IRA) without having to pay the 10% penalty and federal and state taxes if you can return the money into the same retirement account within 60 days. So, if you need emergency funds and you believe that you can deposit the money back into the retirement account in the next two months, this is an option for you.

B.  Another option for withdrawing money from a retirement account without a penalty if you are approaching the retirement age is the so-called *"substantially equal payment method"*; in this method you withdraw equal amount of money every year for, say 5 years. If you start at age 55, you can withdraw equal amounts of money every year for 5 years (until you reach the retirement age of 59.5). With this method you can avoid the 10% penalty, but you will still have to pay federal and state taxes.

C.  Another option for withdrawing from a retirement account without incurring the 10% penalty is if the funds are used for qualified college tuition, to pay insurance premiums if you are not employed or in the event of disability or death.

D.  Look at your income for that particular year: and do some mathematical calculations to estimate your total income. If it looks like by withdrawing certain amount of money from a retirement accounts puts you into the next higher tax bracket (which means that you will have to pay more taxes) try and defer any withdrawals until January 1$^{st}$, so that hopefully you will pay less in taxes. Whenever, you withdraw money from a retirement account that will incur taxes, you may want to have the brokerage withhold the taxes (and send them to the IRS) so that comes April 15$^{th}$ of the next year you will not be liable for taxes. It is not uncommon for people to take the entire amount, spend it and then be left with any extra money for taxes and penalties.

E.  Do Not forget itemized deductions in a year when your income has been low, but expenses have been high: chances are that your income has been lower or low, you can't make the ends meet and therefore, you are reaching for your retirement accounts to withdraw funds for emergency needs. Take advantage of itemized deductions such as medical expenses. If you have medical bills you can deduct them if the total amount exceeds 7.5% of your gross adjusted income. This will lower your overall income, which in turn will lower your tax bracket and hence the total amount of taxes you owe.

F.  Roth Individual Retirement Account (Roth-IRA): Most physicians who are already in practice do not qualify for Roth-IRA, because their income exceeds the upper limit for Roth-IRA contribution. However, if you established a Roth-IRA when you were a resident or a Fellow or before entering medical school, when your income was lower, and you have some of your saved money in a Roth-IRA, withdraw the emergency fund that you need from a Roth-IRA instead of withdrawing from a traditional IRA, a 401K or a 403b retirement account. With the traditional IRA, 401 K or 403 b the taxes are deferred at the time of contribution, therefore, if you withdraw funds from any of these accounts prior to age 59.5 years, it will trigger federal and state income taxes as well as a 10% penalty. If you add up all these taxes for you as a physician, they will be approximately 50%, which means that half of the money that you intend to withdraw will go to taxes. To the contrary, withdrawing money from a Roth-IRA does not because with Roth-IRA you pay the tax upfront (at the time of contribution to a Roth-IRA), and you have already paid the taxes on the money that is in a Roth-IRA account, therefore, you can withdraw money from such an account at any time without triggering a penalty or having to pay federal or state taxes. There is one catch though! The money must have been in a Roth-IRA account for at least 5 years because you can withdraw any funds without incurring penalty or taxes.

**Taxation and Tax issue relevant to you as a physician:**

Albert Einstein once said: "The hardest thing in the world to understand is income tax."

And indeed taxes are not easy to comprehend. The US tax codes are over 4000 pages long and often gets modified. As a physician your affairs are complex and therefore, it may be difficult, time-consuming and inefficient for you to deal with your tax issues. You may want to get help from a certified financial accountant (CPA) for tax issues. Your CPA should be a good resource for you in this respect. Here are some suggestions for year-end tax issues that may help you save some money.

**Year-end tax issues that could save you money!**

A.  Sell stocks, mutual funds or exchange-traded funds that have depreciated and you have lost money on them. The IRS allows you to claims capital losses up to $ 3000.00 a year, which can be deducted from your ordinary income and thus lower the total amount of taxes you pay. However, beware of the so-called "Wash rule" that we discussed earlier. For example, if have purchased 1000 shares or General Electric (GE) at $ 20.00, and the GE stock has dropped to $ 17.00 and you sell the 1000 shares at that price on December 15$^{th,}$ 2010. You cannot turn around and purchase 1000 shares of at $ 16.50 on January 5$^{th}$, 2011 and still claim the $ 3000.00 losses on your taxes for 2010 because you repurchased the same asset within less than 30 days. You could purchase another asset though with the funds that you received from the losses incurred from the deprecation in GE stock such as another stock, mutual fund, or an exchange-traded fund.

B.  If you are employed and you think for one reason or another you will receive refunds from the federal or state governments based on the calculations that you have made on your income and expenses; talk to your human resources/compensation and benefits department and instruct them to withhold less on your last pay check. In that case you get your cash in December (by paying less taxes) instead of having to wait for 8 weeks or more after you file your taxes for the government to pay you your money back!

C.  Increase your contribution to your retirement accounts, whether it is a 401 K, a 403b or other retirement accounts; the more you contribute towards them (up the maximum limit) the less you will to pay in taxes. As of 2014, the maximum contribution if you are an employed physician is $ 17,500.00 a year and up to $ 22,000.00 if you are 50 or older. The additional $ 5500.00 is called catch-up contribution for those 50 and older.

D. You can get a State tax deduction if you contribute towards a 529 plan for a child or a grandchild up to a maximum of $ 14,000.00 per child or you can take advantage of the 5-years plan where you gift the entire amount for the next 5 years all in one year (this year) for a total of $ 65,000.00 per child and get state tax deduction or credit if your state has 529 plans.

E. Charitable contributions: You may make charitable contributions with cash, clothing, furniture, old cars or boats. Vietnam Veterans is one example. Find their phone number, call them and they will pick up all the clothing, and light furniture, etc. from your front porch. They will not come into the house to pick up any items however. Make sure you get a receipt. They usually provide you with sticker with their name on it along with a signature of the individual who picked up the donated items. You may use that sticker as your receipt that you actually did donate items to them. There are other organizations that you can make charitable contribution to throughout the year. This could be your local church or a soup kitchen.The items that you donate have to be in a good usable condition and you claim the fair value of the item at the time of donation for the purpose of tax-deduction.

## State Taxation

**Tax issues when you live in two or more states in one year:**

Because most residency and fellowship programs start in July and many physicians start a new job in July, it is very likely that some of them will live in more than one state during the year of relocation. This means that you will have to file taxes in more than one state.

If you have lived or worked in more than one state, you may need to file multiple state tax returns. You may also have to file part-year resident returns or nonresident returns in multiple states in these kinds of situations.

**If you commute for work in another state**

Many physicians commute into another state to work. e.g. many people who work in Boston, MA, live in New Hampshire. The same situation applies to many Americans who live in contiguous states. In this case you may have to file a resident tax return in your home state and a nonresident tax return in your work state. On your resident tax return you would include all of your income, even the income you made in your work state. This is because most states tax a resident's income from all sources, even those from out of state. On your nonresident state tax return in your work state, you would only include the wages you made in that state. In most states, you'll be able to take a tax credit on your resident tax return for the taxes you paid to your work state so that you are not taxed twice.

How do I file a non-resident state taxes?

First, you will need to figure out how much income you made in the nonresident state and how much income you made in your home state. Most nonresident returns will also use figures from your federal return, so make sure to complete your federal return first.

**How to allocate deductions and income**

In most states, you will list your total income from your federal return in one column and your income as a nonresident in another column. From the totals of those two columns you will calculate the percentage of your nonresident income to total income. We'll call this your "nonresident percentage." Depending on what state you're in, you will use this percentage to allocate your taxable income, your deductions, or your tax liability.

**Taxable Income:** Some states will have you calculate your taxable income in that state as if you were a resident. You would then multiply this by your "nonresident percentage" to come up with your taxable income as a nonresident. The state of Virginia is an example of a state that uses this method.

## How to calculate your deductions:

Other states will have you multiply this "nonresident percentage" by your federal deductions. This amount will be your nonresident deduction amount which you will subtract from the income you made in that state as a nonresident. The State of Maryland uses this method.

Keep in mind that certain federal deductions, such as the deduction for state and local taxes, are not deductible for state tax purposes. You will have to adjust for those differences on your return. You will also be able to add any state-specific tax deductions as well.

## Allocating your tax liability:

Some states, such as Delaware, will allow you to offset your nonresident income by your federal itemized deductions (after adjusting for non-deductible items such as state and local taxes). These returns then have you multiply your actual tax liability by your "nonresident percentage" to come up with your tax liability as a nonresident.

## Filing the Return in Your Resident State

You will also need to file a return in your resident state. On this return you include all of your income, even the income you made in the nonresident state. This is because most states tax the income of residents regardless of its source.

**Credit for Taxes Paid to a different State**

Most states offer residents a tax credit for taxes paid to another state or jurisdiction. Be sure to take this credit on the return you file in your **home state.**

**A CPA can take care of all these issues for you for a handsome fee!**

**Filing a Return for Mistaken Withholdings**

If you are filing a nonresident return because taxes were withheld for the state by mistake and you did not make any income in that state, you would simply report zero income for that state on your nonresident return, resulting in zero tax liability. Your non-resident state then should refund you the appropriate amounts.

**What if you moved during the year (a common scenario for physicians)**

If you moved to another state during the year, you will mostly likely need to file a part-year return instead of a nonresident return. And here is the breakdown for these situations:

A part-year resident is usually someone who has moved into a state in the middle of a tax year while a nonresident has not physically lived in the state. But, as with all things in tax, there are caveats to this general rule of thumb.

**Temporary Moves**

If your move was temporary and you did not make any actions that created residency, like registering to vote or getting a license, you **may** be a nonresident. To be a nonresident you must not move into the state with the intention of making it your permanent residence. An example for this situation would be; you temporarily moved into a new state for a short-term locum tenet (see section on locum tenet in the book) to cover a practice for few months, then subsequently returned to your home state when the locum tenet period ended.

In some states, you will automatically be considered a resident if you have lived in a state for a certain amount of time. Some states may also require that you maintain a permanent home in another state as well.

Whether you are a nonresident or part-year resident, most states require that you pay taxes on any income you made from sources within that state. However, special rules apply to military servicemen and women.

### Members of the Military

In 2009 congress passed a special tax-relief legislation to members of the military and their spouses so that they do not pay taxes in multiple states. Under this act, the military members and their spouses will only be responsible for state and local taxes in their home state where they maintain residency. This tax relief legislation applies only if the family moved because of military service-related orders.

### How to File a Part-Year Resident State Tax Return

If you moved to a new state during the year, you may have to file a part-year tax return in both your old state and your new state.

### Which Form to use?

Most states have forms for taxpayers who were part-year residents, but some use the same forms as full-year residents with special calculations. Sometimes one form is used for both part-year residents and nonresidents. Check your state tax website (or speak with your CPA) to see which form you should use. If your state has a special form for part-year residents (usually denoted with part-year [PY]), that is the form you should use. You will have to fill out a part-year resident tax return for each state you were a resident of during the year.

Do not confuse part-year residency with non-residency. Although there are some exceptions to the rule, in most states, part-year residency means that you actually lived in the state for part of the year, while nonresidents simply made income in the state without maintaining a permanent home there.

**How to divide income between states?**

Part-year tax returns are usually prepared based on your total income for all states, then your tax liability is pro-rated based on how much income you made in each state. Let's start by talking about how to split your income between two or more states.

If you moved to a new state to start a new job, it should be easy to figure out how much income you made in each state. You will get a W-2 or 1099 tax forms (see section of the book titled W2 vs. 1099) from each employer that will tell you how much you were paid. However, if you moved to a new state while still employed for the same institution, it can get more difficult. If you worked for the same employer, but moved to a different state, you are only going to get one W-2 or 1099, which will only state the total amount that you were paid. That means you are going to have to split the income up between the states on your own. There are two main ways to do this.

**Use the paystub or payroll information from your employer:**

This is the most accurate way to come up with the amount of income you made in each state. If you are using a paystub, be sure it is from a pay period that ended around the time of your move.

**Allocate income based on how long you lived in each state:** If your income is relatively the same every month, you can allocate it to each state based on the amount of weeks or months you lived there

For instance, let us assume that you worked for 11 months of the year (you took one month vacation). You moved to your new state and started a new job in early May. This means you would have spent about 8 out of 11 months working in your new state. You would use the fraction 8/11 to allocate your income to the new state. The remaining income would go to your old state.

However, this method is much less accurate than using a pay stub, especially if your income fluctuated during the year. You should only use this method if you are not able to get paystubs, time sheets, or other records that could help you estimate the actual income made in each state.

**Unearned Income and Earned Income, what is the difference?**

The Internal Revenue Service (IRS) defines earned income as income that is from "wages, salaries, and tips", while unearned income comes from non-employment sources. Examples of unearned income are interest from money that is sitting in a bank account or a certificate of deposit (CD), dividends that your accounts have earned from stocks and bonds (in a non-retirement account), social security, and capital gains (which include appreciation on stocks and bonds).

Unearned income is generally allocated to the state you were living in when you received it. For example, if you sold stock at a gain just after you moved into your new state, that income would be attributed to your new state.

However, if your unearned income cannot be attributed clearly to one state you would need to allocate that income to each state based upon the fraction of the year you lived there (e.g. 8 out of 12 months or 8/12).

## What if I Have Both Unearned and Earned Income?

If you have both earned and unearned income you would simply calculate your unearned income in State A, and add to that your earned income in State A, to get your total income for State A. You would do that for each state you were a resident of during the year.

## How to pro-rate tax liability in each state?

Once you determine how much income you made in each state, most state tax returns will then use the percentage of your income attributed to that state to prorate your tax liability. This percentage is equal to the amount of income you made in the state divided by your federal adjusted gross income (your total income in all states). This represents the percentage of your income that was made in that particular state.

This percentage is then multiplied by the total tax amount for that state (which is based on your total income for the entire year) to prorate the tax liability. *The amount of time you lived in the state does not matter here.*

Let us look at an example. James moved from Iowa city, Iowa to Richmond, Virginia to start a new job during the year. His total taxable income for the year was $200,000. He made $160,000.00 in Iowa and the remaining $40,000 in Virginia. Using the tax table on his part-year tax return in Iowa, he has a tax liability of $10,000 based on his total income of $200,000. He would then multiply that $10,000 tax liability by 80% for a tax liability of $8,000. This is because he only made 80% of his total income in Iowa ($160,000 Iowa income divided by $200,000 total income). The same process would be repeated on his Virginia return, using 20% .

## Pro-Rating Deductions

Some states will use this same percentage to pro-rate deductions, which are subtracted from the income allocated to that state. The state tax amount is then based upon that taxable income figure.

Let's look at the same James example, with $30,000 worth of total deductions in Iowa. This deduction amount would be multiplied by 80% ($80,000 Iowa income out of $200,000 total income). This would give James an Iowa deduction amount of $24,000 (80% x $30,000).

To find James' Iowa taxable income using this method, the $24,000 prorated Iowa deduction amount would be subtracted from his Iowa income of $160,000 for an Iowa taxable income of $139,000. His Iowa state tax would be based upon that amount.

## What About Income I Made in the State Before I Moved There?

In the example above, if James had made income in Virginia before he physically moved there, he would also include that income in his Virginia total income. This is because most states require that part-year residents pay taxes on income they made while they were a resident, as well as income received from sources within that state.

## Payments and Tax Credits

On the payments section of each return, you will use the actual amount of tax withheld from your paycheck for each state and any estimated payments you may have made to each state. There is no adjustment made to these amounts.

Tax credits in each state may be subject to special calculations, so read these instructions carefully. Most importantly, *do not forget to take advantage of the credit for taxes paid to another jurisdiction.* Most states offer this credit to part-year residents.

**Reciprocal Agreements: States that do not tax certain out of state workers:**

Reciprocal agreements between states allow residents of one state to work in a neighboring state while only paying income taxes to their state of residency. This simplifies tax time for people who live in one state, but work in another by requiring them to file only one state tax return. If the state where you work and the state where you live have a reciprocal agreement, you are exempted from income taxes on any wages earned in the state where you work. You only have to pay taxes to the state where you live.

Here is a list of states and jurisdictions that have reciprocal agreements:

- **District of Columbia:** If you work in D.C. and you are a resident of any other state you do not have to pay D.C. income taxes on your wages. You will have to submit the exemption form D-4A to your employer.
- **Illinois:** If you work in Illinois, but you reside in Iowa, Michigan, Kentucky, or Wisconsin you do not have to pay Illinois income taxes on your wages. You will have to file exemption Form Il-W-5-NR through your employer.
- **Indiana:** If you work in Indiana and you are a resident of Kentucky, Michigan, Ohio, Pennsylvania, or Wisconsin you do not have to pay Indiana income taxes on your wages. You will have to submit exemption Form WH-47 to your employer.
- **Iowa:** As of 2010 Iowa has reciprocal agreement with only one state and that is the state of Illinois. You will have to submit exemption Form 44-016 with your employer.

- **Kentucky:** If you work in Kentucky and you are a resident of Illinois, Indiana, Michigan, Ohio, Virginia, West Virginia, or Wisconsin you do not have to pay Kentucky income taxes on your wages. Submit exemption Form 42A809.

- **Maryland:** Maryland has reciprocal agreement with the following: District of Columbia, Pennsylvania, Virginia and West Virginia. If you work in one of these states you do not have to pay Maryland income taxes on your wages, but you will have to submit exemption Form MW 507 through your employer.

- **Michigan:** If you work in Michigan and you are a resident of Illinois, Indiana, Kentucky, Minnesota, Ohio, or Wisconsin you do not have to pay Michigan income taxes on your wages. You would submit exemption Form MI-W4 through your employer.

- **Minnesota:** Has agreement with two states as of 2010: Michigan and North Dakota. You do not have to pay Minnesota income taxes on your wages if you work in one of these two states. You would submit exemption Form MWR through your employer.

- **Montana:** If you work in Montana and you are a resident of North Dakota you do not have to pay Montana income taxes on your wages. You will have to submit exemption form NR-2 with your employer.

- **New Jersey:** If you work in New Jersey and you are a resident of Pennsylvania, you do not have to pay New Jersey income taxes on your wages. You would submit exemption Form NJ-165 to your employer.

- **North Dakota:** If you work in North Dakota and you are a resident of Minnesota or Montana you do not have to pay North Dakota income taxes on your wages. You would submit exemption Form NDW-R to your employer.

- **Ohio:** If you work in Ohio and are a resident of Indiana, Kentucky, Michigan, Pennsylvania, or West Virginia you do not have to pay Ohio income taxes on your wages. You would submit exemption Form IT-4NR to your employer.

- **Pennsylvania:** If you work in Pennsylvania and you are a resident of Indiana, Maryland, New Jersey, Ohio, Virginia, or West Virginia you do not have to pay Pennsylvania income taxes on your wages. You would submit exemption Form REV-420 to your employer.
- **Virginia:** If you work in Virginia and you are a resident of the District of Columbia, Kentucky, Maryland, Pennsylvania, or West Virginia you do not have to pay Virginia income taxes on your wages. You would submit exemption Form VA-4 to your employer.
- **West Virginia:** If you work in West Virginia and you are a resident of Kentucky, Maryland, Ohio, Pennsylvania, or Virginia you do not have to pay West Virginia income taxes on your wages. You would submit exemption Form WV/IT-104R to your employer.
- **Wisconsin:** If you work in Wisconsin and you are a resident of Illinois, Indiana, Kentucky, or Michigan you do not have to pay Wisconsin income taxes on your wages. You would submit exemption Form W-220 to your employer.

## New York, New Jersey and Connecticut Tri-State Area

New York, Connecticut, and New Jersey do NOT have reciprocal agreements. If you work in New York and you live in New Jersey, you would have to pay New York income taxes as a **nonresident** and also pay New Jersey income taxes as a **resident** since you live in New Jersey. However, residents of New Jersey (and most other states) can take a tax credit for taxes paid to other jurisdictions.

**Facts and Myths about state taxes**

**Facts:**

**Only Six states base their state income taxes on** *federal taxable income.* **The other 44 states base their taxes on the** *federal adjusted gross income (AGI)* **as the basis for their state income taxes. These states use federal taxable income as the starting point on their state tax returns, which means that their state income taxes can be impacted by changes to federal tax laws that affect federal taxable income. The states that use federal taxable income as the basis of their state tax returns are:**

- Colorado
- Minnesota
- North Carolina
- North Dakota
- South Carolina
- Vermont

**States without an Income Tax**

Only seven states lack a state income tax altogether. They are in an alphabetical order:

- Alaska
- Florida
- Nevada
- South Dakota
- Texas
- Washington
- Wyoming

Two states have a limited income tax on individuals. These states tax **only** dividend and interest income and include:

- Tennessee
- New Hampshire

**Misconceptions about state income taxes**

*I don't owe taxes because I live or work in a state without an income tax*

In order for that to be true you will also have to reside in that state. If you are a resident of the 41 states that have an income tax, you will have to pay taxes to your home state on all of your income regardless of where you earned it, including income you made in a state which does not have a state income tax. Similarly, if you are a resident of a tax-free state, and have worked in a taxing state, you still have to pay taxes to the state where you worked. Unless you are working in a reciprocal state, you will have to pay taxes to the state where you earned your income. You would file a nonresident return to pay these taxes.

*I will pay less tax overall in states where there is no state income tax*

That may not necessarily be true.! After all even these states need revenues to support their government and to ensure that their municipalities function. They have to somehow make up for the state income taxes. They do so by increasing other taxes. Texas and New Hampshire, make up for the lack of states taxes by having higher property taxes. Both states have some of the highest property taxes in the nation. The cost of higher property taxes, sales taxes, fuel taxes, and other taxes could amount to higher overall taxes in some of these states. However, one fact to remember is that property taxes are tax deductible up to a certain income. For most physicians it phases out as their income increases. However, if you are still a resident, the property tax deduction may help boost your disposable income.

## Do Millionaires really pay less in taxes than others?

President Obama (in 2011) gave a speech and made it sound that all millionaires across America pay less taxes than their secretaries. This sentiment was echoed earlier by the Oracle of Omaha, the Billionaire, Warren Buffett, who stated that his secretary pays higher taxes than him. He meant as a percentage of her income of course, but the media as usual did not clarify this issue. Also, Warren Buffett wrote in a New York times earlier that year "that the tax rate he paid last year was lower than that paid by any of the other 20 people in his office". Of course, the media did not elaborate on the word "rate"!

In his White House address on September 18, 2011, President Obama called on Congress to increase taxes by $1.5 trillion as part of a 10-year deficit reduction package totaling more than $3 trillion. He proposed that Congress overhaul the tax code and impose what he called the "Buffett rule," named for billionaire investor Warren Buffett. President Obama's rule was that: "People making more than $1 million a year should not pay a smaller share of their income in taxes than middle-class families pay." He continued to state that "Warren Buffett's secretary shouldn't pay a higher tax rate than Warren Buffett. There is no justification for it".

Furthermore he stated that "It is wrong that in the United States of America, a teacher or a nurse or a construction worker who earns $50,000 should pay higher tax rates than somebody pulling in $50 million."

But is that true? Do Millionaires actually pay less tax than average Americans?

Evaluation and analysis of the data from both private and government agencies tell a different story. On average, the wealthiest people in the US pay considerably more taxes than the middle class or the poor. They pay taxes at a higher rate (35% vs. 10- 32%), and as a group, they contribute a much larger share of the overall taxes collected by the federal government every year. That is not to say that there may be individual millionaires who pay taxes at rates lower than middle-income workers.

According to data from 2009, close to 1500 American households filed tax returns with incomes above $1 million, but they did not pay federal income tax, according to the Internal Revenue Service data. However, this was less than 1 percent of the nearly 237,000 returns with incomes above $1 million.

In 2011, households making more than $1 million paid an average of 29.1 percent of their income in federal taxes, including income taxes and payroll taxes, according to the Tax Policy Center, a Washington think tank. While households making between $50,000 and $75,000 paid only 15 percent of their income in federal taxes and the lowest income households paid even less. For example, households making between $40,000 and $50,000 paid an average of 12.5 percent of their income in federal taxes. Households making between $20,000 and $30,000 paid only 5.7 percent.

Figures available from the Internal Revenue Service (IRS) are a few years old and are limited to federal income taxes, but they show much the same thing. In 2009, taxpayers who made $1 million or more paid on average 24.4 percent of their income in federal income taxes, according to the IRS. Those making $100,000 to $125,000 paid on average 9.9 percent in federal income taxes, while those making $50,000 to $60,000 paid an average of 6.3 percent. The tax policy center estimates that 46 percent of households, mostly low- and medium-income households, will pay no federal income taxes most of the years. Most, however, will pay other taxes, including Social Security and payroll taxes.

President Obama has stated that "…wealthy individuals do not pay their fair share of taxes." This may hinge on the fact that, for high-income families and individuals, investment income is often taxed at a lower rate than wages. Like we have discussed in other sections of this book, the top tax rate for dividends and capital gains is 15 percent (as of 2011). The top marginal tax rate for wages is 39 percent (which is reserved for taxable income above $379,150, as of 2014).

But with such a high tax rate, why do certain individuals and families pay taxes at a lower rate? The answer lies in the tax code, which is riddled with more than $1 trillion in deductions, exemptions and credits, and they benefit people at every income level, according to data from the nonpartisan Joint Committee on Taxation, the US Congress' official scorekeeper on revenue issues.

The matter of fact is that everybody gets some sort of tax break. People at the top, who earn a lot of money get deductions (business expenses, capital gain tax at 15% etc.) and exemptions which lowers their overall tax rate, and people at the bottom of the income bracket also get deductions (property tax deductions, child tax credits etc..) so *that at the end of the year if you make less than $ 45,000.00 you do not pay federal income taxes.*

Treasury Secretary (in 2011) of the USA, Timothy Geithner was pressed by media reporters at a White House briefing on the number of millionaires who pay taxes at a lower rate than middle-income families. He stated that " people who make most of their money in wages pay taxes at a higher rate, while those who get most of their income from investments pay at lower rates". He continued to say: "So it really depends on what is your profession, where's the source of your income, what's the specific circumstances you face, and the averages won't really capture that". This statement summarizes the issue of taxation across the socio-demographic lines.

**Even if you are a millionaire, avoid these common financial mistakes, it will save you money!**

As we state at the beginning of this book, physicians are some of the smartest people around and therefore, we hope that as a physician we will rarely make a financial mistake or acquire a habit that will sink us. However, if we make multiple mistakes, the cumulative effects are likely to have a significant impact on our finances over time. In this section we will discuss some of the mistakes that we should avoid in order to minimize losing money.

*Do you have enough insurance?*

This includes life and health insurance. You may be young and healthy and think that you do not need insurance, however, the older you get the more difficult and the more expensive it becomes to buy insurance.

If you are still a resident or a fellow, buy a life insurance now. Your residency or fellowship program is likely offering you life insurance. When you complete your residency a representative from your current insurance company will likely contact you offering you to continue life insurance and pay the annual premium by yourself. Most financial advisors recommend that you take the offer and buy/continue your current life insurance. If you get life insurance in your mid 20s instead of your mid 50s you are likely to save up to $ 10,000.00 over these three decades. The same is true for health insurance.

*Are you paying too much for your home owner's insurance?*

A study conducted by the Risk department at a major national insurance company found that close to 80% of insurance agents believed that homeowners are paying too much for home owner's insurance. One way to cut back on your home owner's insurance premium is to increase your deductible. For instance if you increase your deductible from $ 500.00 to around $ 2500.00, you could potentially save up to $850.00 a year on your home owner's insurance premium. Of course if you have a nice finished basement with very nice furniture, but it is flooded during one of the winter storms, you will have to pay the first $ 2500.00, but the probability of that happening is low. So, contact your insurance to see if you can save some money by increasing your deductible.

Rashed Hasan, MD, FAAP

*Do not underestimate health care costs?*

You are in the health care field and you know how expensive medical and dental carecan get!. This is more important as you get older and approach your senior years. Evaluate your health and dental care coverage every year to make sure that you have enough coverage in case of a catastrophic event. You may also want to consider getting additional insurance for catastrophic coverage; the AMA offers one such product and the premium is less $ 100.00 per month. This kind of insurance will also cover you and your family in case you get sick or get into an accident overseas and you need to be air lifted back to the US. Also, it has been shown that you may need up to $ 10,000.00 a year for you and your spouse during retirement for out of pocket health care expenses.

*Do not pass up tax breaks*

When you look at your investments do not overlook the taxes that can take a bite out of your portfolio over time. You could easily lose 2-3% per year on the gains on your investments if you do not pay close attention to the tax issue.

So, you need to take a close look at your accounts and identify, which of your investment accounts are tax-free, tax deferred or taxable, then make plans to commit as much of your ordinary income (that you can afford to save) to accounts that are part of SEP-IRA, traditional IRA, annuities or defined contribution plans (read the sections on these topics elsewhere in this book).

In addition, when buying and selling stocks that pay dividends, or managing your mutual funds that pay dividend, read and research on tax rules on the so-called "qualified dividends", which refers to those dividends paid on stocks/mutual funds that you have held in your portfolio for 60 days or more within prescribed windows and that qualify the dividends to be taxed as capital gains and not as ordinary income. Selling stocks even a day sooner can result in paying tax on dividends as ordinary income, costing you 10 percent or more.

*Do you pay late fees on your bills often? If you do you are losing money!*

In addition late fees can eventually adversely affect your credit score! This is more likely to happen if your payments are due at various times during the month. One way to overcome this problem is to have your bills due as close as possible to the day that you get paid or your accounts receivable are most likely to be paid.

You may have to make few phone calls to your utility companies, your credit card company, the company that is financing your vehicle and other service providers and ask them if they could change the due dates to coincide with the date when money is most likely to be available in your account (if you have on line payments) and allow few days for your checks to clear. You or your spouse could create a monthly calendar or bill payment reminder on your cell phone or on a regular paper calendar.

*When you are still young do not invest too conservatively*

Many young investors including physicians have few or no stocks in their portfolio. It is true that the stock market did not do well in the first decade of the new millennium. However, over the long term stocks are likely to beat other assets in performance. Consider increasing your stock exposure when you are still young in order to make the most of the years you have ahead to grow wealth. Otherwise you may slow the growth of your portfolio over time. We are not suggesting that you do not consider other factors such as your current age, your financial situation, your retirement goals and your risk tolerance, but when the stock market is down and there are opportunities and you have the cash, consider investing in quality stocks and you will be rewarded over the span of 30 years or so.

*Do not pay retail price for everything you buy*

This is not an investment by itself, but if you pay the full price for everything it can quickly drain your resources and adversely affect your finances. Nowadays, there are several applications that you can download on your cell phone that will help you compare prices and make a better buying decision. Examples of these applications are PriceGrabber, NextTAg, and RedLaser. If your spouse or significant other is into designer clothing try Belle and Clive website at belland-clive.com. You need to register with your email and get a password to browse items at their website. Also, you or your significant other get used to clipping coupons and use them wherever you shop; it will save you a bundle.

*Do not leave your valuables uninsured!*

If you are a collector of art, jewelry or wine, make sure each item is properly appraised and then shop around to ensure them. Many high-net-worth individuals do not have their expensive collectables insured.

## Your Children

### The cost of raising a child

You probably know that raising a child is very expensive, but new information published by the US department of agriculture in 2012, show that the cost of raising children is rising. The cost has risen by as much as 25% in the past 10 years, which is about 2.5% per year over the past 10 years. The US Department of Agriculture sates that the rise in this cost is primarily due to the rise in the cost of food and to a less extent in health care costs. The USDA reports that families with income greater than $ 99,000.00 (the income bracket in which most physicians fall) are expected to spend around 377,000.00 on each child until they are ready to go college. Of course, this does not include the cost of college education nor the cost of sending your children to private school for their pre-college years!!

If you remain childless, you can save that much per child or spend it on other enjoyments for life. But let's face it, having children is one of enjoyments of life too, besides, if you are lucky they will probably come and visit you when you old and in a nursing home!

For most of us at least, children are the joy of our lives. However, it is worth remembering that once you have children, your life will be centered around them and most of the decisions that you will make will be related to what is most important to them such as where you live, what friends they are going to have, what schools they go to and what extracurricular activities and entertainments are available for them. However, the financial aspects are important and this section of the book is meant to help you pause, think and plan ahead when it comes to having children.

In planning ahead, particularly for physicians, it is important to discuss the implications of having a child. Do you want to have a child while you are still a medical student or you want to wait until you graduate? Do you plan on having a child while you are still in training (residency and/or fellowship) and what are the implications? If you are married to a physician, will both of you continue your training or one of you takes a year or two off while the other one works or continues training?

*A day in the life of a parent:*

You were on call last night in the ICU, you were up all night. Your partner was also up all night because the baby was sick, was very congested and had fever. The baby woke up several times through the night. You arrive home and your partner greets you at the door and says "here, I need a break". The baby appears to have a full diaper. Your partner goes to bed and you are left with this little precious thing with a stinky diaper. You assemble all the tools you need to change the baby's diaper and 5 minutes later "mission accomplished" the baby has a new fresh diaper on, but she is still fussy and crying. You check the temperature it is OK. You assemble the tools you need to make a fresh bottle. The bottle is ready, you feed the baby. The baby takes 6 Oz of formula. You burp the baby on your shoulders and put the baby in her crib. Luckily she falls asleep. You pass out on the couch, but two hours later you are awaken to the sound of a crying baby. You wake up and do the same routine you did two hours ago. This is what you have to do over and over during most the first year of a baby's life, it is probably one of the toughest years when you have a child.

With the arrival of a new baby, your life will change forever! Babies wake up often during the first several months of infancy, some are colicky, which means that you will have to be on call at work and at home. It can be very stressful for you and your partner. Lack of sleep is a certainty during the first year.

The financial aspects can also be significant (also read the section on child care); if one of you is going to be off work and stay home, that translates into a significant drop in your joint income, which can be a significant adjustment if you are still in training. Clarify with your training program or your employer about maternity and paternity leaves and how much of it is compensated.

Also, as soon as you have your first child do not forget to add the child to your health insurance; most insurance companies want you to add the new child to your insurance within one month of birth. Also, inquire about how much will your health insurance premium go up with the addition of one child and if your insurance covers well child care and immunizations. These visits to the doctor can be very expensive if your health care plan does not cover them. Immunizations are even more expensive. If your health care plan does not cover immunization, see if you can have them done at the local health care department for free.

Child care is very expensive and you need to calculate whether it will be to your benefit and the wellbeing of your children if one of you stays home and care for the kids while the other one continue the career path. Also, emergencies do come up when you have kids. Kids get sick and they may get injured; these issues translate into more medical bills.

Other issues to consider, if you are planning to have children has to do with selection of a residency training program or a new job after graduation.

Do you want to be closer to relatives who may help you every now and then with the kids; would you like your kids to be closer to their grandparents?

Are you going to need a bigger place (an apartment or a house) or a safer car? If you drive a FIAT abarth, you may need a bigger car to accommodate the new angel who will be arriving soon.

Also, diapers, wipes, and formulas are expensive and add several hundred dollars per month to your budget. Also, remember to consider buying life insurance and disability insurance so that your loved one is well cared for in case the unthinkable happens to you.

These translates into more monthly costs. You should consider purchasing life insurance that will cover your child and your partner until the child is around 30 years of age. This type of life insurance is usually a term life insurance. As you can see even thought kids are a bundle of joy, but they are expensive. But remember that it is you who decides how much you are willing to spend on them. So, plan ahead and things will work out at the end!

### Chil-care if both you and your spouse work:

Raising children can be a full-time job especially when children are youg. This may be a dilemma if both you and your spouse work. Of course if both of you are physicians and both would like to finish your residency training together, you have very limited options other than a day care, unless you are lucky and have an extended family in the city where you are conducting your residency or the city where you work and your family members are willing to help.

In this section we will discuss issues related to day care including approximate costs, options and tax benefits. Finding a day care that is appropriate for your child can be a monumental task especially in certain cities where the demand is very high and remember is that if you want quality child care you will have to pay top dollar.

*What are your options?*

There are a wide range of child care providers to choose from depending on the local that you reside in. Licensed child care providers include YMCA, Easter Seals, and KinderCare. Family-owned day care centers which are regulated by the local city and states are another option. And finally you can always have your own "baby sitter" a Nanny that comes to your house on a daily basis or a "live-in" such as an au pair. There are also license-exempt centers operated by religious institutions such a church or a temple.

A licensed day care center usually has more children per room and your child will interact with more children. This is likely to make it more affordable, but with the disadvantage of higher risk of upper respiratory infections per month especially early on.

Getting your own baby sitter is more expensive, but has the advantage of having your child stay in your own home. Obviously your child has less opportunity of interacting with other children if you choose this route, but you can find other ways for your child to socialize with other children. The other advantage of this approach is that if you get a mature lady to baby sit your child she will often clean your house too and may even offer to cook your meals so that your dinner is ready when you get home!.

*What is an au pair? Is that an option for you?*

An au pair is a person (usually in their early twenties) who usually comes from another country (European, Asian or Latin American countries) and lives in your house. You provide her/him with room and meals and a weekly allowance. In return, she/he watches (baby sit) your children while you are gone. The work hours for an au pair are usually limited to 40 hours a week and they usually need to have one day off a week. There are various agencies in the US that you can contract with to host au pair in your house.

The terms of the contract are usually for one year and it is renewable for at least another year. The sign up fees (payable up front) are usually significant and range from $ 6500 – 7500.00. This fee includes travel expenses and initial training. Subsequently the monthly allowance is in the range of $750 – 900.00 a month payable weekly. The quality of service will depend on the individual au pair and.

The personal experience with au pairs can be mixed and unpredictable since you are dealing with individuals who are adolescents in their minds. If you get an irresponsible au pair, she/he may not be reliable in providing quality child care, may spend significant amounts of time on TV, computer or other social media devices and may act like another teenager that you have to take care of. One lesson that we have learned from dealing with au pairs is to be firm from the beginning, set very concrete rules and " do not spoil your au pair". Remember the au pair is there as your employer and you should treat her/him as such. People who treat au pairs otherwise, may face difficulties dealing with them.

*What you should look for in a child care?*

Safety is the number one concern. You should also be looking for a stimulating and nurturing environment while weighing in other factors such as quality of the program, location, and cost. There are many child care centers that are less expensive, but are not licensed. They are cheaper because they have less overhead, but the quality may not be what you want for your child.

*What about costs of child care?*

**Cost of child care by region:**

The United States Department of Agriculture (USDA) periodically releases data on the cost of raising a child up to the age of 17 or 18. The costs involved include food, housing and other necessities. According to the most recent data available in 2012 the cost of raising a child is between $ 200,000.00 and $ 300,000.00. The largest of these expenses is housing followed by child care and food. At the USDA website,(www.usda.gov) there is a calculator that can help with calculating child expenses. The cost of child care varies from state to state depending on the region and local, with the northeast being the most expensive, the west coming second, followed by the mid-west. However, there are exceptions that you may want to know. There are mid-western states that rank in the top 10 when it comes to child care expenses. The southern states of the US and the rural areas are the least expensive. Here are the states with the highest child care costs in the nation:

New York:

Everything is expensive in the big apple state and that includes child care with an estimated cost of up to $ 15,000.00 per annum.

Minnesota:

The cost of center-based child care (or day care) is $ 13,500.00 falling slightly behind New York even though it is one of the Midwestern states.

Oregon: $ 11,000.00

Colorado: $ 12,600.00

Hawaii: $ 12,600.00, not bad for a state which is known to be an expensive state to live in.

Kansas: $ 11,000.00 here is another Midwestern state which ranks in the top ten when it comes to child care, so don't be fooled by the location alone!

California: $ 11,800.00. It is hard to believe that you pay only $ 800.00 more in California compared to Kansas.

Illinois: $ 12,100.00

Massachusetts: $ 15,000.00- 19,000. Finding a quality child care for this price in the Boston suburbs is difficult task.

Indiana: $ 9800.00

Wisconsin: $ 10,700.00

*Other data to consider on child care:*

According to data provided by the National Association of Child Care Resource & Referral Agencies, (NACCRRA) the average cost of full-time childcare in 2009 ranged from $4,550 in Mississippi to approximately $19,000.00 in Massachusetts.

For a four-year-old, those numbers fell to $4,050 and $13,150, respectively. In 40 states, the average annual cost for center-based care for an infant was higher than a year's tuition and related fees at a four-year public college, and in every region of the U.S., more than the average annual amount that families spent on food!

So, as you can see child care will eat a major chunk of your monthly budget. Therefore, it is critical that you weigh the pros and cons of one spouse staying home and caring for the child instead of working. This lead us to the next question.

*Do I get tax breaks for child care expenses?*

One source of tax break comes in the form of Child Tax Credit, which as of 2012, is approximately $1,000 per child depending on your income. Married couples who file jointly can earn up to $110,000 and still qualify for child tax credit. For those who make more, the credit limit is modified and gradually phased out. If your annual income exceeds this amount, you may want to discuss this issue with your accountant.

Another source of tax credit is the Federal Child and Dependent Care Tax Credit, which can be larger than the child tax credit according to data from the National Women's Law Center. This is also an after-the-fact credit that families with children under 13 are eligible for. Although it may be used for both in and out of-home care arrangements, you can only claim up to $3,000 annually for one child and $6,000 for two or more children. This tax break provides the greatest assistance to lower income families. Those families who earn over $43,000, can only deduct 20 percent of their eligible expenses as a credit. Obviously, this type of child care credit is most beneficial during your residency and fellowship when your income is likely to be in this range.

Middle-income families (such as yours if you are still in your residency or fellowship) can also get help at the state level. Twenty eight states have tax credits, some for middle income and others for low-income earners only. These provisions may be credits or deductions, which reduce the amount of state taxes owed. You may want to discuss these issues with your accountant early in your residency or fellowship training and also discuss with your training program and your prospective employer (if you have already finished your training and you are looking for a job) about "dependent care" options available to you and your family. Most employers provide dependent accounts that you can deposit pre-tax money in every pay period and then utilize the money for child care/dependent care.

## College funds for your children

The so-called "Qualified tuition plans", are educational savings plans for college and come in two major forms

*Pre-paid tuition plans*: allows you to purchase credit hours at participating Universities and/or colleges for college expenses. They range from full coverage, which includes room and board or partial coverage which includes only tuitions. You purchase whatever number of credit hours (or years) that you can afford and when your child graduates from high school and ready to enter a university the funds will be available. Obviously the fees vary depending on the age of the child at that particular time when you decide to purchase a plan. The younger the child the further away he/she is from graduating from high school the less you have to pay.

*College-savings plans*: These are investments and allow a parent (or a grandparent) to establish an account for the beneficiary (the prospective student in this case). In doing so, the saver will select from a list of investments including stocks, bonds, and money market mutual funds. Examples: the various types of 529 plans (tax-exempt and transferable to someone else for educational purpose) and the unified gift to minor (earnings are taxable and less flexibility in transferring the funds to another person).

In the recent years 529 plans have become synonymous with "a college-saving" plan, however, not everyone is sold on these plans. Let's discuss some of the pros and cons of these plans so that you and your family may make a more informed decision.

As of 2013, Americans have contributed close $ 170 billion into these plans across the 50 states. Part of the appeal of 529 plans is the tax breaks that you get from the state and the money grows in these plans *tax-free*. These accounts also have a smaller impact on a college's financial aid formula than other kinds of investments. The state of Illinois, for example, offers up to a $20,000 annual state tax deduction (for joint filers) for money you contribute to 529 plans, as does Oklahoma. Some states, such as South Carolina and New Mexico, even allow you to deduct the full amount. Other states offer limited or no such tax breaks, and those that do, almost always extend them to in-state residents only. So, you need to do your homework and find out what is the tax status of the state that you are purchasing the 529 plan in.

Furthermore, *you do not have to purchase a 529 of the state that you reside in.* You could purchase a 529 plan for the state of New York even if you do not reside there. You will also have to think about withdrawal restrictions, and restrictions in changing the funds that you invest in and sluggish investment performance of 529 plans, which make them less attractive to some investment professionals. And don't forget the costs associated with 529 plans. These are called expense ratio. Although expense ratios (which is the managerial fees that providers skim off) of the funds in 529 plans have dropped in the last three years, they are on the average between 0.14-0.35 percentage points higher than comparable mutual funds, according to Morningstar studies.

**What are some other investment options for College for your children?**

One big reason to bypass 529s is to find better investment choices. A recent Morningstar study found that all of the age-based investing options in 529s fell short of the performance of their benchmarks, sometimes by as much as 2 percent every year.

With a taxable account, you have unlimited choices. You can invest as much as you want in whatever you want, as opposed to a 529 plan where the options are limited and you can change the holidays for contribution only once.

For example, when you use a taxable account to save for college, you deposit money in an account that is in the parent's name, so any capital gains tax due will be paid by the parent. Some experts consider the 15-percent capital gains tax is not terribly onerous, when in return you get the freedom to use the money as needed. You could for instance buy exchange traded funds (see the stock market section) that mirror certain sector of the economy or industry and aim for growth and avoid mutual funds that have ongoing fees. Some the these ETFs have low volatility and steady growth over time. e.g. Power Shares S&P 500 (symbol: SPY). Other ETFs include: Power Shares Emerging Market Equity Low Volatility, and Power Shares International Developed Markets Low Volatility. If you like the fixed income, one option is iShares Core Total US Bond Market.

**ROTH IRA**

Roth individual retirement accounts (IRAs) can serve a dual purpose, especially if parents are well on their way to saving for their retirement.

Parents are allowed to make withdrawals on their contributions (not earnings) from Roth IRA accounts prior to age 59 ½ without incurring a 10 percent penalty as long as the money is used for higher education expenses. (as of 2013, you can contribute $5,500 to a Roth IRA if you are under age 50, or $6,500 if over age 50.). Parents do not have to pay income tax on that amount, and the money will accumulate tax free just like it would in a 529 plan. The difference is, if the child doesn't go to college, the money can stay in the Roth IRA and can be used for a down payment on a house, disability or retirement. However, some physicians may not qualify for Roth IRA if their income is too high.

## MUNICIPAL BONDS

Municipal bonds are bonds that are issued by municipalities, counties and states so that they may develop their infrastructure and improve the quality of life for their citizens. Accordingly, the yield earned by the investor is tax free (federal tax at least). They are affectionately called "munis". Among bonds, munis make the most sense for several reasons. Parents can take money out of their muni bond investments if they need money for other purposes (such as an illness). You will not be able to do that with money locked up in a 529 plan for your child. Parents can also avoid the so-called kiddie tax because munis are tax-free investments, and the account is held in the parent's name. If a child under the age 18 has more than $1,900 in investment income, part of that income may be taxed at the parent's income tax rate, according to IRS rules.

Sure, muni yields are lower than this year's strong gains in the stock market (in late 2012 early 2013). However, munis are less risky than stocks over the long term, and the tax-equivalent return of munis can range from five percent to six percent depending on your tax bracket. For example, if you are in a 35-39 percent tax bracket (most physicians are), a 3.5 percent muni yield would give you a tax-equivalent return of five percent.

Experts recommend buying the highest-rated muni bonds with principal coming due near the year when the child needs to pay for college. Here is an example: If your child is three years old and you invest $5,000 a year for 15 years in individual muni bonds and earn a compounded interest of four percent, you would accumulate about $100,000 for college. Experts recommend that you should invest in municipal bonds that mature in 15-20 years when saving for college for your children.

**Your Children: Should you continue to consider them "dependents" when they go to College?**

Once your children turn 19, the Internal Revenue Service (IRS) considers them adults and if they earn more than $ 5700.00 annually (as of 2010), they will have to file their own taxes.

What are some of the advantages and disadvantages of continuing to claim your children as "dependents" after they leave home and go to college (or if for some reason they don't want to go college) or start working and have their own income?

*Your children are independent:*

There may be some advantages if your children are working, have an income and consider themselves independent from their parents. One of the advantages has to do with receiving financial aid towards college tuition because the expected financial aid that they will receive will be based on their income and their parents' income. In the vast majority of cases, this means that theoretically they will qualify for more financial aid because their income is lower than one or combined parents' income. The US department of education is the body that controls financial aid for colleges and universities and their criteria for a child being independent from her/his parents are very stringent. The US department of education considers a child to be independent from his/her parents only if he/she is married, has her/his children, is a veteran of a military service, enrolled in a graduate college/university program or he/she is 24 years of age or older. If your child does not meet one of these criteria it will be very difficult for her/him to qualify for financial aid based on her/his income. In this case your child will have to apply for and receive a dependency override from a college or University. It is uncommon to receive such an override.

*You continue to claim your children as "dependents":*

When you are a high-earner and deductions you can receive towards your taxes is a plus. This effect is usually more significant as your income goes higher and higher. The same principle applies to continuing to claim your children as dependents on your taxes. From an IRS-standpoint you can continue to claim your children as dependents if they are full-time students until the age of 24.

*Who is considered a full-time student?* If your child attends college part of 5-calender months each year, you can claim her/him as a dependent.

*Do you gain any tax advantages by continuing to claim your children as dependents?*

The answer is YES. You can write off a number of expenses incurred for your child after he/she leaves home for college, which includes the following:

1. Medical Bills and durable medical equipments: are deductible as medical expenses for the household even though for you as a high-earner it may not amount to significant tax benefits unless and until you have spent considerable amount of money on medical bills for your child. However, the benefits may

be substantial during a year when your child was seriously ill or was involved in an accident and the medical bills were substantial.

2.   Camp expenses, which may include summer camps

3.   College expenses: The tax benefits come in two flavors:

a. Education credit and      b. Tax credit.

The educational credit allows you to receive a $ 2500.00 tax credit per year towards your child's college tuition. However, this tax credit has income limitation. It phases out at an annual income of $ 90,000.00 if you are filing your taxes individually and $ 180,000.00 if you are filing jointly with a spouse. If you are an employed physician it may be tough to qualify for this tax credit because most physicians' income is higher than this range, however, if you have your own practice and you maximize your practice expenses and your retirement accounts; your gross adjusted income may be as low as these income limitations. Alternatively, if you are semi-retired, your income may also fall within this range and you may qualify for this tax credit. The other option is to deduct up to $ 4000.00 per year for educational expenses per child from your taxable income. Again, there is income limitation for this deduction. It phases out at $ 80,000.00 if you file your taxes as a single individual and $ 160,000.00 if you file jointly with a spouse. The IRS rule is that you can claim either one of those two, but you cannot claim both.

4.   You can still claim your children as dependents on your taxes even if they have income, but provided that they don't claim any itemized deductions when they file their own taxes and they pay taxes at their own (lower) tax bracket. The advantage of continuing to claim your children as dependents on your taxes is that if you are single (or divorced), you can file your taxes as "head of the household" as opposed to "single", which will lower your taxes overall. Please talk to your

certified public accountant about these issues every year when you file your taxes since the laws tend to change often.

## *To pay off or not to pay off your mortgage?*

**I am approaching retirement, I have heard that I should pay off my mortgage, Is that true?**

This issue has been discussed elsewhere in the book, but since it is an important issue and most families have a significant portion of their assets invested in their home, we are bringing up the issue again with additional views on the subject.

The conventional wisdom has always been that it is better to get done with your mortgage before you retire, so that during retirement you do not have to make mortgage payments. However, this conventional wisdom may not be absolute during periods of very low interest rate the US experienced in 2010-2014. This period was also characterized by financial uncertainties, housing market collapse, extreme volatility in the stock market and recession. Therefore, the approach to the question of whether you should pay off your mortgage before your retire would depend on certain facts.

*Are you able to replenish the amount of the money that you pay the bank to pay off your mortgage?*

Just in case you need a large sum of cash for another reason, do you have access to the extra cash that you are diverting towards paying your mortgage?

If the answer is YES, then it may be prudent to pay off your mortgage. For example if you have a $ 500,000.00 portfolio of investment that is generating income at 4% annually, and you decide to take $ 150,000.00 out to pay off your mortgage, then the total portfolio value will decrease to $ 350,000.00 and your annual income from the portfolio will decrease from $ 20,000.00 to $ 14,000.00. Furthermore, if the mortgage interest rate goes up in the coming 5-10 years to let us say 8% because of inflation, but your mortgage interest rate is locked in at 4.5%, you will benefit substantially from NOT paying off your mortgage over time. In this case your $ 500,000.00 portfolio may generate up to $ 40,000.00 annually instead of $ 28,000.00 if you pay off your mortgage. So, there are times when it pays to borrow money and mortgage debt is considered by many as "good debt". Besides, it may not be a prudent strategy to tie up a large sum of your money in one investment (in this case your home), because, while it is a nice security to have your home paid off, it will not give you the flexibility with your investment.

*What is your mortgage interest rate?*

Look at your mortgage interest rate and compare it to two things:

1. your historical average mortgage interest rate 2. After-tax return on your investments.

In the first decade of the millennium the interest rate was at historically low levels, being as low as 2.7% and only as high as 5%. This is a very low interest rate compared to 15% mortgage interest rate in the early 1980s. Also, consider the interest rate deduction that you get on your taxes. If you are in the 35-39% tax brackets (which most physicians are), then if your mortgage interest rate is at 4.5%, the mortgage loan is actually costing you only 2.9%. Therefore, if your portfolio of $ 500,000.00 is generating 5%, you are still ahead if you keep your money invested and keep the mortgage and not pay off your home.

*The downside of not paying off your home:*

You will need to make at least 4% on your investment portfolio to make it worth your while. However, in an environment of low interest rate, it is nearly impossible to achieve this goal with very conservative investments such as certificates of deposits (CDs) and bonds. You will have to take more risk because it is hard to find comparable risk-free investments such as CDs. That means that you will have to stomach a loss if you go another route such as investing in stocks with dividends.

## What are other people doing?

It appears that retirees (and this survey included all retirees including physicians) are torn equally between paying off their home or keeping the mortgage. According to a study conducted by Boston College in 2007, roughly 40% of US households who were between 60 and 70 years of age kept their mortgage and decided not to pay it off. Of these, roughly half of them had enough money to replenish their portfolio.

In the same year the Federal Reserve of the US conducted a study which concluded that directing more money towards your low-interest mortgage loan at the expense of continuing to contribute towards your retirement plans is a "costly mistake". Close to 40% of US households are accelerating their mortgage payments instead of saving it in a tax-deferred account. People who decide to direct more money towards their retirement accounts instead of paying more money towards their mortgage yield a mean benefit of 11 to 16 cents per dollar depending on the investment vehicle they choose. Therefore, If you have not retired yet, it may be prudent to allocate more money towards your retirement accounts than to pay off your mortgage. However, *for physicians, remember that one advantage of paying off your mortgage on your primary resident is that the assets will be protected from creditors in case of a law suit* (see the section of the book on "how to protect your assets").

## Retirement

*"Retirement? Isn't it too early to be talking about retirement?"* No it is NOT!

Most physician plan on relying on their retirement accounts as the ultimate source of income during retirement, yet most physicians do not pay enough attention to this important issue. That is why we are discussing retirement following completion of a residency and/or a Fellowship, *because it is so critical that you think about your retirement early, while you are still in training.*

Some of you may have had a job or jobs before entering medical school and already have a retirement account. You should evaluate and reevaluate your retirement plan every time there is a major change in your life and during major milestones in your career such as graduation from a Medical school, completion of a residency and/or a fellowship, securing a new job or changing jobs. If you get married or divorced, these are also times in your life that you should evaluate your retirement accounts. It is also prudent to evaluate your retirement accounts annually in order to keep up with new laws and regulations and to see the performance of your account(s).

A retirement plan has to be a qualified plan under the Internal Revenue Service rules. The word "qualified" implies that contribution to the plan is (tax) deductible, the contributions are allowed to earn income tax-deferred, and protected from creditors (in case of a law suit or if an individual files for bankruptcy in the future).

**Here are some tips for retirement:**

Start early: you don't have plenty of time, if you don't start by 35 you will fall behind and you will struggle to build a descent retirement nest.

Do not think that you will not live long enough to need retirement money. According to national bureau of statistics 80% of male and 90% of female in the US will live until age 65 and 60% of male and 73% of female are still alive at age 75. So if you are still alive and reading this book, there is a very good probability that the above statistics apply to you.

Another myth is that some people say "I won't retire". This may be true now but in 30 years your health may change, your mind set may change and you may want to retire or you may be forced to retire. Recently we came across a very well know surgeon who was still active and wanted to operate at age 72. He was doing a good job for the most part until some of the surgeons and operating room staff around him noticed that he was developing lapses in memory. The hospital became very concerned that this may be detrimental to patient care and he was asked to stop operating and was forced to retire. In most European countries, surgeons are not allowed to operate beyond the age of 70. So you never know what might happen 30 -40 years from now. What new regulations may be introduced that will force even you as a physician to retire.

Pay your debt, but also pay yourself:

Do not focus only on paying off your debt. Your debt may be so large that you may never be able to pay it off in the timeline you have in mind. In the meantime you are losing precious time for investment for your retirement. So start early and contribute as much as you can towards your retirement by maximizing all your retirement accounts and allow time to help with the compounding effects of appreciations, and dividends so that when you are ready to retire at age 65 or 67 you have a nice egg nest.

Do not blindly trust your financial advisor:

Remember your so called "financial advisor" in most cases is a sales person. His/her objective is increase the so called "assets under management" for the institution she/he works for. He could not care less if you really make money. The more clients he/she brings in the higher will be his/her bonus at the end of the year. **"We love physicians [as clients], because they have money and they are dump [financially]" one young "Financial advisor" said [privately talking to his buddies].** It is not an exaggeration, when we say, do not blindly trust "your financial advisor", they may not have your best interest at hand!

### *Understanding the jargons your "financial advisor" or others may use*

As a high earner you will be approached by many "financial advisor" and you may agree to meet with some of them and few my eventually become your "financial advisors". During meetings with them they may use certain terms, complicated terminologies or jargons related to taxes, investments or financial vehicles. They use many terminologies just like we physicians use medical terms, but some terms are more complex, confusing and often contradictory. They may use these terms when soliciting your business to impress you or later when planning or managing your financial matters to intimidate you or confuse you. So, it is prudent to be prepared to face these people! So, here we go:

**Discretionary Trust:**

This is a term that is used often in the setting of asset-protection (read the section on asset-protection). The discretion does not refer to being circumspect or discrete, but rather it refers to the power to decide. This term is used in a setting where an asset such as bonds, an investment property or other assets are put aside for the benefit of another (let's say your children) and a trustee is appointed. The trustee has the right to accumulate the annual income generated by these assets for future disposal instead of paying them annually to the beneficiaries.

**Discretionary account:**

This type of account is common for physicians. It is usually a brokerage account with one of the large financial firms and you have "an advisor" who can trade in your account without securing your approval for every transaction. Usually the advisor trades stocks or bonds or mutual funds (buying and selling) in an account that is essentially your account and contains your money.

**Bottom-Up Investing**

Again, it is figurative. It does not mean buying assets such as stocks, bonds, or mutual funds low or a t the bottom of the price range. It usually means an investment approach based on focusing on a specific company rather than its industry, the economy or market cycles. For example investing in the stock of Citi group, which is a bank stock without paying much attention to the sector (financials) or the category (consumer banking), simply because the person who is managing your money (the person who is managing a discretionary account for you) believes that Citi group has far outperformed others in the same sector and its therefore a good stock to pick (buy).

**Codicil:** is the name for the legal document used to make changes to a previously existing will or trust or both. There is no code to this critical element of estate planning. It must be executed with the same legal requirements such as witnesses. The alternative to a codicil is a new will. The term and concept can come up in probate (court-supervised) proceedings, where there are questions about the validity and/or chronological status of rival documents.

**Disintermediation**

Given the prefix, you might think this term has something to do with being oppositional. But here, the operative meaning is apart or away. As for mediation, well, one guess is as good as another. Disintermediation, in fact, has been practiced in recent years because of the global financial crisis (2008-2012 and ongoing). It is the movement of savings or investment funds away from institutions such as banks into higher-yielding investments in the securities markets, such as treasury bills (see the section on financial aspects of being a physician).

### Efficient Frontier

If your adviser mentions the term: "efficient frontier," it's a reference to the concept that different groups of securities (stocks) have different elements of risk and return on investment and that there is an optimal meeting point on a parabolic chart. Presumably, then, there is such a point for you and your investments. The key word here is efficient, and there is nothing far out about the concept. The efficient frontier concept is said to be a major component of what is considered modern portfolio theory, and is partly responsible for promoting the importance of diversification, i.e. diversifying your portfolio between stocks, bonds, treasury bills, and cash.

### Guaranteed Income Contract

This concept has been coming up more as people opt for annuities, which convert a lump sum into an income stream at a later point, an arrangement that could last for life. In this concept, the contract calls for an insurance company to borrow a lump sum from you (the investor) at a pre-determined interest rate that then produces a pre-determined amount of cash at a specified future date. On a related note, when you annuitize, you are converting a sum of money into an income stream that starts after a certain time period. This is the concept of annuities that you often hear about on television advertisements.

**High Current Income Mutual Fund**

Some financial advisors (that oversee your discretionary account) buy and sell stocks in your account in an attempt to "make you money" and appreciate the value of your portfolio. However, many other financial advisers construct your portfolio with a group of mutual funds, rather than individual stocks, so you will want to know as much as possible about each of the mutual funds you own in order to understand what is happening with your money.

A "high current income mutual fund" sure sounds good, but it says little about its composition. Yes, its goal is to produce high current income, but other kinds of funds are designed to do that as well. The key is that the fund's primary asset is high-yield corporate bonds, also known as junk bonds, which are below investment grade and typically carry higher risk.

So, make sure you understand these mutual funds and you understand the risks because while you may receive high yield, their total values may go down to zero in the future.

**Imputed Interest**

Imputed interest is interest that is not paid but must be accounted for on a tax basis. For instance, if you lend money to a family member and charge zero interest, your advisers or the IRS must decide what the applicable interest rate is on such a loan. If it is 3 percent, then the imputed tax is 3 percent of the sum borrowed and must be reported as income on the tax return of the lender.

Here's a case where it helps to have an adviser who handles both taxes and investments, and maybe even estate planning.

If a significant portion of your investment is in "fixed income" (that means you make money by getting paid interest on your money) should pay special attention. Such interest also applies to certain kinds of bonds, such as zero-coupon bonds: those are bonds that are bought at a sizable discount to their face value but generate a profit at maturity (2,5,10 or 30 years later), which is based on the difference in the purchase and maturity prices.

## Law Of Large Numbers

If you are not happy with your financial adviser's performance who may be managing your discretionary account at a large financial you might hear about this theory. To simplify this term, it means that beating large numbers, let us say large numbers of investors, other money managers or fund managers, is very difficult to achieve. In other words, they will tell you that it is rare for your advisor to out-perform the general market. However, it is unlikely that they will tell you this when they are soliciting your business and before you open an account with them!. For most investors, the law of large numbers makes a good case for the logic of low-cost index funds (read the section on mutual funds) that essentially mirror the market. John Bogel, the father of mutual funds has said that 70% of money managers DO NOT underperform the general market.

## Variable Universal Life Insurance

Life insurance is a complicated subject. It is complicated enough by itself and the industry has made it even more complicated by introducing different products as a form of "life Insurance".

Take this product for example: variable universal life insurance; it combines the standard death benefit and a tax-free savings component. The owner can take the policy's cash value, which is the amount offered to the policy owner by the insurer upon cancellation of the contract and invest it in separate accounts (bonds, stocks), rather than keep it in the insurer's general account. The different investments, of course, yield varying values, thus the "variable." And so in the current world of financial planning, life insurance often seems like an investment.

Another important aspect is that the policy holder has the flexibility of making premium payments of variable sizes from month to month, rather than at a fixed rate.

Like we discussed in the section on life insurance, if you would like to purchase a life insurance that will take care of your loved ones in the event of your death, consider buying "term life Insurance".

## What are some Retirement mistakes you should try and avoid?

If you do not qualify for Roth IRA because your income is above and beyond the adjusted gross income upper limit for Roth IRA, you should maximize your employer matching. Also, if you are self-employed maximize your contribution, which is up to 25% of your net income (income – all your expenses) up to a total of $ 45,000.00 a year (as of 2010). Beyond this you will have to take critical steps so that you don't make mistakes with your retirement plans.

Here are some steps you can take to minimize mistakes:

1.  Utilize tax-saving options: how do you do that?

    Do not withdraw any money from your retirement accounts until you are ready to retire and when you do withdraw, do it gradually, because you are responsible for paying taxes only on the amount that you withdraw. In this manner you will take advantage of not paying a 10% penalty for early withdrawal and your money will continue to appreciate.
2.  Utilize the catch-up provisions for individuals 50 years of age and older: If you are employed and you are 50 years or older you can contribute an additional $ 5500.00 per year (as of 2014) to your retirement contribution for a total of $ 22,000.00 per year. Just like the option in the # 1 above, if you miss this opportunity, you will never be able to take advantage of it again.

3. Never borrow money from your retirement account; it is not a good idea no matter what the reason is: sending a kid to college, buying a house or a condo, etc. your child will probably be able to borrow money to go to college, but if you miss the opportunity you will never be able to catch up, and we are not aware of any loans available for retirement.

4. Do not overestimate your returns: If you have been told and you have believed that the stock market gets 10% appreciation on your retirement portfolio per years, it is an overestimation and you are being unrealistic. The realistic rate of return is closer to 4- 6% per year instead.

5. Make a retirement budget: A safe rate of withdrawal out of your retirement account (when you do retire) is approximately 4- 4.5% of the capital per year. That means if your retirement account is worth $ 500,000.00, you can withdraw $ 22,500.00 per year. If you have 1.5 million dollar in retirement money, then you can withdraw: 22,500 X 3 = $ 67,500.00 per year. So, make a budget for your retirement, cut expenses, and make sure you don't run out of money, because if you do, it is not easy to get a job as you get older.

### When can you take the money out in the future?

If you decide to tap into your retirement account before your retirement age, then you will have to pay a 10% penalty and taxes that equal to your income tax bracket for that particular year. For instance if your income is over $ 375,000.00 (as of 2010) and your federal tax bracket is in the 39%, you will have to pay taxes on the amount of money that you withdraw from your retirement account. In addition, there will be State taxes and possibly local taxes.

However, if you wait until your age is 59.5 years (as of 2010), then there should not be penalties and whatever amount of money you take out will be taxed as ordinary income and is taxed according to your income bracket for that year. So, if you are retired at that time, and you take out $ 50,000.00 out of your retirement account (and you do NOT have any other income), you will be taxed on this $ 50,000.00 at this tax bracket. Notice that in a retirement account you will not have to worry about paying taxes on any gains (appreciations), which is also called capital gains.

### *Do I have to take some of the money out after certain age?*

Yes, A traditional Individual Retirement Account (IRA) are subject to the so called "required minimum distribution", which means that you will have to start taking a minimum amount out of your traditional IRA every years starting in the year that you turn 70.5 years (as of 2010 rules). You must take the required minimum distribution by December 31 of each year.

### How about Roth IRA?

Roth IRA is not subject to required minimum distribution during the person's life. If you decide to covert a traditional IRA account into a Roth IRA account, you will have to pay taxes on the amount that you convert from traditional IRA to Roth IRA, but then you may pass the account on to a beneficiary upon your death without having to worry about any tax issues.

### What do I need to do to manage my retirement plans/accounts appropriately?

*We emphasize that you should periodically review your finances especially your retirement account(s) at every juncture in your career; therefore you need to review your retirement accounts when:*

    *a.   You graduate from medical school and you incur student loans*
    *b.   When you complete your residency*

c.  *When you change jobs*
d.  *And every year thereafter to keep up with new laws and regulations.*

Just because you have a retirement plan or account(s) it does not mean that your retirement in secure. It is important that you consistently (e.g. quarterly if your retirement money is in mutual funds) evaluate your retirement accounts or plans. Financial institutions usually mail out or email statements at least quarterly and here is your chance to evaluate them closely with attention to the following areas:

How much you are contributing to your retirement plans and is that the right amount for you?

Most physicians will be in their thirties by the time they complete their training and are able to contribute to a retirement plan, but if you can try to contribute at least 10% of your income to your retirement in your 20s that is even better. In your thirties increase this contribution to 15% of your income and it should increase to 20% of your income by the time you reach your thirties and forties. Physicians in their 50s should have a more urgent need for contributing to their retirement plans. For those over 50 years of age maximize your contribution to your retirement plans through your employer, if you are employed, and take advantage of the so called "catch-up" contribution.

Diversify, Diversify, Diversify:

If you are employed, the compensation and benefits department at your place of work may give you a long list of mutual funds to select from for your retirement account. The list can be perplexing and you may be confused as to which ones to choose from this long list. Here are some tips:

1.  First of all do not pick any fund that you do not understand
2.  Choose one fund from each category of funds e.g. small cap fund, mid-cap fund, and large-cap fund, a foreign fund that tracks a specific market such as Asian markets, Europe or Latin America. You should also have some of your investments in bonds. One rule that has been publicized is to subtract your age from 100, the number you get is the percentage of your portfolio that should be in stocks. So, according to this rule, by the age of 50, 50% of your money should be in bonds and the other 50% in stocks. Other experts believe, that this may be too conservative and that you should have more of your retirement in stocks. There are websites that you can refer to, in order to find a suggestion for an asset allocation based on your age, your tax-bracket, how much you plan to save every year, and you risk tolerance. A calculator calculates your asset allocation and presents it to you in a nice pie chart based on these parameters in order to create a balanced portfolio. One such website is at http://www.bankrate.com. It is very difficult to predict or time a market. Different stocks in different categories e.g. small cap stocks outperforms other categories such as mid-cap or large cap stocks on different years. Some years bonds outperform stocks, and yet during other years it is best to keep you money in cash. And so if your portfolio is diversified and you own mutual funds in each of these categories, you are less likely to see dramatic swings in the total value of your portfolio. Periodically (such as once a year) look at your portfolio and make adjustments as necessary

Here is one example with suggestions.

Let us say that you have a retirement account that had a total value of $ 50,000.00 in 2009, but appreciated to $ 60,000 in 2010 and the portfolio was follows:

| Portfolio in 2009 | | Portfolio in 2010 | |
|---|---|---|---|
| Small cap | 10,000 | small cap | 20,000 |
| Mid cap | 10,000 | midcap | 8,000 |
| Large cap | 10,000 | Large cap | 10,000 |
| Bonds | 10,000 | Bonds | 10150 |
| Cash | 10,000 | Cash | 10035 |

As you can see that the maximum appreciation came for the outperformance of the small cap funds, which has doubled in value. You may want to move some money from this fund and deploy it to other funds which have underperformed e.g. take the $10,000.00 appreciation from the small cap fund and spread it over the other funds e.g. large cap fund, mid-cap fund and bond fund depending on what is the prospect for the market in 2011. Do your homework and make the appropriate changes. So, now you should not intimated when you sit down with someone from the compensation and benefits department to review your retirement account portfolio. If you have your own practice and have your own IRA account you take the same approach as above.

## Retirement for Women Physicians

Women physicians have to plan better for retirement because they live longer than men and therefore they are more likely to deplete their retirement funds and be left with limited resources when they are old and have limited abilities to generate more income. At least 50% of women in the US are expected to live past the age of 85, some may live into their 90s, but most of them are not planning to live this long according to data from the Society of Actuaries. The data shows that over 90% of retired females and about 90% of those about to retire do not have a financial planning that is necessary to allow them to live a comfortable life for the entire duration of their retirement. Because women live longer than men, they need to plan for inflation, long-term care needs and other health expenses. Inflation on the average has been in the range of 3.5% from 1980 to 2009, but health care inflation has been close to 6% during the same period. The cycle of life is such that our ability to produce a lot more than what we consume increases from our 20s and 30s and peaks at around age of 50 years. Between 50 and 60 years of age this ability declines and so does reliance of others on us to provide for them. Between 60-80 years of age, we tend to be self-reliant and can support ourselves. Past the age of 80, dependency on others starts again, because we no longer produce enough to meet our consumption. Because 50% of women live past the age of 80, re-sources during retirement is a more important issue for them.

Unfortunately, 85% of women who are 85 years or older are wid-owed (compared to only 45% of men) and for many of them the death of a spouse is accompanied by a decline in their standard of living. Women live longer, generally have lower income, but have higher health care costs partly because they are more likely to have longer periods of chronic disability and are more likely to need a nursing home or other types of long-term care. The expected average value of the cost of lifetime long-term care for a woman is more than twice that for a man. So, if you are a woman physician you need to take all these factors into consideration and plan better for your retirement starting in your younger years instead of planning on working longer than you expect because this may not be a solid option in your older age. You may not be able to work due to illness, disability or the need to provide care for another family member.

## Specific retirement plans

*Most of the following retirement plans do not (will not) apply to you if you intend to be an employed physician in a large health care orga-nization and you receive a fixed salary with benefits (also see W2 vs. 1099 section).*

## Simplified Employee Pension-Individual Retirement Account (SEP-IRA):

The Simplified Employee Pension (SEP)-IRA allows contributions of a fixed percentage of salary (up to 25% of income) to individual IRAs of most employees, including the physician(s) who own the practice. As of 2010, the upper contribution limits for these plans are $49,000, with another $5,500 "catch-up" contribution for participants aged 49 years and older.

The IRS requires that a fixed percentage of compensation be used to calculate the amount of pension contributions, and this percentage must be the same for owners/physicians and other employees in the practice. This makes the SEP a relatively expensive plan in terms of employee funding. There is no component of salary deferral by employees, and all plan funding is immediately "vested", which means that it belongs to the employee immediately and if they leave employment with your practice they can take that money with them.

Most corporations require that you work for them at least 3, but most require 5 years of employment before the employee becomes vested. However, the advantage of the SEP plan is the minimum amount of paperwork and ease of set up. Generally, SEP-IRA plans are used by smaller practices, which may not have outside employees other than family members. SEP-IRA tends to work well for physicians who are independent contractors with health care systems such as emergency medicine physicians, contingent physicians and physicians who work on a part-time basis or provide locum tenens services to hospitals. However, an independent contractor with an income of less than $170,000 can also deposit more pre-tax money in the so called Self-Employed 401(k) plan (described in more details below).

**The Savings Incentive Match Plan for Employees IRA (Simple IRA):**

This is another plan that is easy to set up and administer. It allows companies with fewer than 100 employees to open individual IRA accounts for their employees. The employees may defer salary in amounts of $10,000 to $13,000 (depending on age), with an employer "match." All the money in the plan is immediately vested. The match is generally a dollar-for-dollar matching contribution of up to 3% of the employee's salary.

For example, a practice owner with a compensation of $100,000 would be able to defer up to $13,000 (if age 50 or older), and then have the company match up to 3%, or $3,000 more. One distinct feature of the plan is that the 3% match has no limits. For example, a physician with a small group of employees and an annual income of $400,000 can put away $13,000 in salary deferrals and another $12,000 (3% of $400,000) of match at no employee cost.

A SIMPLE IRA plan is a good choice for small businesses such as a medical practice in which the owner (which is most likely to be you the physician) is highly compensated, and few employees wish to defer salary. Its disadvantages are in the immediate vesting for the matched funds, and relatively low total amounts of contributions compared with other qualified plans.

### 401(K)/PROFIT-SHARING PLAN

This is by far the most common type of qualified plan in existence. These plans have 3 components:

**1) 401(k) salary deferral.** In 2010, employees may defer $16,500 (if under the age of 50 years) and $22,000 (for individuals 50 years or older), depending on their age. This money, and earnings on it, are not subject to federal income tax until withdrawn in retirement, and are immediately vested.

2) A "match." This is an optional part of the plan in which an employer may contribute a matching amount to give employees an incentive to participate. Matching funds are usually subject to vesting on a time schedule (often 3-5 years of continuous employment), and can be of any amount as long as there is not a defined benefit plan in place.

3) Profit-sharing. Like the match, this is a discretionary contribution by the employer of up to 25% of W2 payroll. The profit-sharing component is usually subject to a vesting schedule to encourage employee longevity. Note that the profit-sharing contribution is not the same as a match. A match is only present if the employee makes a salary deferral, whereas the profit-sharing contribution is independent of employee behavior.

In addition, there is a self-employed 401(k) option for small practices that have no full-time employees other than the physician and spouse. It operates in much the same way as a standard 401(k) plan, but with little expense and much less paperwork.

## DEFINED BENEFIT PLANS

These plans are becoming less and less common as the concept of pension disappears. Defined benefits plans are based entirely on company contributions to a fund (no employee salary deferral) that is actuarially designed to produce a set benefit amount at retirement. All the risk for providing the promised benefit rests with the employer. The advantage of this type of plan is in allowing a much higher contributions on a pretax basis, but the disadvantage of these plans is higher administrative costs.

These plans work extremely well for high-income businesses employing a single individual who is nearing age 50 or over. In addition, physician practices that employ a spouse or physicians of different ages can often use a defined benefit plan in conjunction with a 401(k)/profit-sharing plan to great benefit.

Note also that maximum contributions to a defined benefit plan preclude contributions for the same business to a profit-sharing plan. While it's possible to make less than the maximum contributions to a defined benefit plan and also some profit-sharing contributions, this calculation is usually quite complex and changes yearly. However, making the maximum contribution to a defined benefit plan does not preclude a 401(k) salary deferral and match by the employer of up to 6% for this deferral.

## DEFINED BENEFIT 401(K) PLANS

In 2010 new rules were introduced where employers may elect to provide a plan that offers some of the benefits of both defined benefit and 401(k) salary deferral plans. As of 2010 the details are still evolving, but basically the plan seeks to provide funding equal to 20% of an employee's salary. In order to qualify, employees must contribute at least 4% of their salary into a 401(k) salary deferral plan, which the employer then matches equally.

### Combining Plans:

You can also combine plans. For instance you may combine a defined benefit plan for an older physician or physicians, along with a few of the employees. The employee cost of the defined benefit plan is proportionally lower for younger and lower-paid employees. The remaining employees and younger physicians use a 401(k)/profit-sharing plan. This allows the older physicians to increase their annual pretax contributions significantly, while participants in the defined benefit plan are still allowed to make a full 401(k) salary deferral in addition to a 6% matched contribution.

Multiple plans may also be used for a physician's practice when the group owns multiple businesses. For instance, a physician may practice on a regular basis, but have a separate consulting firm that involves locum tenens, or giving educational lectures to groups of physicians around the state or the country. Any contributions made to the above plans may be used to shelter income from both businesses. However, the salary deferral side of any combination of plans must be aggregated, and may not exceed the annual limit ($16,500/$22,000) in 2010, but up to 25% of compensation for W2 income can be put into a profit-sharing plan in either business to maximize contribution and shelter the money from taxes.

**Let us look at some examples to clarify some of the specific examples of retirement account:**

**Example 1.** John Doe, MD is a family physician in a thriving practice and he has 5 employees, one of them is his wife. Dr Doe has established a profit-sharing plan with a local brokerage company that manages the account for him free of charge. Dr Doe's annual income is $ 260,000.00 and he has been deferring 15% of this income into the profit-sharing plan every year for a total of $ 39,000.00. He will also have to make 15% contribution to the 4 employees (excluding his wife; see below) which totals $ 110,000.00 for a total of $ 16,500.00.

Dr Doe pays his wife $ 62,000.00 in order to be able to make $ 9,300 (15% of $62,000) contribution towards her retirement. However, he will have to pay an additional $ 9,300.00 in social security taxes for his wife. *Should Dr Doe do things a little bit differently?*

**Here is a suggestion for doing things differently:**

Dr Doe could implement the following changes to his and his employees' retirement plan:

- Lower his wife's salary to approximately $ 20,000.00 annually, this will save him approximately $ 6000.00 in social security taxes.

- Change to a 401 (K) profit-sharing plan managed by a financial institution, which will involve some costs, but this cost should be under $ 3000.00
- His employees cost for this plan will drop from 15% to 6%, which will add to a savings of close to $ 9,000.00 (15% of $ 100,000 = $ 15,000.00 vs. 6% of $ 100,000.00 = $ 6,000.00).
- Dr Doe and his wife can now contribute a combined amount of approximately $ 66,000.00 to their retirement plans.

The key is to review your plans, talk to financial advisors and accountants and customize retirement plans that suit you and your practice the best. In doing so make sure you hire an independent financial advisor who can give you an advise that is best for you and not for the financial firm he/she works for.

**How can I save more money for retirement and reduce my taxes ?**

A cash balance pension plan and other forms of defined benefit pension plans can be great ways for practices that can afford them to dramatically increase retirement savings while reducing taxes. As an additional benefit, the plans provide essential asset protection for doctors, and the significant contributions they permit could offer a great way to catch up if you have not saved enough in the past or if your retirement account balances have been affected by investment losses during the recent economic turmoil.

**PENSION ACT INCREASES PLAN POPULARITY**

Although still rarely used by physicians, defined benefit plans slowly have become more popular since the enactment of the Pension Protection Act (PPA) of 2006. The PPA permits small businesses to have cash balance plans and allows medical practices to sponsor both 401(k) profit-sharing and defined benefit plans to take advantage of the unique characteristics of each and benefit from the combination of the 2. The PPA explained how to cross-test the benefits of both types of plans and weight the contributions more heavily toward the doctor-owners if the demographics are suitable for this plan design.

Some benefits of defined benefit plans under the PPA:

- **Flexibility.** Historically, defined benefit plans were thought to be fixed and inflexible. The PPA brought a new funding method to the table that gives rise to a range of funding options. Proper plan design and this new funding method could result in significant year-to-year funding flexibility, which previously was not permitted in defined benefit plans.
- **Larger, more predictable contributions.** As a result of these changes, practice owners now may make substantially larger tax-deductible contributions to their retirement plans. The plan designs are doctor-friendly in that they allow a contribution level that fits the needs and cash flow of the business. This increased funding flexibility also can make contribution totals more predictable from year to year.

## IMPORTANT CONSIDERATIONS

One thing to know when deciding whether to pursue a defined benefit plan for your practice is that such plans work best when the average age of physicians in the practice is at least 10 years more than the average age of staff members in the practice. This is because an actuary determines contributions based on the age and compensation of each plan participant. The law permits greater contributions for older workers because fewer years exist for their plan funds to grow and fewer contributions are anticipated until they reach retirement age. When the doctors are older than the staff members, the lion's share of each contribution dollar funded benefits the physicians.

Another consideration is that defined benefit plans require the services of an actuary in addition to a plan administrator. Instead of paying $2,000 to $5,000 for annual plan administration, you likely will spend $5,000 to $6,000 to operate the plan. These higher costs must be factored into your decision but usually are minimal relative to the benefits achieved. If you believe you are able to contribute at least $100,000 per year for yourself, then have an actuarial study performed to compare the defined benefit plan structure with that of your current plan to help you assess whether a change is warranted.

**You have inherited an IRA, how should you approach this retirement money?**

An important change in the law regarding an inherited individual retirement account was introduced around 2010. Prior to passage of this act, when a plan participant died, a spouse who was named as a beneficiary could roll the account into her (or his) own IRA, had the ability to stretch the benefits of appreciation over his or her lifetime, and even pass them on to next generations (his or her children), thereby deferring income taxes for decades. However, if the beneficiary was not a spouse, but a child the tax was levied either in the year of the participant's death or no later than the end of the fifth year following the participant's death.

The new act has changed this provision and allows a non-spouse beneficiary to receive the inherited IRA and stretch out the payments in a fashion similar to that available to a spouse.

To determine whether a defined benefit pension plan or a combination of plans is right for you, and to determine whether your current plan provides for an inherited IRA, you should consult with a pension attorney because details of these plans are complex and are beyond the scope of this book.

**What if you are 50 years of age and older?**

As of 2014, individuals who are younger than 50 years may defer $17,500 into a 401(k) accounts or 403 (b) account. With matching and profit-sharing plan contributions, the total can be increased to $49,000. Those 50 years old or older can defer an additional $5,500.

In comparison, if you are in your mid-50s, you can contribute and deduct $200,000 or more, just for yourself, in a properly designed cash balance plan or other form of defined benefit pension plan.

## Transitioning to retirement as a physician

Many of physicians believe that they can work long hours for many many years to come. Some believe that they are invincible. "I am healthy, I eat well, I exercise, my cholesterol and blood glucose are within normal limits and I am in my late 50s. I even had a stress test recently and everything was fine", said one physician talking to family members.

However, life is unpredictable. You still could have coronary artery narrowing and a plaque could get dislodged unexpectedly and all of a sudden you have a heart attack. If your medical profession involves significant amount of exposure to radiation such as interventional cardiologists and interventional radiologists you could develop sub-capsular cataract that may interfere with your vision and you may not be able to perform the duties you used to perform several years earlier and then you suddenly recognize that you are at a cross-road in your life. You will have to think about making changes in your career.

A spouse or a family member may get a serious illness and may need your attention, which may also demand changes and your career. These changes that may involve financial adjustment. If you are employed, you will have to negotiate with your employer about making changes to your schedule, including modifying the pattern of your practice e.g. doing only diagnostic radiology if you are an interventional radiologist or doing non-invasive cardiology if you are an interventional cardiologist. If you are in a private practice group with several other physicians and you are part owner, then you will need to have a lengthy negotiation to reach at an agreement that will serve both you and the practice best. Here is one option on how to approach this delicate issue if you are in a private practice and considering smoothly transitioning to retirement:

1. You could elect not to perform invasive procedure and not to take calls for the practice, but practice non-invasive radiology or cardiology. For this change in the pattern of your clinical practice to work well with your group, there must be enough physicians in the group to cover the calls which can be labor-intensive with fields such as intensive care, cardiology, orthopedics, and obstetrics and gynecology. You should make sure that the practice has enough physicians so that there are no hard feelings between you and other physicians in case there is shortage of manpower to cover calls. Or the practice may consider a younger physician in a year or two who is willing to take calls for the same salary.

2. In return the practice may ask you to sell your share in the practice to younger physician members of the practice. The proceeds from selling your share may be spread as payments to you over a period of 5-7 years so that you some additional income as you transition to retirement.

3. Another alternative is if you become a salaried employee of the practice and receive a paycheck every month with rooms for negotiation with regard to the exact compensation. Often your salary will be lower since now you are a senior member and you do not take calls, which means that the younger physicians in the practice will have to take over the burden

of additional call nights and weekends. Also, since you know have an employee contract, both parties should agree on clauses pertaining to the termination of the contract. You should emphasize to the physicians in the group that your continued presence in the group will translate into continued referral by physicians in the community to your practice since you are probably well known in the community.

4. Most often the contract in such a situation is renewable annually or less commonly every two years, and each party is allowed to terminate the contract with an advanced 120-day notice.

5. Essential benefits such as health insurance, malpractice insurance, disability insurance, and life insurance are negotiable, but since you probably already have these benefits through the practice it is probably more efficient for you if the practice continues to pay for these benefits because if they are cancelled and you had to go out and purchase these insurances, the premiums may be much higher than the current premiums.

6. Other benefits such as pager and cell phone expenses, car allowance, Society memberships, Journal subscriptions, and CME expenses should be mutually agreed upon and should be open for negotiation.

7. In order for this agreement to work long enough until you are ready for full retirement; there must be ongoing mutual respect and collegiality among the partners and between you and the partners, otherwise, past resentments and difficulties are sure to raise their ugly heads again and disharmony may arise. Also, you have to be productive enough to cover your salary and compensation and benefits so that the current owners of the practice feel they got a good deal and everyone is happy and content.

**Final words on retirement for you as a physician:**

**Strategies recommended by "financial advisors". Do they work?**

The general recommendations by "financial advisors" is to save certain amount of money (depending on your income) every month, invest over a long period of your working years (30-35 years) and hope that your investment will appreciate over time so that you will have a good nest egg for retirement. This strategy may or may not work depending on one major factor. Your retirement must appreciate considerably over the last decade or so of your working years, otherwise you may not have enough money for a comfortable retirement. Many people who were close to the retirement age and lost money in the financial meltdown of 2008 can relate to that. If your portfolio of investment does not perform well during the early years in your career, it might be easier to recover because the total amount invested is not as much and over the subsequent several years your portfolio may recover, but if the same happens during the later years of your career when you are closer to retirement it may not and you may end up in a disastrous situation because you will not have enough money for retirement.

Since most people including physicians have their retirement money invested in the stock market, you like many others are relying on the stock market appreciation, dividends that your portfolio receives from the stocks in your accounts and any interest rates that you may receive from money in savings accounts, certificates of deposits (CDs) or money market accounts over time. In this process you are relying on the power of compounding over time to help boost your retirement money. Realistically for most people, you are relying on your money to almost double during the last decade prior to your retirement in order to have enough money for a comfortable retirement.

Most Americans have annual income of $ 30,000.00 or less. So for an average person who is in her/his mid-20s and has an annual income around that figure and who saves about 8-10% of her/income annually over a period of 30 years and assuming around 6-7% appreciation in the investment and approximately 3% increase in annual salary (for inflation) the total amount saved for retirement is expected to be approximately around $ 500,000.00. Most people (as of 2010) are aiming for a total retirement amount of one million dollar in order to live comfortable during retirement years. Therefore, between the age of mid 50s until the retirement age of 65 (as of 2010) the investment will have to double, which is very difficult to achieve assuming a rate of return of 6-7% . The 6-7% appreciation (and not 10% appreciation) is a more realistic rate of growth. As you can see for the average person it would very difficult to reach this financial goal by the time that person retires. Luckily as a physician your income will be or is significantly higher than the average person and this should allow you some flexibility in managing the funds allocated to your retirement.

You should be able to save a significantly higher amount each month (the percentage of your income that you save may not be much higher) so that you will not have to deal with uncertainty of missing your goals for retirement. Start early saving for retirement. The earlier you start the sooner you are likely to reach the critical money level you will need for the compounding effect to accelerate your portfolio towards the retirement financial goal so that you do not end up in a predicament towards the final years of your retirement. To accomplish this you will need to save more than many retirement calculators suggest. Make an effort to save more money early in your career, assume a more conservative return on your investment especially towards the latter years of your career e.g. 5% rate of return instead of the more audacious rates of 8-10% and assume that your career will be 40 years ± 10 years. The bottom line is this: save more each month and assume that you will a more conservative portfolio with less risk.

**How much money you will need for retirement?**

You may have read about various formulas to calculate how much money you will need for retirement. There are also websites, which ask you to plug in numbers and it will give you a certain amount that you will need for retirement.

One simple formula is this: Add all your savings (cash, stocks, bonds) and multiply the total amount X 4% = your annual income during retirement.

If you believe that you have (or will save) $ 2,000,000.00, multiply it by 4/100 = $ 160,000.00 annually = $13,300.00/month + whatever you will receive from social security every month= your total monthly income. Don't forget that you will have taxes on this income at that particular tax bracket. Interesting, a recent survey that involved may participants from around the world about how much money you need to be happy? Most participants stated that they will need $ 160,000.00 a year to be happy.

# Insurance

**Disability insurance:** When you are a resident, the residency program will provide you with limited disability insurance usually through one of the companies in the insurance business. However, when you are getting close to graduation from residency you may want to discuss with the same company about extending that disability, but with higher monthly income in case of disability.

After your graduation, most prospective employers cover your disability insurance, however the compensation in case you do become disabled is somewhat limited. Therefore, it is a good idea to get your own disability insurance, in that way you know exactly what would be the monthly payment to you and your family in case you do become disabled and your family is taken care of. Some Insurance companies sell disability insurance that specialty specific so that for example if you are a surgeon and you do become disabled and are not able to perform your duties as a surgeon, but can practice in other fields you may still qualify for monthly payment as part of your disability.

Over the past two decades or so insurance companies have restricted the total monthly payments you can receive as a disabled physician to approximately $ 10,000.00 per month. In other words you will not be able to purchase excessive disability insurance i.e. more than $ 10,000.00 per month (in case you do get disabled) by purchasing several disability insurances from several companies. Like other insurances, insurance companies communicate with each other. In case you become totally incapacitated you may also qualify for social security disability if you have worked for at least 10 years and paid enough social security taxes during these years. Also, explore a specific type of disability insurance which will cover you if you are not able to perform the tasks of your specific field in medicine e.g. If you are a surgeon and you sustain a serious injury to your hands, you may not be able to perform surgical procedures, but you may be able to continue to practice medicine in another field. In this case the insurance will pay for the difference in your income between practicing surgery and let's say family medicine.

**Life Insurance:** Life insurance is a type insurance that pays your family a certain amount of money after you die. There are various types of insurances, but the one that most experts recommend you purchase is the "term life insurance".

With term life insurance, you decide on the amount of life insurance, the term of the insurance usually 10 or 20 years and accordingly you pay a monthly premium. For a physician with a family (a spouse and children) it can range from 0.5 to 2.0 million dollars.

You may purchase a term life insurance for $ 1,000,000.00 for a term of 20 years. This is the type of life insurance you should buy for yourself and perhaps your spouse. If you die within the term of the life insurance, your family will receive $ 1,000,000.00. May experts recommend that if your goal is to make sure that your family have enough money to live in case you die unexpectedly, term life insurance is the type of life insurance you should purchase.

There are other types of life insurance that go by different names such whole life or variable life. With these types of life insurance you still pay a monthly premiums, but the funds are invested over time and in case of your death your family will receive the balances in the account (instead of a specific amount such as $ 1000,000.00) based on how well these investment have performed. This is obviously riskier and most experts do not recommend that you purchase these types of insurances.

One disadvantage of term life insurance is that the terms of insurance are limited e.g. 10 or 20 years and if you live beyond the term of the life insurance you are no longer covered. For instance, if you purchase of 20-year term life insurance when you are 30 years old, by the time you reach 50 the term of that particular insurance will expire and you are no longer covered should something happen to you. Therefore, it is imperative that you have alternative plans for your loved ones when the end of the term life insurance is approaching.

## Long-term care insurance, do you need it?

As a physician who is a high-earner you should have a disability insurance policy, a term life-insurance policy and a retirement account that will allow you to live comfortably during your golden years. But what is long-term care insurance policy? and do you need to purchase long-term Insurance care for you and your spouse?

A long-term care insurance policy like any other type of insurance is a form of protection, in this case against the potential of a financial disaster resulting from a severe and unexpected injury or debilitating illness or you live until you are very old and you need someone to care for you. This insurance will pay for care that you may need either at your own home or at a licensed senior care provider. When the care is provided at home, the insurance will pay someone to help you with activities of daily living such as preparing meals and feeding you (and/or your spouse), bathing you, doing your laundry and helping you with daily exercises in order to avoid stiffness or contracture in your joints.

*Where do you buy a long-term care insurance policy?*

Most policies are sold through individual insurance brokers, with the rest sold through employers, professional associations, and other organizations such as the American Medical Association (AMA), the American Academy of Family Physicians (AAFP), the American College of Physicians, and the American Association of Retired persons (AARP).

*What are the variables in such a policy?*

There are several variables to a typical long-term care policy.

First is the length of waiting period between the time of the first claim and when benefits actually begin, which is similar to that of a long-term disability policy and it ranges from 30 to 90 days.

Second is the amount of the daily benefit, generally determined by the cost of nursing home or in-home care in a particular region.

Finally, there is the duration of the policy.

Whereas insurance companies used to routinely write policies with lifetime benefits, the increasing number of claims in recent years has caused most insurance companies to sell policies with limits on the number of years for which they will pay claims. Close to 50% of policies sold in recent years (as of 2010) are for only 3-4 years after the first claim is filed. This is an important issue to discuss when you are purchasing a long-term care insurance.

*What are your options when you purchase a long-term care policy?*

Again, there are a number of variables. For instance with some policies the policyholder may receive the specified dollar amount in the coverage, regardless of the amount of service provided. Other policies use a reimbursement form, in which the caregiver bills the policy-holder who then submits the bill to the insurance company. Most plans will pay the full amount of coverage only to a licensed professional. So, you could have a licensed professional help you with activities of daily living for part of the day and then have a family member come and help you for the rest of the day. The insurance company will compensate the non-professional the balance of your indemnity.

Another option to consider is an inflation rider, so that reimbursement keeps up with increases in health care costs since living expenses continue to go up annually and often faster than the consumer price index and we are not certain what the cost is going to be 15 years from now. Another option that you may have to explore when purchasing a long-term care policy is to buy the option to upgrade your policy in the future to keep up with any future innovations in care in the future.

*Is there a good age to buy a long-term care policy?*

Close to 50% of policies are sold to people between the ages of 55 and 64. This is the age when people are contemplating retirement, have the disposable income to purchase a policy, and are still able to medically qualify for policy underwriting.

*What is the cost of a long-term care policy?*

Because of the many variables that go into policies, their costs differ widely.

According to the AALTCI, annual premiums among the 55-to-64 age group for policies sold in 2009 ranged from $794.00 to $8,824.00, with a mean price of $2,300.00. Most of the decision on coverage, is based on the individual selecting a policy and is based on what she/he can afford to pay. In reality, you can spend about as much as you want on a policy if you get all the bells and whistles on it. e.g. You could probably purchase a policy that is for 6 years for you and your spouse for an annual cost of approximately $ 5000.00

**A word of caution!**

Although long-term care coverage has been gaining popularity, experts caution that it's not for everyone. You should look for insurance if you are trying not to pay for care yourself or have assets you want to pass on to heirs. If you have assets of $2 million or more you probably have enough to self-insure.

## Bankruptcy

During the economic crisis of 2008, the number of people filing for bankruptcy protection soared across all age groups and what was interesting is that the fastest segment of the population seeking bankruptcy protection was the senior citizens i.e. those who were 65 years and older. For many physicians, bankruptcy carries a stigma of personal and professional failure and shame. However, sometimes, bankruptcy is the only option whether you are a physician or another professional, and under these circumstances it is not necessarily a bad option out of the financial trouble that you are in.

One main question that anyone or a physician in this case has is: Will they take my house and all of my retirement money and leave me with nothing?

The answer is : NO

You can keep your home: Most states have homestead exemption laws, which protects your home equity from creditors. The amount that is protected varies from state to state and ranges from $ 250,000.00 to $ 500,000.00.

In the state of Massachusetts, for instance, you are protected up to $ 500,000.00, which means that you can live in home that is worth up to half a million dollar if it is your primary resident. Most states will also allow you to own one car. In addition, your retirement accounts and your social security money are also protected up to approximately $ 1,000,000.00 (yes you are reading the number of zeros correctly; up to one million dollar) so that you continue to have a stream of income from your retirement accounts and from your social security benefits if you qualify.

Credit card debt and medical bills on the other hand are legally classified as "unsecured debt", consequently these debts will be "discharged" when you file for and complete a bankruptcy procedure. This would mean that you are more than likely not have to pay them or pay only a percentage of them. What often happens though is that the original lender could sell your debt to another entity and that entity may attempt to collect as many cents on a dollar as it can.

Another concern that many people including physicians have when they are thinking about filing for bankruptcy protection is that bankruptcy is a very difficult process; you will be dragged through courts day in and day out and is likely to be one of the most humiliating and traumatic life experiences!

You should not be afraid of filing for bankruptcy for these reasons because the reality is that this is for the most part not true. Most debtors who do file for bankruptcy protection do not appear before a judge in a court. Close to 90% of people who file for bankruptcy never go to court or face a judge. Most or nearly all of the interactions is with your attorney. You often have to appear at one meeting with a "trustee" and this occurs usually six months after you are done with the bankruptcy protection, a process often referred to as "you have been discharged from bankruptcy protection".

*When do you know that you should file for bankruptcy?* When you are at a point in your life where you are unable to handle your bills or you are basically living off your credit card for day-to-day living expenses and those credit card balances continue to pile up. Like we discussed earlier, you should not have unreasonable worries that the creditors will take everything you own and that you will be homeless. That usually is not the case. Most people can live in their own home and often can get the creditors off their backs.

### Should you file for bankruptcy if you are a senior citizen and/or a retired physician?

If you are at a point where you are not able to handle your bills and it is a task to get through another day, and answer is probably yes. With the financial crisis of 2008, seniors including physicians lost a substantial portion of their retirement account because of the significant drop in the stock markets. The interests rate has been very low for several years and therefore, people like seniors who live on fixed incomes (from interest on bonds or dividends on stocks) have had their income drop, while at the same time living expenses have continued to rise and medical expenses have continued to escalate.

Therefore, it has become more common for some senior citizens to live off credit cards for an extended period of time. For physicians, use of credit card may not be for their entire daily living expenses, but for discretionary expenses in order to be able to maintain a good quality of life or a senior citizen may need to use a credit card to cover the cost of necessary health care and prescriptions.

A senior citizen physician who is having financial difficulty to the point that she/he is living off credit cards should consider bankruptcy if this is the only option out. Some seniors particularly physicians are ashamed of admitting that they have financial problems. It is this sense of shame and stigma that holds some of these senior physicians from filing for bankruptcy. However, some experts on bankruptcy suggest that as a senior citizen thinking about filing for bankruptcy you should not be afraid that you are going to lose your home, your retirement money, your car and basically be homeless.

That is not true. Actually, you should be able to keep your home, your retirement money, one car and live comfortably without the hassle of creditors. Hopefully, you would have learned a lot and you are wiser this time and try and live within your means. Because believe it or not you may even be able to get a credit card, even after bankruptcy, but the interest rate will probably be much higher so you need to act responsibly. If you have your home, your car, your social security benefits and hopefully some income from your retirement plans you should be able to live comfortably without having to borrow and go into debt again and bankruptcy will stop the constant drain on your limited resources.

**Tips for physicians who are approaching their senior years:**

If you are approaching the age of 55, you are technically approaching your senior years (you probably have already received a membership application for the AARP). You need to make plans for your "golden years". These plans are particularly important for physician who are single: divorced and alone, widowed, or never married. Consider the following:

If you become ill or incapacitated, someone will have to care for you. This could a spouse, a life-partner, a friend, a child, or someone else. This person will need to know what your wishes are with regard to your health and wealth. You put all this information in a "Well and Trust", which are documents that make decisions for your body and your assets when you are gone or in case you become incapacitated. It is critical to establish a well and a trust when you are under the age of 55. However, surveys have shown that only 35% of people have one. And so we are in a situation where seniors never communicated about their health and wealth, the children do not know where anything is and they do not know what their desires were. Therefore, some experts in this field recommend writing a letter around one of the holidays to chronicle "this stuff". Tell your story and your wishes and desires and where everything is and include details of the following:

1. Every time you opened a retirement account, bought a life insurance, or annuity you must have listed a beneficiary or beneficiaries. Who are they and what proportion each one gets. These designations are contracts that must be executed. If the beneficiary was your ex-spouse, but you forgot to change it, he or she will be entitled to the benefits in case you unexpectedly die.
2. Get another professional to review your will and trust to make sure that all your wishes are accurately stated.
3. Plan for inflation with regard to your retirement

Once you have done all that, Plan for fun during your retirement: traveling or pick up a hobby that will keep you occupied during retirement and have a back up plan for long-term care, cuts in social security and at least some tentative plan to have a part-time job.

## Employment following graduation from residency/ Fellowship, W2 or 1099?

You successfully secured a position in residency, you have moved to your preferred city and it has been several months into your residency. It is not too early to start thinking about what you would like to do after you complete residency.

What settings you would like to work in. Hospital-based medicine or an ambulatory setting?

And the bigger questions:

***Would you like to have your own private practice or you would like to be employed?***

If you are employed by a hospital, a health care organization or a groups practice, you will receive a W-2 tax form at the end of the year.

On the other hand physicians who are self-employed or independent contractors will either get a 1099 tax form or they will have to file their taxes as a corporation.

There are advantages and disadvantages to having your own private practice or being an independent contractor vs. being employed. Here is a discussion about the pros and cons of each:

*Being an employed physician:*

In some cities in the US, private practice opportunities are limited. In these locals, physicians will have to align themselves with one of the large health care organizations that provides health care to that region. You are an employee of one of these organization or a hospital, you are offered a contract that is usually limited to 2-3 years and renewable upon mutual agreement. But your employer has the right not to renew your contract at the end of each contract period. You go by their rules and regulations. You receive a salary and benefits, which usually includes health insurance for you and your family, disability insurance, limited life insurance, retirement matching (which means that your employer contributes certain amount each year towards your retirement), CME expenses reimbursement, CME days off (usually one week), and 3-4 weeks of vacation annually.

You receive a pay-check the same way it is during your residency. The pay -check includes your gross salary minus the federal, state, and local taxes. Because taxes are withheld up front usually you don't have to worry about owing taxes at the end of the years when you file your taxes and you don't have to keep track of professional expenses for tax purposes unless those expenses exceed 2% of your gross adjusted income. In certain respects, there is "less headache" from a tax standpoint.

Your employer usually takes care of managing the practice and also takes care of all the federal and state regulatory hurdles. You are unlikely to have to deal with third party payers such as insurance companies. Some physicians like this type of practice. Your main focus is to take care of patients and follow the rules and regulations of your employer. With the widespread of managed care organizations and the reimbursement cuts for physicians, it has become more difficult for physicians to practice on their own in a private practice setting. More and more physicians are choosing to work for an organization instead of having to deal with the headaches of managing a practice in addition to practicing medicine. **As of 2013, there are also speculations that the passage of health care reform may further limit the ability of physicians to practice independently in a private practice setting.**

If you are an employed physician, you may lose your independence and the ability to have a say in everything. These are left to the administration in your hospital or your health care organization. Employers are often willing to take suggestions from you, however the larger the organization the less likely it is that your voice will be heard. The bottom line is that you are not the boss, you have a boss that you have to report to.

*What are some of the advantages of being an employed physician?*

You will have protected time off, which is difficult to achieve in many private practice settings. As a salaried (employed) physician, you will often be allotted 4 weeks of vacation and 1-2 weeks off work for CME. During these periods, the employer is required to cover your practice with other physicians, either from within the health care system or physicians who work on a temporary basis (Locum tenens). In addition, you may be off on most national holidays except for being on call on some of these holidays. Sometimes you may also receive the support of a nurse on call who will screen your calls so that you will have to answer only a small percentage of all calls from your patients. In contrast, if you are in a private practice, especially if you are a solo practitioner, and you decided to take two weeks of vacation, you will have to provide coverage for your practice during that time period and also find someone to manage your practice; otherwise you will have to be on call for any contingencies during your vacation.

With the widespread of electronic health records (HER) it may be advantageous to be employed by a large health care organization where you can access patients' HER at various locations in the clinics and hospitals. Some physicians who work in these settings state that they are able to access patients' records and discuss care with other physicians with ease. They state that you don't have to pull paper charts and then try to read other peoples handwritings, which are not easy tasks. EHR will also allow physicians to analyze data pertinent from a quality assurance point of view. e.g. the rate of influenza vaccine administered during the influenza season to high risk patients.

*Ok, how about some of the disadvantages of being an employed physician?*

- You are not the boss, you have a boss that you have to report to, and this inherently limits your autonomy

– You get a monthly salary: Gross income – taxes (federal, state, and local taxes as well as social security taxes). You are NOT eligible to deduct any of the expenses related to your profession such as travel, lodging and fees involved with CME programs (unless the total annual costs exceed 2% of your adjusted gross income, but even then the deductions are limited). In contrast if you are in private practice all the expenses associated with your profession including: License fees, professional association membership fees, CME expenses, your business mileage, meals, and others are deductible from your total gross income. If you and your accountant manage your "itemized deductions well", you may pay substantially less taxes overall and be able to save more.

– The contribution towards your retirement is limited to the total federally allowable amount. This amount has been steadily going up. As of 2013, it is $ 17,500.00. The employer can also choose to contribute towards your retirement by adding certain amount of money called "matching" every month. You need to discuss with your employer matching during your contract negotiation both in terms of the total amount and the period of time it takes for you to be vested. Most employers have clauses in your contract that states that you will have to work for that particular employer for a minimum of 3 or 5 years before you qualify for the amount that is matched by employer. What that means is that if your employer has a minimum of 5 years for you to be vested and you leave that particular job after 4 years, you will lose the entire matching contribution from your employer.

– If you are self-employed in private practice you will have to keep track of your taxes, which means that you will need to hire an accountant and perhaps a tax attorney. The accountant (which should be a certified public accountant [CPA]), will keep track of your income and will suggest to you to make estimated tax payments every quarter. You will have to pay taxes on your net income = gross income – expenses.

– Expenses may include the following:

Office: rent, utilities, computers, billers and any other equipments etc.

Cars: either the annual business mileage or the monthly car payments if you have leased vehicles

Professional expenses including license fees, CME and other educational conferences important for your professional development.

– Gross income – Expenses = net income, The advantage you have with being in private practice is that you can contribute up to 24% of your net income towards a self-employed individual retirement account (SEP-IRA). So, let us use an example of Doctor John Doe who has a gross income of $ 600,000.00 per year from his practice.

– His expenses add up to $ 350,000.00, therefore his net income = 600,000 – 350,000 = $ 250,000.00. He can contribute 25% of the net income (up to a maximum of $45,000 as of 2010) towards a SEP-IRA = 62,500, but the maximum allowable amount is $45,000. Therefore, his taxable income has come down from $600,000 to $ 250,000 (because of his practice expenses) and then to $ 205,000.00 because of his SEP-IRA contribution. So this physician who is in private practice will pay federal, state and local taxes as well as social security and Medicare taxes on the a net of $ 205,000.00.

– If he was an employed physician and was receiving a monthly salary of let us say $ 17,000 for an annual income of approximately $ 205,000.00, he will pay taxes on the entire annual income. This is because if you are an employed physician and you receive a W-2 tax form at the end of the years (which specifies your gross wages and the taxes withheld) you don't qualify to deduct any expenses associated with your practice (your employer takes care of those) or your professional expenses (unless they exceed 2% of your adjusted gross income).

***So, what would you like to do? have your own Private practice, or be an employed physician?***

As you advance through your residency you need to think about this over and over and look at both options in terms of life style and from a financial standpoint, but here are certain points to remember:

— If you end up working in a University-based academic institution, you are usually employed and you very rarely have the option of being in a private practice in these settings.
— From a financial stand-point, analyze your potential income and your retirement contributions under both circumstances and ask yourself the following questions:
— Will I generate enough income from a private practice to cover the expenses associated with the private practice including the office rent, utilities, staff, etc., and then end up with a net income that is greater than my income if I was an employed physician?
— Do I like to deal with the hassle of managing a practice on my own and deal with federal, state, and insurance regulatory hurdles in addition to practicing medicine. What about the coverage for my practice in case I get sick, have a family emergency, or if and when I would like to take a vacation. How easy it is to find coverage for my practice during those periods?
— Or you are saying to yourself, I just want to practice medicine and don't want to worry about the hassles of dealing with regulatory agencies and insurance companies and dealing with office staff and their issues. In that case, you may be one of those physicians who prefers to be an employed physician.

**Current trend: Employed vs. your own practice:**

In the first week of November, 2010, the Wall Street Journal published an article about this issue. The article stated that based on a survey performed by a large Medical Group Management Association Survey, one of the largest physician recruitment agencies in the US, concluded that the share of practices that were owned by hospitals increased to an all-time high of 55% in 2009, up from 50% in 2008. This percentage was up from only 30% five years earlier in 2003. Merritt Hawkins, the biggest US physician-recruiting firm, reported that the share of its physicians' searches that were for positions with hospitals (meaning the practice was owned and operated by a hospital) hit 51% for the preceding 12 months. This was up from 45% a year earlier and from only 19% five years earlier.

On the other hand the overall number of searches for physician groups and partnerships has dropped during the same periods. Some younger physicians are seeking more regular hours of a salaried position, while avoiding to deal with issues such as the longer hours involved in practice ownership, battling with insurance companies over payments, and soliciting and often chasing patients for their insurance copayments.

With the new health care law (of 2010), a new health care model is emerging. This has been labeled as the "accountable-care organization", in which the health care provider (employed by a hospital or a health care organization) shares the financial benefits of efficient care.

Because this process is supposed to save money and resources, hospitals are seeking to position themselves for new methods of payments by employing physicians. In this new system, a larger third-party payer such as Medicare, will pay a finite sum of money to a health care organization and that particular organization has the responsibility of providing care for a specific number of patients, let us say 5000 Medicare patients. The care provided to these patients will include preventive care, ambulatory care, hospital care, and surgeries or other procedures. This model is likely to lead to more physicians being employed because it would be very difficult for a groups of physicians to be able to care for a very large number of patients, say 5000 Medicare patients, on their own.

As of Jan 2010, It is not clear with this model how the specialists who are already in private practice will be reimbursed. For example if an orthopedic surgeon performs a hip replacement procedure, on a Medicate patient, and he/she is part of this large health care organization, how she/he will be reimbursement for this procedure and how much?

However, what is clear is that since the bottom line is to cut cost, the end result will be fewer dollars paid to the physicians and the possibilities that physicians will be able to practice as solo practitioners are reduced.

More recent data published in 2011 show similar trend. The total number of physicians employed exceeded 100,000.00. Data available from 2010 show that 91,000 physicians were employed full-time and 24,000 were employed part-time for a total of 115,000 employed physicians.

Three quarter of health care organizations surveyed in 2011 said that they increased physicians staffing level in 2011 and that they were planning on hiring more physicians in 2012. Perhaps, health care organizations are preparing themselves for the new health care reform. They are trying to increase their physician referral base in order to increase admissions. From the physician side, flat third-party reimbursement, increased practice costs and more desirable life-style is driving physicians to look for employment rather than having to manage their own practice and the financial complexities associated with it.

*Financial issues associated with owning your own practice:*

Due to the combined effects of declining reimbursements and increasing expenses associated with running a private, physicians continue to be under tremendous pressure if and when they decide to own their own practice or are thinking harder about establishing a practice following completion of a training program.

According to data from the Medical Group Management Association (MGMA) published in 2008 based on 2007 data, the costs for operating a practice increased from 58% in 61% over the preceding decade. During the same period, revenues from multi group practices increased by 5.5%, which was a full percentage point (6.5%) lower than the median operating cost for running a successful practice. Specific practices including Obstetrics and Gynecology, Pediatrics, and family medicine saw similar trends during the same period. The increases in operating costs were due to increases in salaries for office staff, medication supply costs, and professional medical liability in- surance premiums. In most cases these increases in expenses involved in running a practice were in addition to the student loan payments that physicians are responsible for.

## How much do I need to run my practice?

People say "it takes money to make money". That is true for any busi- ness, but how does that fit into a medical practice?

Even after funding a practice start-up, it still takes money to keep the practice running. You can have a full patient schedule, but without cash, you can't pay your bills. Even if you have a concierge style cash- only practice and don't accept insurance reimbursement, you still have to rent the office, hire staff, and buy supplies in advance in order to see that cash-paying patient. You may have to periodically renovate the office, or fix broken equipments in your office. To accomplish this you may either use your own money (current cash saved) or use OPM = other peoples' money, through borrowing, usually from a bank.

In business terms, the money you owe is called long- or short- term liabilities. The money spent to run a practice is referred to as working capital. Working capital equals your current assets minus your current liabilities. Having positive working capital means that your practice is able to pay off its short-term liabilities such as payroll, supplies, and rent.

Having negative working capital means that your practice is unable to meet its short-term liabilities with its current assets including cash, accounts receivable, and inventory. The worst-case end-result of ongoing negative working capital is bankruptcy, when you can no longer pay your bills.

**Things to watch for in your assets and liabilities:**

The period between having positive working capital and bankruptcy can be quite complex, and certainly stressful. Having it be stressful is better, though, than having it go unnoticed. Paying attention to your practice's working capital ratio can give you an advance "yellow flag" warning that something is going wrong, hopefully in time to fix it.

For example, noticing that the accounts receivable due more than 90 days are climbing, while the checking account balance is dwindling, should prompt you to look into the reasons for this phenomenon. Other warning flags may include your bookkeeper coming to you with concerns or the need to dip into your practice's line of credit to put money into the practice to make payroll.

Working capital can be used as a barometer of a practice's operational efficiency. Accounts receivable that are increasing also increase working capital and on the surface would appear to be a good thing. But if your accounts receivable are increasing because your collections activity has slowed—as is common in this economy—it can mean trouble.

Money that is owed to the practice cannot be used to pay current bills. Accounts receivable more than 90 days old may not really be an asset, as the older they get, the less likely it is that they will ever be paid and thus converted into cash. So if a practice is not operationally efficient, that will be reflected in the working capital. Having a lot of your working capital tied up in accounts receivable instead of cash is inefficient and can lead to trouble, as there are better uses for your cash. The same goes for having your cash tied up in equipment that is not being used efficiently to create profits, like that hair-removal cosmetic laser you never got around to marketing effectively (even though you and your colleagues are now largely hairless).

## How much money you really need?

Increased productivity, such as expanding hours or adding an additional provider or ancillary services, can increase working capital needs. When a medical practice increases its productivity, the accounts receivable will likely increase as well. It will take time to collect the accounts receivable, so in the meantime the practice may need extra cash to pay current bills.

One way to forecast how much more cash is needed is to calculate last year's working capital (assets minus liabilities) and divide the amount by last year's charges. Then multiply the ratio times the projected future charges to calculate capital needed.

Here is an example:

let us say your assets are $ 200,000.00 and your liabilities are $ 80,000.00. Therefore your working capital is $ 120,000.00. The previous year charges were around $ 600,000.00 therefore, the ratio is 120,000/600,000 = 20%. If the projected future charges are $ 160,000 then the extra capital needed would be = 160,000 X 0.20 = $ 32,000.00.

Most medical practices are labor-intensive and you do not need to have a lot of capital tied up, upfront (provided you do not purchase expensive equipment such a LASIK machine to perform ophthalmological procedures) and therefore, employees salary and building rents are the largest portions of your expenses. You may have to pay the first month of rent up front (plus security deposits), but employees do not need to be paid up front! They get paid towards the end of the month and therefore, you will have at least one month to come up with the capital to pay employee salaries, because the way third-party payers i.e. insurance companies operate, is they often pay you for your services within 2-6 weeks after you submit a bill (even though they have up to 120 days to pay you after you render a medical care).

It is this fortunate fact that most insurance companies make the payment within 2-6 weeks that makes it easier for you to run a practice with less upfront capital. However, it is still not soon enough before your staff expect to receive their paycheck (which is usually within 2-4 weeks, depending on whether you decide to pay them every two weeks, or monthly). Therefore, you should have enough cash on hand to pay your staff before your accounts receivable have any funds in them.

The cost of running a practice goes up every year just like other commodities we purchase for our day-to-day living. At the same time reimbursement from medical insurance companies have been declining over the past two decades. Therefore, expect to work harder or work smarter by instituting cost-cutting measures frequently.

Balancing the cash income and outflow is often referred to as revenue cycle management. Revenue cycle management is very important in labor-intensive businesses like a medical practice. It can often be deployed with minimal capital. Proper use of capital to invest in strategies that yield a return on investment without additional physician labor also improves working capital.

Here are some monthly benchmarks to keep track of:

- Total accounts receivable: no more than 2x monthly charges;
- Accounts receivable over 90 days: less than 10% of total accounts receivable;

- Cash balance: always enough to cover 2 weeks of regular expenses;
- Line of credit balance: as low as possible;
- Owner salary or draw: regularly paid, not missed;
- Variables happen (e.g., when there are 3 payroll periods in a month), but any change of direction for 2 months or more should be investigated.

**Identify and address the following issues in order to make the financial aspects of your practice as healthy as possible:**

There are some simple analyses you can do to check the capital health of your practice.

Perform these exercises every few months to look for trends and make every effort to optimize them:

**Current assets/liabilities ratio of greater than 1**

Your current ratio is calculated by dividing your current assets convertible to cash in less than 1 year (I would exclude any accounts receivable over 90 days) by your current liabilities to be paid off in less than 1 year (including payments on long-term loans). A current ratio above 1 or more is considered healthy.

**Debt ratio of <1**

Your debt ratio is your total debt/ your total assets. A ratio of < 1 is considered healthy.

**Dividends >$1**

Dividends are your return on investment (and return on working capital) for ownership of your practice. Dividends are calculated by adding up your discretionary earnings, which include: personal gross salary, plus profit, retirement plan contributions, and any benefits paid by the practice to you such as health care insurance, life insurance, disability insurance, car allowance, and continuous medical education benefits. From this subtotal subtract the cost of employing a replacement physician to see your patients as if you were disabled, and could own the practice but not work in it. The result is called dividends, or a return on equity (ownership) rather than a return for your personal labor.

If the result is $0 or less dividends, you are earning less as a practice owner than you would by quitting and taking a job with someone else as the employer. This indicates a $0 return on working capital. If your dividends are $ 0.00, your practice has only asset values and your practice is not earning you more than you would receive from being employed and your investment cash is not making you any money.

If you exclude personal preference as a factor and look at it purely from a financial standpoint, one option would be to sell the practice and deposit the money in a savings account. In the health care industry, a medical practice commonly sells for 2 to 3 times dividends.

What if you have declining working capital i.e. cash? Here are some strategies for your practice to free some working capital to invest in your practice:

- get your working capital out of accounts receivable by improving co-pay, billing, and collections performance;
- either you and your billing staff take billing and coding courses so that your coding becomes more efficient, which will hopefully result in better compensation.
- evaluate whether there are tests and procedures that could be done in your office that you currently commonly refer to specialists or outside diagnostic services

- if you are usually booked at least 2 to 3 weeks in advance for noncurrent visits, consider employing a midlevel provider, or drop your worst-paying insurance plan
- when moving to an electronic health record (EHR) system, consider renting rather than purchasing a system. Also, as of 2010, look into incentives for using HER offered by various government agencies including Medicare.
- when replacing or adding expensive instrumentation, talk to your accountant about financing the purchase rather than investing cash or leasing;
- talk to your accountant before borrowing against your accounts receivable, or further investing in your practice.

Paying attention to working capital and some of these benchmarks can help keep your practice healthy with the cash flow you need.

**Additional steps to make your practice more efficient:**

*Get paid for your hard work i.e. Billing for the care you provide to patients.*

When you see a patient in a clinic or a hospital, how do you get paid for it?

Unless you have a concierge service or your practice plastic surgery where most of the services or procedures are not covered by health insurance and your patients pay cash, most physicians will have to bill the insurance plan for the patient and hope that they will be reimbursed for the services they have provided. How is that done?

You would ordinarily need a billing service, which consist of one or more "billers", who have knowledge and experience in billing insurance companies. You will have to provide them with the relevant information including: patient's demographics, patient's insurance company/plan, the level of service you provided and any procedures you performed on the patient.

If you talk to physicians who practice in Canada, they will often tell you that the billing system in Canada is so simple that the physician herself/himself can do the billing at the end of the day. In the US, however there are over 400 different third-party payers and there are over 400 different ways of billing for the services that a physician provides. This is because each insurance company has a different set of guidelines for submitting and processing the billing. This leads to inefficiencies in the system, which is associated with extra costs estimated to be in the vicinity of $ 300-400 billion (yes with a "b") dollars.

There is no shortage of data and information available about how administrative complexities bog down the healthcare system and that the need for a different claims management system for each insurer, places a substantial administrative burden on physicians' practices and adds a huge, unnecessary cost to our healthcare system. Here are some examples:

According to information from the American Medical Association (AMA), the cost of inefficiency in the billing system including processing, payment and reconciliation is estimated to be between $ 20 to 200 billion dollars, which translates to consumption of 10-14% of physician practice revenues by the most conservative estimates.

The AMA's 2010 National Health Insurer Report Card found that the health insurance industry has about an 80% accuracy rate for processing and paying claims, but close to $750 million in unnecessary administrative costs could be saved if the industry improves claims processing accuracy by as little as 1%. Increasing the accuracy rate to 100% would save up to $15 billion annually.

The American Academy of Family Physicians AAFP also concluded that simplifying procedures for billing could the health care system in the US $ 300 billion dollars annually.

A recent study by a team of researchers at Massachusetts General Hospital is a good illustration of the inefficiencies associated with the current billing system. These researchers analyzed the billing system of a physician's group affiliated with a large urban academic teaching hospital. They discovered that close to 13% of claims were initially rejected. With considerable staff time and effort, 80% of these claims eventually were paid.

They also found that by standardizing the medical billing system and using a single set of payment rules for multiple payers in a single claim form with standard submission rules would save significant staff time and could save U.S. physicians about $7 billion annually.

Some pieces of good news in this area include the following:

1.  The secretary of the U.S. Department of Health and Human Services has been given the responsibility of establishing transparency and consistency in claims processing and to solicit input on electronic standardization of this process. The deadline date set to accomplish this goal, was January 1, 2012.
2.  There are calls for a voluntary coordinated nationwide approach to key administrative process when it comes to billing including the following: a universal credentialing form to eliminate repetitive paper work; adoption of industry-wide standard for interchangeable electronic data in determining and verifying patient insurance coverage; standardizing health care patient identification card; and improving coordination of prior authorization process for certain specialties.

One can only hope that the insurance industry will get more serious about this issue.

The USA spends 30% of health care expenditure on administrative costs compared to 8% for other industrialized nations. A significant amount of money could be saved by fixing the billing system in order to make it more efficient. Part of our healthcare cost problem is that administrative costs are so convoluted and expensive, and a lot of that has to do with standardization.

You can get involved in this process, which is an important issue for all physicians. Every little step in improving the billing system will translate into more efficiency for your office. In the meantime, when it comes to billing, contracting with a biller who works for you based on commission is better than hiring people who get paid a fixed salary to do the billing for you. The commission for billing ranges from 5-10% of net amount collected. Experience has shown that when you give your billing business to an entity that works for you based on commission the billing becomes more efficient, the accuracy rates increase, and the overall revenues increase because the more you collect, the more the billers make.

Before we proceed with the next section, let us clarify some terminologies in the new health care ear, so that it is easier for you to understand the discussion involved around this topic.

**Q: What is an Accountable Care Organization (ACO)?**

**A:** An ACO is an organization of healthcare providers that agrees to be accountable for the quality, cost, and overall care of Medicare beneficiaries who are enrolled in the traditional fee-for-service program who are assigned to it.

For ACO purposes, "assigned" means those beneficiaries for whom the professionals in the ACO provide the bulk of primary care services. Assignment will be invisible to the beneficiary and will not affect their guaranteed benefits or choice of doctor. A beneficiary may continue to seek services from the physicians and other providers of his or her choice, regardless of whether the physician or provider is a part of an ACO.

**Q: What forms of organizations may become an ACO?**

**A:** The statute specifies the following:

- physicians and other professionals in group practices;
- physicians and other professionals in networks of practices;
- partnerships or joint venture arrangements between hospitals and physicians/professionals;
- hospitals employing physicians/professionals; and
- other forms that the HHS secretary may determine appropriate.

**Q: What are the types of requirements that such an organization will have to meet to participate?**

**A:** The statute specifies the following:

- have a formal legal structure to receive and distribute shared savings;
- have a sufficient number of primary care professionals for the number of assigned beneficiaries (to be 5,000 at a minimum);
- agree to participate in the program for not less than a 3-year period;
- have sufficient information regarding participating ACO healthcare professionals as the HHS secretary determines necessary to support beneficiary assignment and for the determination of payments for shared savings;
- have a leadership and management structure that includes clinical and administrative systems;
- have defined processes to a) promote evidenced-based medicine, b) report the necessary data to evaluate quality and cost measures (this could incorporate requirements of other programs, such as the Physician Quality Reporting Initiative, electronic prescribing, and electronic health records, and c) coordinate care; and

- demonstrate that it meets patient-centeredness criteria, as determined by the HHS secretary.

## How to protect your practice and your assets from the big brothers?

If you are an older physician reading this book, you probably recall the era of the 1980s, when hospitals were aggressively buying practices of physicians who were in practice for cash up front and perks believing that by doing that they can control flow of patients and in the process become bigger and bigger and control the health care in certain locals. The cycle repeated itself in the 1990s when practice management companies and to some extent hospitals were out there buying private medical practices. Some of you may remember in the early 1990s when talking to one of the front desk clerks of one of the practices saying " all of a sudden" physicians were not seeing as many patients as before", we had to turn away our patients who have been with us for years, simply because physicians in the practice started limiting the number of patients they saw every to 20 patients a day". "I think that is because, they get a salary now; and they no longer have an incentive to work as hard as they used".

Then several years later, the practices became less and less efficient, the hospitals and health care organization did not make as much money as they were anticipating and the thought that the Mammoth medical groups will control health care ended. Then hospitals started telling physicians they will no longer pay their salaries and pay for their practice expenses. Some organizations ask physicians to take their practices back for free and they did. Some physicians file law suits against hospital for breach of contract. If you are a younger physician, ask some of the older physicians to tell you these stories or their stories, you may find them very interesting and history often does repeat itself if we do not learn from it.

So, as you can see the healthcare has seen major changes in the past few decades. These changes have often resulted from changes in the economic climate or new legislations and have been based largely on the assumption that big business can profit from controlling physicians' methods of management, referrals pattern, and oversight of patient treatment plans. Also, Wall Street motivated by intense desires for profit and Hospital and health care system under pressure from Wall Street in constantly increasing profits have often imposed paradigm shifts on medical practices willing to accept their premises and terms. Part of the "business strategy" for these entities has been to persuade physicians over and over (roughly every decade or so) that joining large healthcare systems is an inevitability. In many cases physicians who believed that they had a foresight and that their decisions were prudent agreed to change from smaller physician-owned practices to larger corporate Health system or Health organization. These shifts were often motivated by misrepresentation of facts and data coupled with modest amount of cash up front. However, when the thesis did not materialize, as was the case in 1980s and 1990s cited above, the losing party in the process were the physicians who returned back to their practice demoralized and with a significantly less total net worth financially.

Now in the new millennium, physicians are being promised that in the age of the internet, where "everything" is in the tip of your finger, we can create a system whereby physicians, hospitals, insurance carriers, and the government can all "plug" into, to improve and coordinate health care. Based on history, we as physicians will have to be careful with yet another suggestion in changing health care delivery. We, the physicians who are the health care providers and who are medically, morally, ethically, and legally responsible for rendering care to our patients will have to make decisions on how this new paradigm shift will be implemented instead of leaving it in the hands of Wall Street, the insurance corporations and large health care organizations. We should insist that this process will work best if and when independent physicians and independent multispecialty physicians groups participate in the process as venture partners rather than employees (directly or indirectly) of large health care organizations so that we as physicians are not subjected to pressures to join large health care systems because of fear of being left behind.

There are a number of signs that indicate that there may be a major shift towards " big Medicine" in the horizon. Among the ingredients in the Patient Protection and Affordable Care Act that was passed in 2010 and will be implemented in 2014, is a move or encouragement for a move towards large health care systems. The Government sees that these large health care organizations are key to providing quality and efficient health care by sharing information and providing a full scope of "coordinated medical care".

Consequently, hospitals, insurance plans, and Healthcare Medical Organizations (HMOs) perceive that they are under pressure to acquire or partner with medical practices in certain specialties. Recent changes in Medicare reimbursement for inpatient services such as cardiac catheterization and some diagnostic services add to the momentum. At the same time, the "anti-kickback laws" makes referral more difficult and dictates that being employed would be the only means by which a healthcare system can control the decision-making and referral pattern of its physicians. Thus, executives and administrators are seeking ways to increase collaboration in all aspects of patient care and treatment.

Another entity that will be established to play a dominant role in the practice of medicine is the so called accountable care organization (ACO), which are expected to be in full effect in 2014. As a further incentive, the ACOs will provide Medicare cash bonuses to large integrated health organizations composed of medical groups, hospitals, and outpatient facilities that treat 5,000 or more patients with favorable outcomes.

The thesis here is that the entire medical system may enjoy the same risk-sharing profits and rewards, for efficient care as primary care physicians in managed care organizations have been earning for many years. It is expected that many private carriers and HMOs will be involved in these ACO systems, which will include outpatient testing, treatment, hospital services, and home healthcare services. Physicians should get involved so that physicians groups will be part of the equation and not leave these ACOs in the hands of hospitals and large Health Care organizations.

Physicians should also get more recognize so that they are best compensated by controlling ownership and operations of these organizations. They should also put in their maximum input into the large health organizations so that they are based on sound models and professionally designed management systems that are loyal to the physicians while being accountable to all players in the system.

As the world of healthcare moves toward big medicine, it is crucial for physicians to plan ahead, understand their options, and take steps to strengthen their bargaining positions at the negotiating table. In past transitional times, physicians who prospered the most, were those physicians who either remained unaffiliated or those who hammered out cash-rich deals with livable escape clauses. There are reasons to believe that history will repeat itself. Therefore, as an independent physician you need to remain vigilant, participate in meetings and in negotiation and do your homework before giving up your most valuable assets to the Large Health Care Organizations as the health care system evolves again in the 2010-2020 era.

**Other issues to consider during a transition in Health Care:**

**Be cautious when you are asked to "invest in a project ":**

Physicians should be cautious about investments that require significant overhead or long-term commitment. When opportunities do arise, it's advisable to pursue available joint venture options or structure an arrangement with a quick and inexpensive exit strategy that will allow others such a health care organization or an insurance entity to bear most of the risk with capital losses. Some signs that physicians need to evaluate carefully include the following:

When you are asked to invest, remember that outward signs that a practice is successful do not always guarantee that a practice is healthy and has a profitable bottom line. Make sure that you review the tax documents for the practice for the preceding three years and have an experienced certified public accountant evaluate these documents. Also, compare any data with benchmarks relevant to the practice and other groups in the area.

If you have carefully considered the previous advice and have decided that a hospital network best suits you, it's important to understand the situation you are entering into in order to maximize your position within the larger network. Here are additional issues to consider:

## PROFITABILITY: THE KEY TO SUCCESS

In each transition we have witnessed, a medical practice's profitability has been the primary factor in determining its success, so maintaining strong revenues and controlling overhead should be top priority for practices. We have never seen a physician group experience stellar success because it bought the most beautiful building, had the most expensive testing or treatment equipment, or took the most time off.

On the other hand, working effectively with referral sources, meeting patients' needs, taking advantage of service and reimbursement opportunities, and responding to market demand, while honing a good reputation for intellectual achievement and inventiveness, make a significant difference. It's also crucial to have qualified, trustworthy employee(s) who understand medical practice finance and management to ensure appropriate billing and coding and to monitor the staff's overall effectiveness.

In our experience, smaller practices tend to be more profitable per owning physician (with the possible exception of multi-office, single-specialty practices) as long as they are managed well and overhead and revenues are controlled by each office.

## WORKING WITH OTHER MEDICAL GROUPS

Participation in large medical group organizations has advantages and drawbacks. Advantages include better market access and bargaining power with health plans, resulting in better reimbursement, unified computer networks, electronic medical systems, and sometimes a reasonable balance of power within the group.

Larger groups also may attract more sophisticated management personnel and often enjoy economies of scale in the cost of ancillary operations and facilities. Experience shows that this model can work well with single-specialty groups. Size also can provide negotiating leverage, particularly when the group can move patients to competing hospitals.

On the other hand, we've seen clients join large group practices and encounter much higher per-physician overhead, along with expensive and sometimes ineffective management. Also, a "large-herd mentality" can result in a less competitive position than some smaller groups enjoy. Additionally, the success of single specialty groups generally does not extend to multispecialty groups unless one specialty is clearly in charge.

## HAVE AN EXIT STRATEGY

Doctors who join large groups should be mindful of the "divorce clause." If a large group medical practice breaks up, those members who are able to move to an independent or more profitable practice will be in a much better position to keep their patient bases (and independence) if they have negotiated the right to continue practicing in their geographic areas without significant interruption.

Oftentimes, non-compete covenants can be negotiated to provide the doctor with a buyout right or the right to consider the clause non-effective under certain circumstances.

We've seen significant differences in the treatment of physicians leaving hospitals or corporate systems, depending on the nature of the non-compete covenant and other contractual leverages that were negotiated.

## IMPACT OF ACOS

It is expected that by 2013, the benefits of ACOs with 5,000 or more patients will be implemented. Physicians participating in these plans likely will see higher compensation and access to additional marketing and referral patterns. It appears that hospitals, insurance carriers, and other healthcare systems are open to networking into these systems to unify healthcare administration and control costs. The rules will not require that all 5,000 patients be handled under one medical group or entity, so medical groups should not have to legally integrate into one large group or healthcare plans in order to participate. However, there will be expensive and time-consuming changes to computerization, common protocols, and electronic health record coordination that practices will need to undertake to participate in these organizations. This is where the large companies may have the upper hand, because these systems will be costly and likely will require large information technology teams to monitor and maintain them. Computer system businesses make quantum leaps each year, however, so these systems could be available to all ACOs, whether the controlling organizations are hospital systems, insurance companies, or large physician practices.

Although the ACO system rules may cost doctors and potential sponsoring organizations significant lost time and effort in meetings and other coordination efforts, it is important to prepare for them and begin seeking parties with whom to share management system organizations sooner rather than later. It's likely that some entre-preneurial and astute medical groups in each specialty will work to bring physician groups into networks to fulfill the ACO requirements without having to be a part owner or an employee of a hospital, health plan, and/or HMO system.

Also, some software and consulting platform companies will pros-per by providing systems services to hospitals, healthcare plans, and medical practices. It is not too early to be in discussions with other practice groups and institutions about future planning, but with a view toward working from a position of strength and opportunity rather than one of fear or uncertainty.

**Be Cautious, Do not sign up right away, but negotiate hard:**

The first offer provided to a physician by the hospital, healthcare plan, HMO system, or group practice almost always will be negotiable. Many physicians do not realize the benefits they can gain through appropriate negotiations and proper communications, including more thoughtful provisions, better financial concessions, contingency es-cape clauses, and long-term, more balanced relationships.

When negotiating, beware of false deadlines, misrepresentations, and unfounded assumptions. Arguing politely over what works best and over legal and business terms is a common business practice that can lead to a much better structure for all involved parties. Don't ever believe that "this is our contract and it is nonnegotiable." Don't do business with anyone who tries to foist that type of arrangement on you.

**How can you protect your practice from auto accidents liability**

If you drive a vehicle that you lease through your practice, but it is insured on your personal auto-insurance policy, what happens if you get into an accident and you are sued. Can the law suit involve your practice?

A business owners' insurance policy written for a physician's practice often contains protection for vehicles rented on practice business and the so called "non-owned" autos (employees driving their own vehicles while on practice business). The practice-lease arrangement, however, makes a vehicle an "owned" auto under insurance policy definitions, negating coverage under the business owners' policy. However, there are ways to protect your practice from liability related to auto accidents and here are some examples:

A. If your insurance carrier allows it, add your practice entity as an "additional insured" on your personal automobile policy. If you choose this option, make sure your personal policy has enough coverage to support both your exposure and the exposure of the practice in the event of an accident. Keep in mind that a practice entity with significant assets or receivables creates a deep pocket for a plaintiff's attorney, and that sharing your coverage may mean less protection for you personally.

Your practice still may be liable in the event of an accident while you (or any other employee of the practice) are traveling on practice business. As long as such accidents occur with a "non-owned" vehicle, however, your practice will be protected by its business owners' policy.

**Branding, How to apply it to your practice?**

*What is a brand?*

The first steps in aligning employees with the practice brand is conveying to them what the brand really means, Most health care facilities have an opportunity to help staff understand the brand and what it means in very concrete ways. So if a medical practice says that extraordinary care is its key brand attribute, what does this mean in terms of a day-to-day perspective to the employees? What actions will employees exhibit to reflect this brand and how they will communicate it to patients and their families? Also, a brand should be broken down into very real and manageable terms for practice staff. To say you provide extraordinary care or exceptional service or you are patient-focused doesn't mean a whole lot to staff unless they can see it in what they do day to day.

Employees can play an important role in making the brand "real" to the patients and family members they encounter every day. They have, in addition, the opportunity to play an important brand ambassador role as they interact with people in their personal lives—friends, family, neighbors. You want employees to advocate for the practice and its services, but you also want employees to advocate for the patients. If you trust your employees and allow them to be your ambassadors, that can do a whole lot for the brand. Knowing employees' role in branding gives you the opportunity to understand what the key access and service differentiators are for a good brand.

**The process:**

Arguably the greatest impact in any service organization such as a health care facility, comes through interactions that patients, their family members, and others have with your staff. The Staff include the receptionist (who is the face of your practice), the office manager, the nursing staff, and of course you the physician. Branding a medical practice (a clinic) or a health care facility is more complex than branding a tangible product such as a car, a computer, or any other product. For a practice, branding may be affected by factors that may seem innocuous such as the tone of voice of the receptionist answering the phone, comfort of the chairs in the waiting room, the presence of a flat screen television in the waiting area, the programs that are played on the television, the color of the office's walls and carpet or hardwood floors. Many marketers focus on how they convey their brands through communication vehicles such as television advertisements, Internet Web sites or billboards using the company's logos and other materials. However, for a brand to become popular and endure, it must be understood easily, internalized, and acted on by employees at all levels so that the practice or the health care facility lives up to expectations of the patients and their families.

**Reinforcing and protecting a brand:**

Once a brand identity has been established, physicians must ensure that brand is reinforced by all members of the practice. The role of the employee is critical. Employees have to understand and accept the brand identity. Every employee who interacts with patients has a potential impact. Those employees who do not interact directly with patients may interact with friends, family, and community members. Therefore, employee must be involved in the process of protecting the brand on a regular basis. If they are not brought in, then they may be sending subtle messages that conflict with what you are trying to accomplish. In a medical practice a lot of communication happens between employees and patients in the examination room, before the physician goes in there, therefore, it is important for everyone on the team to be on board and understand what the physician is trying to accomplish and why. Even the look of employees can have an impact on your brand. If you yourself, the physician, and one or more of your staff are physically unfit or overweight, then patients who are overweight are less likely to come to your office, especially with issue related to obesity. Attitude of the staff also comes into play. If potential patients call and are greeted with someone with an annoyed tone of voice and a big sigh, it does not send a good message to reinforce your message. All of these issues need to be considered in developing a strong brand, beginning with hiring and continuing through training and establishing expectations for employees and their interactions with patients.

How to create and maintain a strong brand identity:

*Constant positive reminder:* which involves efforts to provide your employees with daily reminders of your brand promise. Tactics might range from distributing culture cards for employees to keep in their wallets for easy reference, to making culture a key aspect of new employee orientation.

*Addressing key barriers to communications:* which might include communications from the physician leader to reinforce key messages, hosting practice-wide "culture days," or finding ways to recognize brand ambassadors and their stories e.g. recognition as employee of the month.

*Training and Education:* Training and education are important to the process of ensuring that employees can serve effectively as brand ambassadors. The most successful companies are those that have the best brand ambassadors and where training is built into the culture. You should provide your employees with the necessary tools they need to do the best they can on a regular basis. Strengthening the brand through your employees requires engagement and buy-in. It can be a team effort that creates excitement. If staff members understand why, and that they are part of that process, then they know they're being dealt with more respectfully and they're more likely to come along with the vision. Thinking about the desired brand image and how to support it through training of employee and their positive interaction with patients before new patients start to call can transform a practice or a health care system into a competitive and successful brand name.

**Your office Manager:**

Among other reasons to have an office manager for your practice is to have a person that your staff, patients and their families can go to if they have issues or complaints they would like to address. In some respect it may diffuse some issues and/or divulge them from you to someone else, so that you can focus your attention on patient care. However, we are not suggesting that you abdicate your leadership entirely to an office manager, because if you do, you are likely to run into problems with and in your practice. The problem is that not all mangers are created equally. The question you should ask your self is "Do I need an office manager?". You can have good office management without a manager and bad office management with a manager. You can have a good manager under bad management, but it is far rarer to have a bad manager under good management. Often, when we find a bad manager, we also find physician leadership that has abdicated management responsibility.

If you do decide that you need an office manager, it is important you understand the roles of an office manager and that you define these roles clearly from the outset. Here are some of the duties of an office manager:

**A source of information about your practice:**

An office manager is commonly the collector and the custodian of your office's information and you should be able to turn to him/her for data (financial or otherwise) about your practice. He or she should understand how to gather and transmits information between outsiders (hospitals, insurance companies) to the staff, and physician leaders in the practice. She/he should also be knowledgeable in policies and procedures that would meet state and regulatory requirements such as the Health Insurance Portability and Accountability Act, the Occupational Safety and Health Administration, Medicare and Medicaid, managed care organizations, and labor laws. She/he can also organize files and retrieves the practice's clinical and nonclinical data and personnel records.

**Managing relationships:**

An office manager could play as an intermediary with the people in your office and your practice. She/he should be able to manage and support relationships with patients, your staff, hospital staff, vendors, advisers, outside services, and colleagues. He/she should act as a symbolic figurehead liaison and a leader, whether he or she has been granted any real authority. The office manager should inspire staff members to do what is necessary to please both patients and providers with great performance, and to look for ways to improve this relationship.

**A decision maker:** Office managers make and implement decisions so the physicians do not have to. Many office managers have responsibility for finding, hiring, training, and firing staff and vendors. They might decide where and when to recruit new providers. They handle disturbances and crisis with staff and patients and between providers. Office managers also allocate resources, decide staff schedules and vacations, and may decide whether a practice can afford a new device or equipment. Some office managers may also have entrepreneurial authority to negotiate leases, contracts, and add ancillary services. They commonly decide agendas and lead meetings. A great office manager may be able to make decisions that affect the business-health of the practice.

**Billing collection:**

One of the primary duties of an office manager is billing and collections, and perhaps staff scheduling. If accounts receivable are high, accounts payable are late, staff members are unhappy and turnover or attrition rate are high, patient visits frequently run late, and the office manager's office and desk are covered with piles and piles of papers, then you should come to the conclusion that the office manager is not managing and perhaps you the physician are not managing your office manager well. This should be a red alarm to you, because one of the biggest costs in a medical practice business (and in any other business) is employee incompetence. When the incompetence is related to the management skills of both the owners and the office manager, the result can be economically disastrous. This should be a wake-up call for you.

So, if you do decide to have an office manager and next time you hear someone in your office saying "I want to speak to the manager", which is often a prelude to escalating a complaint, you will, hopefully can refer them to your office manager and you continue to focus on patient care. However, you need to continuously evaluate whether your office manager is performing her/his duties, other why have one in the first place. We are saying this because many practices, especially smaller practices, often face administrative difficulties even though they have an office manager. This is because in these practices the office manager either has been working in that office for a long time and therefore, has be granted that position based on "seniority", or the office manager is the wife of one of the senior physicians and does not perform any of the essential functions discussed above. One of the worst situations for a practice to be in is when a physician opens a new practice and he/she employs his/her spouse as the office manager, with neither having private practice, medical office, or management experience. Remember that management is a complex, but a learned skill, just as is medicine. If the manager does not have the training or the experience, management is likely to fail.

*What is the solution?*

If you have a small practice of let us say 1-3 physicians and each one of you are willing to participate in the management and decision making of the office, then you probably do not need an office manager. These practices are small enough, and simple enough, that the physicians should be the managers executing management duties. Either one physician can be the managing physician (and be compensated for it) or management duties can be officially divided among the physicians. For example, one physician handles finances and statistics; another, staffing; and a third, systems and vendors. If a practice has more than five staff members, instead of an office manager, there can be "team leaders," typically divided into "front and back" or "reception and medical assistant" teams. A practice can avoid many of the problems of the "sort-of-office-manager" by officially placing management duties as the responsibilities of the physicians.

In those small practices, not having an office manager also can result in lower overhead. A recent study found that employees with the title of office manager are paid one-and-a-half to twice as much as a receptionist or medical assistant. This should not dissuade you from hiring an office manager if you believe that your practice really needs a good office manager with clearly defined responsibilities. Adding an office manager does not mean giving your best employee a title and dumping management on him or her (that is, "bump and dump"—yes, this error is common enough to even have a name!). You can't expect him or her to add administrative duties to an existing work schedule and continue to perform well at the current job. Often this leaves the doctors disappointed and the employee frustrated. However, with proper training, mentorship, and support to learn and develop management skills, it is possible that your favorite employee could be a good office manager—but not overnight. It is also likely that he or she would suffer the envy of other staff and not have the authority with the owners as would an experienced new employee. This is one reason practice management consultants often have more success than do your own staff members or spouse in getting you and your staff to change behavior. The sociological and authoritative relationship is different.

Some practices try to overcome the office manager issue by leasing staff. However, most consultants find that poor physician management is not overcome by leasing staff; it frequently results in significantly increasing labor costs.

**Quality Improvement, A constant process:**

There is a fairly simple technique to manage a small practice with or without an office manager. As a group, the physicians and staff meet for an hour, once a week, to discuss practice issues. One person acts as a scribe.

At the first meeting, everyone suggests as many questions needing answers, problems experienced, and ideas about practice improvement as possible, without critique or further discussion or analysis, until all questions and ideas are exhausted. The scribe lists all these points on wall charts or posters (pads of self-adhesive posters are convenient) that will be brought to subsequent meetings. The group then prioritizes the topics for discussion, then discusses the issues in order, and memorializes the outcomes to a practice "operations manual." The prioritization step is critical; otherwise, discussion is easily sidetracked.

At every subsequent meeting, attendees report on results of the last meeting, add new points to the discussion list, prioritize the discussion, and then proceed with discussion. The result is that over a period of time, the practice adopts a management process known as "continuous quality improvement." The operations manual becomes a valuable resource on which staff members can rely for management decisions and as a training tool for new staff so that the intellectual properties of the practice are not lost due to staff turnover.

**Should you open your own pharmacy in your practice?**

In general, pharmacies are marginally profitable, but the upside is that they're a great convenience for your patients. The big advantage of having a pharmacy in or near your office is that it substantially increases your patients' medication adherence because they are more likely to have prescriptions filled right there in front of you. It also reduces the need to offer samples. From a legal standpoint, the real question is whether you intend to open a retail pharmacy in which anyone can walk in, or a dispensing pharmacy in which you provide drugs only to patients whom you are treating. That's an important distinction, because most states allow the latter but some do not allow the former. Then, there are issues in getting recognized by pharmacy benefit managers, which are companies hired by health plans to manage subscribers' pharmacy benefits. Additionally, there will be regulatory issues under state law, so check with your state medical society. Finally, if a physician is dispensing controlled substances, there are additional legal issues.

**Should you Incorporate?**

Business owners including physicians who own a medical practice often elect to incorporate their practice(s) because it may provide tax advantages and it may also limit their personal liability exposure. From a liability standpoint, the total liability may be limited to the assets of the corporation (as opposed to the entire assets of a physician) and from the a tax standpoint, incorporation may allow the physician to decide how to distribute the profits made by a practice more efficiently and more flexibility with retirement options so that the total amount of money that is tax-sheltered is maximized. However, you as a physician/businessman or woman, you need to understand that there are different types of Corporations, each with its own legal and tax consequences. An examples of the type of Corporation that you need to be familiar with as a physician is the so called "personal service corporation (PSC)". You need to know about this because under some circumstances, the Internal Revenue Service (IRS) *has the right* to designate your incorporated practice as a PSC, which would mean that you could be taxed at a higher rate than other forms of corporations.

## How did PSCs come into being?

A Personal Service Corporation (PSC) is a type of corporation for which the main activity is the performance of personal services, typically by employee-owners. PSCs are a subcategory of professional corporations, which are corporations formed for the purpose of engaging in a licensed profession. All PSCs are professional corporations, but not every professional corporation is a PSC.

Professional corporations began at a time when physicians, attorneys, accountants, therapists and other licensed professionals operated almost exclusively as sole proprietorships or partnerships, and they were taxed at a higher rate than corporations.

To rectify that, Congress and the IRS began allowing professionals to incorporate and thereby enjoy the same tax advantages as corporations, although without the benefit of a corporation's limited liability.

The lines between the different forms of business organizations have blurred in recent years, however, as more tax advantages have become available to sole proprietorships and partnerships and more liability protection has been granted to professional corporations.

As greater numbers of professionals incorporated for the sole purpose of sheltering income, Congress subsequently reduced the incentive to incorporate as "qualified professional services corporations" and taxing them at a flat rate of 35%.

## What is the difference between Corporation and PSC?

As we indicated above, every PSC is a professional corporation, but not every professional corporation is a PSC.

According to the IRS's rules, for a business to be considered a PSC it must be organized under state law and then pass two federal tests: the function test and the ownership test. The function test requires that substantially all (95%) of the business activities of the corporation involve services within specific occupations in the fields of health, law, engineering, accounting, actuarial science, consulting, or performing arts.

The ownership test requires that substantially all the professional corporation's outstanding stock be held directly or indirectly by qualified people, defined as either (1) employees who are currently performing professional services for the corporation; (2) retired employees who did so prior to their retirement; (3) their heirs or estates.

Thus, for example, if a doctor has non-medical business activities under his or her practice's corporate umbrella, such that less than 95% of the corporation's activities are related to medicine, the corporation is not considered a PSC. A professional corporation organized under state law that does not qualify as a PSC is treated as a general partnership for federal tax purposes.

### So, What? What are the tax consequences of being a PSC?

PSCs are taxed like regular "C" corporations but, as noted previously, at a flat 35% rate rather than at a graduated rate, depending on the level of income earned.

What do you mean by a graduated rate? US taxation is a graduated tax system with different tax brackets. What that means is that if you earn $200,000.00, you are taxed at a rate of 10% for the first $ 8500.00, 15% for your income between $8500.00 to $ 34,000.00, 25% on your income between $34000,-83000.00, 28% on your income between $83000 - $174,000.00, and 33% on the balance of your income.

The PSC files a corporate tax return and issues a form K-1 to all shareholder/employees to show their individual shares of the corporation's profit or loss. Any income retained in the PSC is subject to the corporate tax rate, whereas any salaries paid to employees are considered tax-deductible business expenses.

Like most small corporations, PSCs are likely to pay out all income earned by the business to shareholders in the form of salaries, bonuses, and fringe benefits, thus reducing corporate taxable income to $0. Of course, the shareholder/employees still must pay personal income taxes on the income they receive

**What are some of the nonfinancial benefits?**

In spite of the punitive rules and flat tax rate, the use of the PSC remains popular, often for non-financial reasons. For example, physicians may find protection from certain kinds of vicarious liability. Also on the plus side, organizing as a PSC includes tax benefits and transferability of ownership. A PSC also is subject to special tax rules, including the ability to use the far-easier cash method of accounting.

From a financial perspective, one of the main advantages of incorporation is that it permits the closely held medical practice to distribute among family members—in the form of salaries, fringe benefits, and dividends—the income earned by the principal shareholder of the corporation, or to retain such earnings in the corporation. In addition, incorporation may allow the physician to establish substantially more generous retirement plans (far more than the allowable amount of $16,500.00 per year as of 2011) and other fringe benefits for herself or himself.

**What are some of the disadvantages of a PSC?**

As discussed above, the principal disadvantage of PSCs stems from the flat corporate tax rate, which can be as high as 35% as of 2011. Retaining earnings within the medical practice rarely will make sense due to the higher tax bracket, and this higher bracket may reduce the practice's flexibility in distributing income to shareholder/employees. Also, if dividends are not paid regularly and earnings are retained, they could become subject to the tax on accumulated earnings. To the contrary, most regular corporations can "split income"—adjust the amount paid out to shareholder/employees—so that both the practice and the individual can gain the most favorable tax bracket possible.

## RISK OF DOUBLE TAXATION

Finally, professional corporation shareholders may face the problem of double taxation upon liquidation of the practice. Income from the sale of real estate or equipment might accrue to the practice, where it would be taxed at the corporate rate.

If this income then were distributed to shareholders as dividends (because the practice was no longer in business and thus could not pay it out as salaries and benefits to employees), then it would be subject to taxation again as personal income.

## GROUP PRACTICES

Physicians in group practices often are concerned about liability exposure for the malpractice of their co-owners. Although a PSC, limited liability company (LLC), or S corporation may shield a physician's personal assets, the assets inside the group still are at risk. For this and other reasons, physicians often form multiple personal service corporations when practicing as part of a group.

Generally, each individual forms a separate PSC in which the individual physician owns 100% of the stock in a practice-wide PSC. The practice then organizes as a firm under one of the following methods:

1.  Each physician owns stocks in an S corporation, and in turn the corporation contracts with the separate PSCs for professional services.
2.  Each PSC owns a partnership interest in a practice which is organized as a partnership
3.  Or Each PSC is a member of a bigger practice organized as an Limited Liability Corporation or LLC.

## PROFESSIONAL ADVICE IS IMPORTANT!

If you're thinking of incorporating, it is important to seek the advice of experienced attorneys and accountants. They can help you decide whether to incorporate as a PSC or some other form of corporation, and if the latter, how to structure your corporation to meet the function and ownership tests and avoid subsequently being designated a PSC.

Incorporation can bring many benefits to a medical practice. Just remember—the IRS is watching, and if the IRS designate you as a PSC it could mean a big jump in your tax bill.

### Make cash flow analysis part of your financial plan

The IRS-imposed limits on tax-deferred retirement plan contributions ($16,500.00 per year if you are employed, and 25% of your net income up to $ 40,000.00 per year if you are self-employed as of 2011) may not be adequate to enable you to reach your retirement savings goals. Additional savings may be necessary to enable you to maintain your standard of living during retirement years. A comprehensive financial plan is essential to attaining this goal, and cash flow planning and analysis are key to making such a plan work.

Do not confuse cash flow analysis with budgeting. Budget implies keeping various spending categories within pre-specified levels, whereas cash flow analysis is a detailed delineation of household expenditures and income, usually done on a monthly basis.

## CASH INFLOWS AND OUTFLOWS

Categories and sources of cash inflows might include salary, bonuses, investment income, self-employment income, royalties, and child support. Knowing the various categories, and how much comes from each, can help you plan for a change in financial circumstance.

Such information also is useful in tax planning. For example, there may be years when it would be better from a tax standpoint to defer a bonus into the following year.

Similarly, it is essential to identify categories of cash outflows. These categories might include debt service, living expenses, itemized deductions, insurance expenses, retirement contributions, savings or investments, taxes as well as the detailed expenses within each category.

## DISTINGUISHING BETWEEN OUTFLOW AND EXPENSES

Identifying outflows in this manner helps distinguish between household expenses and outflows. Taxes, retirement contributions, and savings/investments are considered cash outflows rather than household expenses.

A cash flow analysis, in short, separates household expenses from other outflows. Performing this kind of analysis is helpful to the process of planning discretionary spending and forecasting retirement spending needs.

In the absence of a concrete financial plan, the excess cash inflows that are not needed to support necessary expenses such as mortgage payment or rent, utilities, food, insurance premiums, and taxes can be spent on vacations, recreation, renovations, clothes, and luxury items. On the other hand, implementing a comprehensive financial plan quantifies long-term goals so that you can determine the levels of savings required to support such goals, including and, most commonly, college savings and retirement savings.

## IDENTIFYING SAVINGS REQUIREMENTS

The financial planning process helps identify the annual savings requirements for each goal, and a thorough cash flow analysis will identify the availability of sufficient cash surpluses to support these savings requirements so that you have adequate funds available to reach these milestones.

Physicians, especially early in their career, often believe that they do not have enough money left over at the end of the day to contribute to college or retirement savings accounts. A detailed cash flow analysis will help you find areas where you might reallocate spending to reach these and other long-term goals.

## AVOID COMPROMISING FUTURE GOALS

You may also covert any cash that might be available beyond what you need to support long-term goals to discretionary spending items that can enhance your current lifestyle, knowing that in doing so you are not compromising future goals.

If you are able to identify and quantify your lifestyle goals, then you can allocate the cash resources toward them so that, if properly managed over time, you attain your goals and have a peace of mind.

**Resources available to you as a provider (physician) to help contract with Insurance companies so that you can increase your pool of potential patients:**

1. National Society of Certified Business Consultants (http://nschbc.org).
2. Healthcare Billing and Management Association (http://www.hbma.org)

## Other patterns of practicing Medicine:

## Working as a locum tenens

*What is locum tenens?*

Locum tenens refers to the process by which physicians work for a hospital or a clinic on a temporary short-term basis often to cover the practice of a physician or substitute for a specialist in a hospital setting where the full-time physician is on vacation, attending a medical conference or a leave of absence for health reasons, or family reasons.. etc. In fact "locum tenens" is a Latin phrase, which means "to substitute for". In the US many physicians work as locum tenens providing services to hospitals and clinics on a temporary basis.

*Is locum tenens a good choice for you?*

If you are not sure what you would like to do or where you want to work after completing your residency or Fellowship, one option you have is to work as a locum tenens. Half of health care providers surveyed in a locum tenens survey stated that the main reason for choosing to work as a locum tenens is the flexibility in the schedule. Indeed when you are a locum tenens provider, you can choose which days of the month you are available to work and which location you would like to work. Other reasons for providing locum tenens service is the opportunity to travel to various cities and states, having some extra income and gaining clinical experience because as a locum tenens provider you will work under different circumstances in different locations. Working in different locations may also provide you the opportunity to become familiar with certain geographic locations, practice settings, income levels, administrative issues and therefore, it is a way to help you decide where you would like to settle and practice on a permanent basis in the future.

Why do hospitals and clinics use locum tenens?

Physicians and other healthcare providers who are employed full-time or own a practice need to take time off every now and then for vacations, health issues, or family issues. During these periods it is important patient care continues. Instead of hiring more full-time physicians that may be necessary for most the years, they hire locum tenens to provide health care for short periods of time such 1-2 weeks.

How do I find locum tenens positions?

Often, you will have to contract with a locum tenens agency; an agency that connect physicians with hospitals or clinics for this purpose. Occasionally, you may be able to find a position through word of mouth.

How much do they pay?

Usually they pay well. Payments are either on hourly or daily basis. In addition the locum tenens company or their clients (hospitals or clinics) pay for the airfare, accommodation, and car rental expenses. A survey of locum tenens anesthesiologists for 2007-2009 showed annual income in the $ 350 thousand range. One advantage of working as a locum tenens is you are considered an independent contractor, what does that mean? That means you will get a 1099 (and not W2) at the end of the year. Remember 1099 income is more tax efficient because you can write off all your expenses and therefore, you are taxed on your adjusted income i.e. gross income – expenses. Therefore, if you are smart (but legal) with your taxes you net income could be higher.

**Social Security Benefits? When it starts? How much do I get? Is it going to be available when I retire?**

If you are an employed physician and you receive A W-2 form at the end of each year, and you will notice on your biweekly pay stubs that a certain amount is paid to Social Security Administration. You will notice the same thing on your bi-weekly pay stub when you are a resident. As of 2010, 6.2% of the first $ 106,800.00 of each employee's taxable income goes to social security. Any earning in excess of that amount is not subject to social security taxes. So, if your annual income is $ 250,000.00 (very realistic for a physician) or $ 400,000.00, you will pay a total of $ 6621.60 per taxes social security taxes. Because there is a cap on the total amount of taxes you pay to social security every years, there is also a cap on the total monthly payment that you will receive when you reach the retirement age. As of 2010 this monthly payment is capped at approximately $ 1850.00 per month.

In addition 1.45% of your income goes to Medicare and there is no cap on income with Medicare taxes. Employers have to match both social security and Medicare taxes, in other words employers must pay 12.4% + 2.9% of each employee's income to the government every year. So if you decide to have your own practice after completing your residency and you will certainly have employee that is the % that you will have to remit to social security and Medicare every year.

After you work for at least 10 years and you have paid social security and Medicare taxes for at least 10 years you have earned enough credits to qualify for social security and Medicare when you retire. Social security calculates your benefits at the time of the time of your retirement based on best 10 years in terms of income. After you have worked for at least 10 years you should receive an annual statement from Social Security Administration stating that you have earned enough credit to qualify for benefits and it will also states your benefits at the time of retirement and in case disability. If you believe that you have worked for at least 10 years and you have paid taxes during those

10 years, but you have not received a statement from Social Security Administration you may want to contact them. As of 2010, it is projected that Social Security benefits will be available until year 2045.

*I got divorced from first husband of 15 years who had significantly lower income than me, but I am remarried now, will my ex-husband be eligible for spousal social security?*

Your ex-husband can collect Social Security spousal benefits as long as you were married for at least 10 years, he is now unmarried, he is 62 years old or older (as of 2010), and the benefits he is entitled to receive on his own work record are less than the benefits he is receiving based on your work record. The amount of benefits your divorced spouse receives has no effect on the level of benefits you or a future spouse may receive.

### What is on the horizon for Social Security Benefits?

As of July 2011, Lawmakers were considering changes to how Social Security is adjusted for inflation. Ordinarily, when inflation rises, retirees' social security checks keep pace with small increases. But if some lawmakers get their way, those raises may be a whole lot smaller in the future.

In 2011, there has been intense ongoing debate between the Republicans and the Democrats about the current US deficit (which is approximately 98% of GDP for the US, the lowest of any industrialized nation). As part of this deficit-reduction talks, White House officials and Congressional leaders on both sides of the aisle are advocating changes to the way inflation is calculated when it comes to Social Security Benefits. What is being proposed is measure inflation with the consumer price index, a metric that would likely make inflation look slower than the current measurement does. That would result in smaller Social Security increases for seniors and may negatively impact seniors and their family members who help them out financially.

It is estimated that 60% of seniors rely on Social Security for at least half of their retirement income. Under the new calculation, the rate of inflation would grow at an average annual rate of about 0.3% less, on average, than under the current calculations, according to the Congressional Budget Office. If Social Security uses the new measurement to determine cost-of-living adjustments, the average retiree would receive about $18,000 less in benefits over 25 years, according to The Senior Citizens League. Or, under the new calculations, after 10 years, a 73-year-old would get a check that's about 3% smaller than he would get under the old calculations, according to the Congressional Budget Office. This would be (hopefully) should not be a major problem for a high earner such as you (a physician), but it may affect some of your family members or your parents who are less fortunate than you and have limited resources. It may affect you indirectly however, if you are supporting a family member because lower benefits are part of the point. As of 2011, using the slower-rising index is being billed by many including President Obama's fiscal responsibility commission and the Bipartisan Policy Center, as a way to generate much-needed savings to help deal with the country's mounting debt crisis. Their argument is that this plan will results in an estimated $112 billion over 10 years.

The critics state that the new proposal only makes a bad system worse. The current measurement of inflation is supposed to account for the spending habits of adults of all ages, including only a small proportion of retirees, however, it doesn't reflect the true inflation seniors face. For example, many older people spend a large share of their budgets on items like health care, whose prices have risen about twice as fast as overall prices, according to a 2010 paper published by the Congressional Research Service.

To be sure, almost everyone agrees that the current Social Security system is unsustainable, and the current debate over the deficit has turned up the pressure. Social Security has become a target partially because of the significant cost of the program. In 2011, the government will pay out an estimated $600 billion in Social Security, survivor's benefits and related expenditures; this number is projected to rise to more than $1 trillion in 2020, according to a report from the Social Security Administration.

Whether the new measurement will be adopted remains unclear. Some experts think at least some Social Security cuts will go through, at least in part because President Obama has warned that unless an agreement on the current debate to extend the United States' borrowing limits is reached, Social Security benefits cannot be guaranteed starting on Aug. 3. For some retirees, the proposed switch could mean more belt-tightening. For pre-retirees, it could mean saving more earlier to make up for lower benefits. On top of that, it would become more important to protect a retirement portfolio from inflation hikes, experts say. That includes considering investments that rise or keep pace with inflation, such as dividend-paying stocks, Treasury Inflation-Protected Securities, or floating-rate loan funds (see the section on financial aspects of being a physician) and avoiding low-yielding certificates of deposit, which are likely to lead to less buying power for a senior citizen in retirement.

### I qualify to receive Social Security benefits at 62 next year, should I delay receiving it?

As of 2011, the age for receiving social security benefits is 62. If you have other sources of income that will maintain a standard of living that you would like to maintain, then it is not a bad idea to delay receiving social security benefits, because the longer you delay it the more will be your monthly benefits (pay check). This is will beneficial to you if you are healthy and you are expected to live for the next 20 years as it will ensure that when you stop working you will receive a bigger check every month. On the other hand if you have health issues and you are not expecting to live for the next 20 to 25 years then it is probably not a good idea to delay receiving social security benefits.

### The "fiscal Cliff " of 2012 and Social Security:

Following the presidential election in November 2012 the discussion about the so called "fiscal cliff" negotiations was revived by the two major political parties in the US. A major point of argument between the Republicans and Democrats was around Social Security benefits as one of the major component of what some call "entitlement programs". In a poll conducted by Pew Research Center in 2012, about 50% of the Americans believe it's not likely there will be enough money in Social Security and Medicare to maintain current benefit levels into the future. Under current government estimates, Social Security could face funding shortfalls in approximately two decades if the revenues and the payouts from the Social Security remain the way they are now, simply because the aging U.S. population is living longer compared to when this program was first established in the 1960s when the life expectancy for the US population was shorter. That sounds like a disheartening scenario for workers who are currently paying into social security and worry that they won't get as much out of it once they retire. However, "experts" say that there are ways to fix Social Security and that there are politicians in the US Senate and US house of representative who could work together and come to an agreement because this has been done before. In the mid-1980s, then President Ronald Reagan, worked with Democrats in Congress to oversee an overhaul of the nation's retirement safety net. Experts say there are two ways to fix Social Security: increase revenue or reduce benefits; both of these options are perceived as painful to certain groups of politicians and their constituents.

## Increasing the revenue

Under the current rules, the maximum taxable earnings for Social Security (as of 2012) is about $110,000.Most physician's income exceeds that amount and therefore, they are taxed only on the first $ 110,000.00 of their income. If you are employed you will notice on your paystubs that your employer takes out money for Social Security for the first $ 110,000.00, after that amount this deduction stops. Some argue that an easy fix would be to simply raise the cap on Social Security taxes to include higher wages. For example one proposal is to raise the cap to $ 200,000.00 since the income of people in this range has gone up and there has been growth in wealth in the top income scale. However, others say it is unlikely that politicians will propose raising taxes on high earners now, when many expect those taxpayers to already see increases as part of the fiscal cliff negotiations.

Another option would be to add an across-the-board increase in payroll taxes that go toward Social Security. Although that would help solve the system's future funding woes, experts say it's also likely to be a hard sell in these tough times because Americans may already be facing higher payroll taxes in 2013. For the past two years (as of the end of 2012), Americans have enjoyed a payroll tax holiday that reduced the amount of money they paid toward Social Security, but that could end in the coming year.

Politicians may be nervous about proposing any reform to Social Security that costs more or results in fewer benefits, but Americans seem to accept that some changes are needed. For example, in the Pew poll we referred to above, 2/3 of Americans polled also said they would support raising payroll taxes on high-income earners, while about half of them said they would support reducing benefits for high-income seniors.

Just 38 percent said they'd support raising the eligibility age for Social Security Benefits.

## Reducing Benefits

One of the few parts of the fiscal cliff negotiations (as of the end of 2012) that President Barack Obama (the sitting president for the period 2012-2016) and House Speaker John Boehner (Republican) seem willing to compromise on involves a change in the way Social Security increases are calculated going forward.

The proposed switch to calculating cost of living increases using the chained Consumer Price Index (reflects how expensive things are) instead of the current method would result in smaller annual Social Security raises. That's because that method assumes that people change their spending habits when prices go up.

Proponents say the switch could save billions of dollars and is a more realistic method of how Americans really adjust to rising cost of living..

But opponents say the chained consumer price index is not a good way to measure the needs of older and disabled Americans, because their expenditures are disproportionately focused on things like health care and medications. Families may adjust what they eat if the price of certain food items goes up, but families who need health care and medications for certain medical problems cannot make adjustments. One of the longer-term options for reducing benefits is to simply tell people they have to wait longer to get their full benefits. By extending the age at which you can get full benefits, proponents argue that Social Security would be keeping up with trends toward longer life expectancies, but opponents, say that a closer look at the data show that the bulk of improvements in life expectancies have come from wealthier Americans. They say a broad-based increase in the age at which people can get benefits would punish less wealthy Americans, who haven't seen such big life expectancy gains.

Another suggestion has been to decrease benefits for middle- and high-income individuals (such as physicians) while maintaining the current system for the poorest Americans. Proponents of this argument say that if wealthy people are told to expect less Social Security, they have more leeway to prepare for it than poor people. Physicians for example may say if you cut my Social Security benefits I'm going to react by saving money and working longer, one expert said, "That's good for the economy." Other options that have been brought up include reducing Social Security benefits available to spouses. Some critics argue that's growing outdated now that more women work and earn their own Social Security payments. So, stay tuned for the ongoing debate on Social Security Benefits.

## Marriage

**Marriage:** If you are already married, we wish you the best. If you are not and you are contemplating marriage, recognize that marriage is a constant work, it is not an easy task, and another full-time job. When married, the two of you need to be patient with each other, appreciate each other, help each other out and when differences and conflicts arise try to resolve them peacefully. Going through residency is very stressful for the marriage, duty hours are long, and the work and training is stressful. Your spouse needs to know that ahead of your start date and he/she needs to be understanding and supportive. You will have to learn how live on a budget since the resources are limited. This leads us the first step in the marriage process, the wedding.

**The wedding:**

Most people will have some sort of a ceremony "The wedding" day. There is probably no other situation in life where love, money, and family converge to create an intense hurricane, which sweeps away the common sense. This can lead people to spend an exuberant amount of time and money for a wedding. The fact is that there is an industry out there which profits considerably from this process. This industry profits from your (and your spouse-to-be) fantasies, dreams, and expectations and therefore, it is in the best interest of this industry to take advantage of these dreams and fantasies in a way that tilts the (financial) scale in their favor. Just to give you an idea the cost of American weddings currently average between $27,000.00 – $35,000.00 and it is estimated that in 2011, approximately $23 billion will be spent on weddings. In addition another $ 20 billion will be spent on gifts related to the wedding and the events leading to it and approximately $ 8 billion on travel and other expenses related to honey moons.

It may be true that as a health care provider you are a high-earner and you can probably afford all that money, but it is realistic for you to understand that researchers in this field have demonstrated that the expenses associated with wedding is one of the most manipulated processes. This manipulation is based on an inelastic demand function. Wedding planners and vendors bet on your expectation that this is the only time you'll do this in your life and they price your wedding accordingly. Therefore, here are some tips that you may want to follow as you make your way through this hurricane:

*First comes first "The ring":*

Obviously, before you pop the question you will have months if not years to think about the most important element that follows the question "Will you marry me?", the RING!

*What do you need to know about the engagement ring?*

The first step of the many financial commitments that you will embark on is the ring. This is a large and rare financial transaction that you will have to make wisely and you should do your best to avoid scams. You may want to brush up on your knowledge about diamonds and rings. If you have a trusted friend who is a woman or a sister, they could be a good resource for you. Your mother could be a great resource too, however, if you want to surprise everyone then you will have to do the home work on your own. So, you could head to the internet. There are various websites, but BlueNile.com is one of the most reputable one and the largest online retailers of engagement rings. You do not necessarily have to purchase a ring from this website, but the educational information that you can gain from this website is valuable and here is a breakdown of what you should look for in an engagement (diamond) ring:

Cut: refers to the cut of the diamond. This is the most important feature of the diamond in an engagement ring. The cut affects the degree of sparkles that emanate from a diamond ring. The better the cut, the more sparkly and the more amazing the diamond appears. To avoids scams have the seller put it in writing the quality of the diamond cut using a recognized and popular grading terms such as the GIA (The Gemological Institute of America) or the AGS (American Gem Society Laboratories). Other important features of the diamond in a wedding ring are: Color, Clarity, and Carats. The final feature decides the size of the ring: a 1.5 Carat ring is larger than a ¾ carat ring. Most people go for something around one carat.

*The Wedding Budget*

Having a budget for a wedding is as important a financial decision as buying a home, or car and so treat it that way. Your wedding budget needs to fit into the picture of your overall financial goals. Any time you're going to spend a large sum of money, assess if you are on the same page with tradeoffs. For example what else we could do with our lives instead of the money we put into this wedding? While we know wedding costs can spiral out of control, capping the budget is ultimately very doable. The most common budget pitfall is not talking or asking close family members such as your parents or older siblings.

**Getting married or you are already married, what does it mean to you?**

If you are not married yet and you plan on getting married in the future you need to know the following:

- From the financial point of view, marriage is a business part-nership. It does not matter if you are a physician (a high earner), but your spouse stays home and has no income. Assets that are accumulated during the marriage are joint property. Any assets that you brought to the marriage separately are usually yours to take away, but if you have been married to someone for a long time (usually 10 years or longer) the boundaries may become blurred. Therefore, if you still like to protect the assets that you have accumulated prior to marriage you may want to think about prenuptial agreement.
- If you put these separate assets into a joint account, they may be considered joint property
- Consider making a list of your assets, including bonds, stocks, mutual funds, pension plans, bank accounts, and pending tax refunds if you want them to remain your sole property.

*The Marriage Penalty*

Like we have discussed in other sections of this book, marriage is a combined financial entity as far as the government is concerned. As such, you and your spouse will face some income-tax adjustments. You can choose to file your taxes jointly or separately as a married cou-ple. Experts in this field suggest that almost always better to file jointly, unless it's an unusual situation such as the situation where one spouse has significantly higher medical expenses-more than 20-25 percent of their income-and the other has none. Or if you believe that your spouse is committing fraud – you wouldn't want to sign their return.

Whether you file jointly or separately, either way, you'll pay more taxes as a married person. In America it's cheaper-strictly from a tax code perspective- to be single. The "marriage penalty" originated in 1969, when Congress tried to eliminate what was then an advantage for couples.

As of 2011, the marriage penalty affects taxpayers who jointly earn $156,000 or more. The chart below compares what single-filers and married filers will pay this year.

*Should you keep Something Separate?*

You may not want to drop your own credit. You want to keep it separate and you should receive your own credit report.\ It is not uncommon that one spouse has troubles, and the other one does not have any troubles with her/his credit report or score. With separate accounts, your sweetheart's past credit history has no impact on your credit profile. Only when you open a joint account will information be shared on both credit reports – usually when you plan that first big purchase. For instance, if you buy a home together, your spouse's negative credit history could impact your mortgage rates. Work to improve it before you buy a high ticket item such as a house. As you can see it would helpful to have few meetings (before you get married) where you bring your credit report and score, tax returns and have an open discussion about the financial situations to avoid any unnecessary financial surprises.

# Divorce

Yes, Divorce. It is more common than you think. In some locals in the US, divorce rate is about 60-65% depending on the year. So it is a reality that may happen to anyone. You have worked hard over the years and have set aside a good size retirement account through your retirement account with your employer (called 401 K if your employer is a for-profit organization or 403b for non-for-profit organizations) or a self-employed retirement account (SEP IRA). Physicians are high-income earners and consequently their retirement accounts are larger than the average person. Here are some common questions that may come up with regard to your retirement account in case you do have to go through the painful process of divorce.

Any assets that you have accumulated in your retirement account (s) during the years you were marred is considered marital property. Yes, it is not all yours. Most employers do not require spousal consent for you to take some of that money out or borrow against it, but some do. By now you should (I hope so!) have asked your Human resources department at your place of the work about their rules regarding this issue.

When you get divorced, you will have to split the retirement account assets with your ex-spouse. If you are a physician and your spouse is not, chances are you are the main bread-winner and he/she is not. If you are the money maker in the marriage as soon as divorce papers are filed your spouse's attorney will file a motion with the courts ordering that your retirement account be flagged with your employer so that you cannot cash it out or borrow against it. Some employers will comply with that, others will have to comply with the court order.

How do you split the retirement assets? Your spouse or his/her lawyer will file an application (courts call it "a motion") called "qualified domestic-relations order or "QDRO", which is a decree or property settlement order under state law that assigns part of the retirement account (usually half of the total assets if you have been married for at least 10 years) to the spouse. A piece of good news here is that your spouse can cash out the retirement account assets without paying the 10% early withdrawal penalty. However, he/she will have to pay income tax on that money. If your spouse does not want to pay taxes, she/he may roll over the money into an individual retirement account under his/her name and have a full autonomy over the account in the future. The money is now his/hers.

## Other divorce Issues:

When most couples say "I do" during the wedding ceremony, they never imagine that their happily-ever-after could turn into a disaster that could end up costing a lot more than just heartbreak. For those potentially parting ways, there are some important pecuniary points to ponder.

*Litigate or Mediate?*

The actual costs of the divorce generally surprise most people. First there is the retention fee (the fee you have to pay an attorney or a law firm to accept to be your attorney). This is followed by bills for "services" they provide to you as you go through the divorce. The way attorneys operate is that once they know that you are a high-earner, they start to charge higher (higher end of fees for services) fees for all the "services" they provide and so the bills start accumulating. One of the authors knows colleagues who spent in excess of $ 100,000.00 going through divorce. Therefore, in order to cut costs some experts recommend mediation since it is a very cost effective way to resolve the divorce process. When couples pursue traditional litigation, two attorneys are paid to negotiate and then, possibly, go to trial. In mediation, a neutral third party works through decisions with the couple. With mediation the cost could be in the vicinity of $ 7000-10,000.00 in most states as opposed to $ 50,000- $100,000.00 with litigation. You can save even more money by careful planning before visiting your mediator.

For instance by going in to see the mediator prepared and having discussed how everything would be divided, you may be able to keep your visits to a minimum and at $350 an hour. On the other if you are not prepared you may spent $3,000 in legal fees if you as a couple spend your time fighting in an attorney's office over an issue that is worth $ 1000.00 or less. Think of the divorce as a business transaction and you will save a lot of time energy and money.

*Your current resident*

For most couples, the biggest asset they own jointly is a home. In most cases, either one person leaves or the property is sold to pay for new housing. That alone can make a big difference.

When you're married, there's one pot of money that pays for all your household expenses. When you divorce, the pot of money stays the same but suddenly must support two households. It is difficult or impossible to maintain your standard of living. For those who can't afford to maintain two residences, a new, albeit uncomfortable situation has arisen in which divorced couples are living together rather than suffer additional financial hardships.

The average expenses associated with divorce in the US can around $ 15,000.00 (but like we said above it got reach $ 100,000.00). A young couple with children wanting to divorce may not have the money to pay for it if they are still going through their residency or fellowship training. If you add to that the expenses associated with one of the partners moving out to get her/his own place the total cost could be considerable. That may be one of the reasons behind the phenomenon of couples staying together after the divorce. Of course this arrangement has its own drawbacks, but it has some advantages. For instance children can stay in the same residence and they may feel that things that are more stable. The housing collapse that occurred in 2008 and has continued until the writing of this book in 2011 may have contributed to this phenomenon too. Houses are either not selling or are not worth the amount a couple paid for it. therefore, rather than sell the house and take a considerable loss, come couples have decided that it is smarter to live in the same house and hold out for things to improve.

So, as you can see that it is way better if the two of you negotiate and work things out instead of having a bunch lawyers decide for you. Most of them are interested in how many hours they put in and charge you high fees for these hours. One of the authors was chatting with a man who came to his house to do some renovation in his house and the subject of divorce came up. He said he got divorced some 10 years ago. His name was Fred. So he started to talk about his divorce. He said I have told my ex-wife, "every time we disagree and fight over an issue, we pay the lawyers $ 5000.00", so it is cheaper to negotiate and reach a settlement with regard to property, cash, retirement accounts, the house, and the kids. Fred was a simple guy, but he was right about this issue. Fights between ex-spouses benefit only the lawyers.

Once you and you ex- reach an agreement on an issue either one of you can file a motion and go to the court representing yourselves. Most courthouses have a library next to them (the Law library) and the have very knowledgeable librarians who are very helpful in finding the correct forms, help you with instructions to fill them out and how to file them at the court. There are also websites that can help you with the process such as www.Divorce.com and www.DivorceOnline.com.

*There are also expensive necessities, like health care.*

Prior to the Patient Protection and Affordable Care Act, also known as the Health Care Reform Bill, signed into law March 23, 2010, many spouses who were dependent on their partner for healthcare coverage found themselves scrambling to find private health insurance following a divorce. While COBRA (Consolidate Omnibus Budget Reconciliation Act) is an option, it is usually very expensive and is only available for 36 months after the divorce is final.

Spouses with pre-existing conditions often have a very difficult time getting insured and if they do, costs can be substantial. The bill provides immediate access to insurance for those who are uninsured because of a pre-existing condition through a temporary high-risk pool, making healthcare coverage less of an issue in terms of divorce.

Another area of contention is who is going to pay for the healthcare of adult children of divorcees, who find themselves unemployed, back at home and uninsured. Effective September 2010, the PPACA requires that group health or individual plans continue to provide dependent coverage until 26 years of age, making it a bit less pricey for parents who are divvying up the costs of co-parenting.

*Other "small issues"*

Many couples are so focused on the obvious big-ticket items, they often forget about some of the smaller possessions they accumulated together in happier times. Things such as artwork, antiques, club memberships, season tickets and frequent flier miles are all considered marital property.

Hidden costs abound when it comes to divorce and can devour previous dollars. One little-discussed but very real expense is the cost of getting the children to and from each parent in shared custody situations. Make sure you document who is doing the dropping off and picking up the kids. With gas prices tipping $4 per gallon, the cost of shuttling children back and forth adds up quickly if you are still in your residency or fellowship.

Other covert costs include counseling for spouses as well as children and the additional expense of extended day care, should parents needs to increase their work days such as moonlighting to make ends meet.

*What is your exit plan?*

Coming up with a post-divorce financial plan is key. For some, a one-time settlement may have to last the rest of their lives. It is important to come up with a plan to figure out how to cut expenses while making the most of those resources. Divorce is really about managing risk both in terms of handling income from spousal or child support as well as dividing a portfolio of investments. When you have child or spousal support, these are very insecure forms of income and they change at any time depending on the financial situation of the parents. Another issue is illness and disability. Any parent can become disabled at any time. In fact the younger you are, you are more at risk for becoming disabled than you are for dying. So, make sure you adequate life and disability insurances that will cover expenses for your children until they grow up.

Investment accounts: which usually contain a blend of stocks, bonds and mutual funds should not just be divided by default. Even if the instruments might be valued equally, one party is usually less tolerant for risk and that should be taken into account when pulling apart a portfolio. Likewise, if one investment has a gain, while another has had a loss that should be distributed according to which party can best manage the tax consequences.

By going into divorce with eyes wide open, recognizing the costs and potential financial challenges that can occur, spouses can make smart financial decisions about how to proceed and plan for their single futures.

**Divorce check list:**

1.  Assets you owned before the marriage are usually yours to take away, but if you have put them into a joint account, they could be considered joint property. Also, if you have been married for more than ten years, they may be considered joint property.
2.  Make a list of your assets, including mutual funds, bonds, stocks, retirement accounts (401K or 403b), bank accounts, frequent flyer points, time shares.
3.  Consider making copies of important family photos (believe some couple do fight over photos and sometimes there is no resolution to it)
4.  Do not leave your primary residence before you talk to an expert such as an attorney, unless there is a danger to your

life. You may be ready to end the marriage, but your finances may not be ready.

5. If you are on your spouse's health insurance, see your doctor and ask her/him to do all the necessary laboratory or images before the divorce is final. Ask your spouse to carry the children on her/his insurance if possible. Get your own individual Health insurance.

6. Fix your car

7. You will have to decide who gets the house, who can afford to live there or you both leave the house and sell the house.

8. If the assets that you have are not easily tapped, make sure you have enough cash flow for living expenses for you and your children (if any).

9. Do not clean joint bank accounts, defer compensations or bonuses from your job because if the court investigates and finds out you will not look good in front of the judge. You can open a new account under your name only and you have subscribed to direct deposit of your salary, make sure you contact your employer to stop any direct deposits into the joint account.

10. If you have joint debt, each person is liable for the full amount until the balance is paid. The same is true for taxes. So, do contact the Internal Revenue Service (IRS) to inquire about outstanding taxes that have not been paid. The same is true for any capital gain taxes. If one of you has made money that involves capital gains taxes, you are both liable for it.

11. Certain debt that one of you brought into the marriage such as student loans travels with that person

12. Freeze all your credit reports

13. Do you have to pay alimony. Alimony is the monthly payment you make to your ex- in order for him or her to maintain the same standard of living that she/he has enjoyed during the marriage. This varies from state to state and is often at the discretion of the judge and what the two of you agree on.

Alimony is taxable to the receiver and tax-deductible to the payer. Child support is not

14. Each state has formulas for child support that is based on the percentage of parents' income and the number of children you have together. But the formula is standard and is published at the State Government's website. These formulas are modified periodically, but the child support amount can be changed only by a court order (One parent my request modification of the monthly child support amount by filing "a motion" with the court)

15. In most states, a custodial parent cannot cut back visitations for the other parents if child support has not been paid.

16. Change the beneficiaries for your retirement accounts, bank accounts, and other accounts. Do this before the divorce is final. If you don't your ex- will the beneficiary in case of your death. If consent must be signed from your spouse, secure it before the divorce is final.

17. Name Change: If you would like to change your name, follow the normal procedures in your state.

18. And finally, if you have been married for more than 10 years, your ex- can receive social security benefits, when he/she reaches the qualification age even if you are now remarried, provided that his/her income from social security at the retirement age is less than what she/he would get based on her/his employment history or he/she does qualify for social security benefits.

## Ways to create income during retirement

During earlier years you were investing for growth and the objectives were to grow your nest egg as much as possible so that you can maintain your standard of living and live comfortably during retirement. Once you retire however, you may have to convert that nest egg into a predictable and hopefully reliable source of income. This process may be more challenging than investing for growth where the rate of return may vary from period to period or even from year to year. For examples, during periods of time where the interest rates are very low (such as the period around 2011-2012) it will be impossible to have any significant returns on your nest egg because bond yields and interest rates on certificate of deposits may be below inflation rate and close to zero. During these periods your purchasing power may be diminished significantly. During these periods you will need to seek strategies other than investing in bonds and CD in order to have a consistent income that will help maintain your standards of living.

Here are some strategies that a retired person may use in order to have in income during retirement:

Annuities: (also read about annuities in other sections of this book):

*What are annuities?*

Certain types of Life Insurance policies which generate monthly payments in exchange for an upfront deposit of cash are called annuities.

*Are there different types of annuities?*

Yes, Fixed and variable types

*The fixed version type of annuity:*

Offers guaranteed payments over a certain period of time e.g. 20 years or for as long as you are alive (for life). This is in exchange for an upfront deposit of cash. The length of payment will depend on how much you are willing to pay. Because you have to commit a large sum of cash up front, the biggest risk with annuities is that you lose the liquidity power. You no longer have the cash in case you face a financial emergency or you would like to invest in other vehicles. You give your money a giant insurance company and they pay you certain amount monthly for a certain period of time or for life. Also, it is worth keeping in mind that once you commit the cash and give it away to the insurance company, you will never get that capital back even if you die shortly after you purchase the annuity. You spouse will not be able to get the capital back unless you purchase it jointly with survivor benefits. The other issue with annuity is that because the return (monthly or annually) is fixed, your purchasing power may diminish over time if inflation rises. Also, fixed income annuity can be costly and often require an investment in the six figure range if you would like to secure a monthly income large enough to be a significant supplement to your monthly expenses. However, fixed income annuity does exactly what you need it to do: it creates a pool of money that will last as long as you live. So, if you are healthy and you live long enough it has some advantages of secure income for the rest of your life.

Inflation adjusted rider: Some insurance companies offer this option but you will have to pay extra for it. Experts suggest that it is well the higher price because it give some insurance that inflation will not eat into your monthly or annual income should inflation get out of control during certain periods of time such as the early 1980s in the USA.

*Variable annuities:*

Variable annuities allow a person who retired to choose a rate of return by investing the annuity by selecting accounts that invest mainly in mutual funds. Payments can begin immediately but often delayed for a certain period of time. The value of your payment is not guaranteed. Your payment will depend on how well your investment perform over time. However, these products do provide death benefits (unlike the fixed annuity, see above). If you die, the beneficiaries that you select are guaranteed to receive an amount of money equal to at least what you have invested.

## Reverse Mortgages (Home equity conversion mortgage)

If you own a home and you have paid off your mortgage and you are at least 62 years of age you may qualify for the so called reverse mortgage. In this process you covert a portion of the equity you have in the house into cash and you receive a monthly payment. Usually, the total amount that you can withdraw over time in limited to ≤ 50% of the equity that you have in the house. There are no income restrictions and therefore, even if you still practice as a physician and have significant income you can still apply for a reverse mortgage. More importantly, the income that you receive (usually from a lender) is not taxable. The income also does NOT affect your social security income or your Medicare benefits. With reverse mortgage, you DO NOT have to repay the money that you receive as long as you continue to live in the house as your primary resident. However, if and when the surviving borrower dies or if the house if sold or is no longer used as the primary resident the money must be paid back. If you have a lot of cash tied in a house and you need cash this may be an option for you so that you can meet you daily living expenses obligations. Reverse mortgage is offered by private lenders as well as the federal government. They offer a variety of products that vary in their method of payments. For instance you could receive a large one-time lump sum of cash or you may select to get paid monthly over time.

*Beware of fees!*

Some of the issues with reverse mortgage are the fees and the expenses associated with the application process and which may be buried into the mortgage. Some lenders charge a mortgage origination fee and may also charge for insurance. So, shop around for the products that are associated with least expensive fees. The fees can range from $ 3000 to $ 5000.00 on a $ 100,000.00 reverse mortgage. So, you are talking about a 5% fee here, but it could be as high as 15% if you don't shop around.

## How about stocks that pay dividend?

Blue-chip stocks that pay a consistent dividend (also read the section on stock market) can create predictable cash flow. Historically, these assets have been less volatile that the broader stock market, but they also offer a smaller return. There are handful of the so-called "blue chip" picks that have consistently increased their dividend over time. Most of the these stocks are part of the Dow 30 stocks and include the stock of the following companies:

Abbott Laboratories symbol ABT
Coca cola (KO)
Johnson and Johnson (JNJ)
McDonalds (MCD)
Proctor and gamble (PG)
International Business Machine (IBM)

If you do not wish to invest in individual stocks, you can consider certain funds with good dividends such as the Vanguard dividend growth fund (VDIGX). This fund has produced a consistent average return of 3.1 over the past 5 years despite the turmoil in the world and US economies and the turmoil in the stock markets. Depending on your situation and your risk tolerance, some experts suggest that you may allocate as much as 50% of your equity exposure to the stocks of quality companies who have solid balance sheets, pay a good dividend and who have a track record of increasing their dividend over time.

## Would you like to get TIPs?

Treasury inflation protected securities or TIPs

These are still popular among retirees who are seeking a safe and consistent income despite the very low yields in recent years due to the prevailing low interest rate environment. TIPs are exempt from State and local taxes and they are designed to keep pace with inflation. This is critical because inflation reduces the purchasing of physicians who have their major source of income coming from a fixed income. For example a portfolio that is worth $ 100,000.00 today may be worth only $ 65,000.00 25 years from now if the inflation rises at an steady rate of 3% per year. Experts recommend that you should have a portion of your retirement portfolio in TIPs somewhere in the neighborhood of 20-30% and TIPs are best held in tax-sheltered account so that you can lower your tax burden. You can invest in mutual funds or in exchange funds (ETFs) that mirror TIPs. Examples of mutual funds are the Vanguard Inflation protected securities fund (VIPSX) or the Harbor Real return fund (HARRX). IShares Barclays TIPS bond (TIP) is an example of an exchange traded fund that mirrors TIPs. You may purchase any of these funds or ETF through your stock broker.

## *What are the best places to retire as a physician?*

That will depend on your priorities. You need to set some criteria for your place of retirement and make a plan spans that over several years before you make a final decision about your place of retirement. Are expenses important to you? Are taxes important to you? Or you have saved enough money and the expenses are not as important to you and you just want to live in a nice place regardless of expenses and taxes. Sometimes, the best way to find out about your future place of retirement is to actually visit the place and spend some time in the local to become familiar with place and get a feel for it to see if it actually suites you, your significant other and your goals for your life after your retire. Obviously, the climate is very important. If you are not a winter sport enthusiast, a place such as Hanover, New Hampshire may not be the place for you to retire. If you have children and they already have or are planning to have children and you would like to see your grandchildren often, you may have to compromise and live in a state with the grandkids close by.

For most of us expenses and taxes are important and we would rather not spend excess money on paying various types of taxes during retirement.

The federal taxes will be the same regardless of which local you reside during your retirement, however some states have exemptions for income from social security and government and private pension funds as well as private retirement accounts up to a certain limit each year. Since most of your income during retirement will be coming from one of these sources, it is prudent to investigate which states and local are more tax-friendly. Property taxes can be a bigger concern depending on where you live because it can fluctuate considerably from state to state and from city to city within the same state. And finally, remember that local sales taxes will take a bite out of your income every time you purchase something.

According to Kiplinger magazine (October 2010 issue), there are 35 states that do not tax social security income. Here is a list of the 15 states (presented at random) which DO TAX social security income and you may want to avoid them, unless you don't mind paying extra taxes:

1. Montana
2. North Dakota
3. Delaware
4. Minnesota

5. Iowa
6. Nebraska
7. Kansas
8. Colorado
9. Utah
10. Kentucky
11. New Mexico
12. Virginia
13. Connecticut
14. Rhode Island
15. Vermont

Most Pension-friendly states:

1. Alaska
2. New York
3. Pennsylvania
4. Massachusetts
5. Vermont
6. Michigan
7. Illinois
8. Tennessee
9. Alabama
10. Mississippi
11. Louisiana
12. Texas
13. Florida
14. Kansan
15. South Dakota
16. Wyoming
17. Nevada
18. Washington

Least pension-friendly states are:

1. California
2. Nebraska
3. Rhode Island
4. Connecticut
5. Vermont

Property taxes may be the highest dollar amount you have to pay a retired physician. What is worse about it is that the amount is fixed and is not progressive unlike other taxes. You may not have an income, but still you will have to pay property taxes for the full value of your home. The above states are considering most friendly when it comes to real estate taxes.

Top states with the lowest real estate taxes are:

1. Arizona
2. Louisiana
3. New Mexico
4. West Virginia
5. Alabama

And here states with the highest real estate taxes:

1. California
2. New York
3. New Jersey
4. Connecticut
5. Illinois

Remember that every time you decide to buy something, sales taxes will take a big bite out of your wallet; here are the top states with the lowest sales taxes:

1. Virginia
2. Kentucky
3. Wisconsin
4. Hawaii
5. Wyoming

And here are the states with the highest sales taxes:

1. California
2. Rhode Island
3. Indiana
4. Mississippi
5. New Jersey

And even better, here is a list of states which have NO SALES taxes:

1. Delaware
2. Vermont
3. Alaska
4. Oregon
5. Montana

If you decide to work during your retirement to supplement your income, here is a list of states with no income taxes:

1. Alaska
2. South Dakota
3. New Hampshire
4. Florida
5. Texas
6. Washington
7. Nevada
8. Tennessee
9. Wyoming

Here are some examples of states when it comes to how you will be treated as a retiree:

**New York:** The state of New York does not tax social security income. It also does not tax income from other sources such the military, New York state or local cities' pensions as well as some other civil services pension income. Private pension income is exempt from state taxes up to $ 20,000.00 per year for individuals who are 59.5 or older. The sales tax is 4%, but there are additional local sales taxes that could be as high as 5%. Food and prescriptions are exempt from taxes. The state law allows the local municipalities to grant senior citizens a reduction in property taxes as deemed appropriate. There is no inheritance tax, however estates valued at more than one million dollar must file a tax-return.

**Michigan:** Michigan does not tax social security income, nor it does military, federal and state pension funds income. Private pension funds are exempt up to $45,000.00 (as of 2010) for individuals and up to $ 90,000.00 for married couples if they are filing jointly. The state has a flat income tax rate of about 4% and the sales tax is set at 6% statewide. Food and prescription drugs are exempt from sales taxes. Properties in Michigan are assessed at 50% of their cash value and the millage (approximately x amounts of dollars for every $ 1000.00 of the assessed value) varies from one municipality to another. At the high end are those municipalities that have a millage of 45 i.e. you pay $ 45.00 for each $ 1000.00 of the assessed value of the house. So, if live in a good neighborhood in Michigan and own a property that you purchased for $ 500,000.00, the assessed value for the house would be $ 250,000.00 and your property taxes would be (250 X 45 = $ 11,250.00 annually). In some municipalities, seniors may be exempt from the portion of the property taxes that goes towards the local school taxes. There is no inheritance tax in Michigan.

**California:** you probably believe that California is one of the most desirable places to live. That may be true for some parts of California. However, people who live in California pay one of the highest taxes in the state of the union. Social security income is exempt from taxes, however all other types of pension income are taxed at a rate close to 11%. Sales tax is around 8%, but the local taxes can push the sales tax north of 10%, but luckily food and prescription drugs are exempt from taxes. Property taxes are based on the 100% of the assessed value of the house, but this tax is capped at 1% of the cash value of the house. So, if you buy a property for $ 500,000.00 you property taxes will be capped at : 500,000X 0.01= $ 5000.00 per year (compare this calculation to that of a house in a really nice neighborhood in Michigan!).

Like we discussed before, there are factors, other than economics that some people may consider when it comes to a place to retire in as a physician. The year-around climate, public services, proximity to your children or grandchildren, family and friends, safety, and the atmosphere in the city that you live in. Do you like to live in a metropolitan city during your retirement, a college town, a suburb or the country side? Do you like to be close to the ocean. Luckily in the US we have one ocean to the east of us (the Atlantic ocean) and one to the west of us (the Pacific ocean). Here is a list of cities listed by money Magazine in September 2010 as the places to retire.

**College towns:**

If you like college towns, here are few cities that have been rated as one of the best places to live by Money Magazine:

*Ann Arbor, Michigan:*

Ann Arbor is the home town for the University of Michigan and the University of Michigan Medical Center with a population of a little bit over 100,000 of which 25% are over the age of 50. Ann Arbor has the highest doctor to patient ratio in the nation and the University of Michigan is considered in the top medical centers in the nation. Michigan does not tax social security income, nor it does military, federal and state pension funds income. Private pension funds are exempt up to $45,000.00 (as of 2010) for individuals and up to $ 90,000.00 for married couples if they are filing jointly. The state has a flat income tax rate of about 4% and the sales tax is set at 6% statewide. There are plenty of functions for different seasons of the years ranging from theatres, to festivals, art shows and competitive college sports that the University of Michigan participates. Winters are long and harsh, if you are not used to living in a cold environment, but spring in nice, summer is beautiful and the fall is very colorful. The city is very diverse and packed with highly educated individuals and families. The University offers varieties of courses for seniors and there are plenty of continuous medical education courses that will help you meet the requirement for your medical license.

## Durham, North Carolina

Durham is where Duke University is located. A college town with a population of slightly over 200,000, of which 25% are over 50 years of age. The state of North Carolina does not tax social security income, but as you can see from reading the previous pages it is not one the top states that is considered tax-friendly and does have a state income tax of 7.75% and the rest of taxes are in the middle of the road category. The climate is moderate all year around with no extremes of temperatures. The median home price in Durham is in the neighborhood of 160,000.00. There are plenty of opportunities in the city for attending concerts, interesting restaurants, and may golf courses on the outskirt of the city. There is a large seniors learning center which has a large number of members. Duke University Medical Center is one of the best in the nation. If you like the college town atmosphere, this is a nice place to live in.

*Hanover, New Hampshire*

Is a very small college town with a population under 10,000.00 and is the home for Dartmouth College. New Hampshire does have income tax or sales tax and it does not tax retirement plan income, however income for interests and dividends are applicable for any income in excess of $ 2400.00 per individual and $4800.00 for couples. Seniors 65 years of age and older may receive exemptions for the first $ 1200.00. The climate is very harsh in the winter with significant amounts of snow falling each and every year. Therefore, it you are a winter-sports enthusiast, this place is probably not for you. Housing are expensive with a median price of a house in excess of $400,000.00, but if you are willing live outside the city by about 20 minutes, you may be able to find more affordable houses. Dartmouth college has a senior learning program that has been in existence for several decades.

*Austin, Texas*

Austin is the capital of the great state of Texas with a population of about 800,000. It is not a small college town, but is the home to the University of Texas. 22% of population are over 50 years of age. The city has a lot to offer ranging from southern hospitality at the myriad of restaurants in the city to art and music. Being in the southern part of the US, the climate is moderate year around and people who have lived in Austin say that you can walk around with a t-shirt all year round. However, don't expect to see the four distinct seasons that you would see in Ann Arbor, Michigan. There is a center for performing arts in the city and the Austin International Folk Dancers has been around for over 50 years and you can learn cultural dance at that center. The University of Texas also offers the "Road Scholar" travel educational odyssey for retirees. You can also, attend lectures and other continuous medical education seminars at the nearby medical centers. Texas is considered a tax-friendly state, there is no state income tax, and does not tax social security income or income from other pensions.

**The Kentucky Derby:**

*Lexington, KY*

Lexington, KY. With a population of close to 300,000 people (1/3 of them are over 50) this University town is famous for Kentucky's famed horse race; the Kentucky Derby in Churchill Downs, which is only 90 minutes away from the center of this city. The city also offers many options for retirees such as restaurants, a Farmers market and the Kentucky Theatre. Since 1964, The University of Kentucky has offered locals 65 and older free access to University classes that have open space. The state of Kentucky does tax social security, has a 6% income tax, is not considered pension-friendly, but the has one the lowest sales taxes.

**Warm and dry:**

*Tucson, AZ*

Is a city of the southwestern part of the US with a population of close to half a million people, 28% of them are over 50 years of age. Tucson is the home of the University of Arizona. Most people have the impression that Tucson, AZ is a dessert with limited greenery and it is hot a dry most the year. What most people do not know is that Tucson is surrounded by mountains from all four directions! You can even go skiing at one of these mountains; Mount Lemmon. The city has enough world-class golf courses designed by World leader s in golf such as Jack Nicklaus, if you are an avid golfer. The University of Arizona at Tucson offers courses on a variety of subjects. The city is rich with historical places for you and your spouse to explore and restaurants which offer some of the best southwestern cuisines. Arizona is not one the states that is considered pension-friendly, does tax social security (as of 2010), has an income tax of approximately 4.5%, but has one of the lowest real estate taxes.

## How about a Cow-Boy Town?

*Prescott, AZ*

Prescott is located approximately 100 miles north of Phoenix with a population of around 40,000, of which 50% are over the age of 50. That tells you that this city is a retiree destination. The city has the older Rodeo and several hundred buildings are registered on the national register of historic houses. Even though Prescott is in the desserts of Arizona, the city is located at a 5000 feet elevation, which gives the residents the luxury of experiencing 4 distinct seasons. Prescott has a very large national forest, miles and miles of trails, several quality golf courses and offers a number of festivals annually including outdoor concerts, film festivals, and craft shows.

## The Pacific Northwest:

*Bellingham, WA*

With a population of around 80,000 (30% over 50 years of age) located between Vancouver (Canada) and Seattle, Washington (that is the state of Washington). There is a harbor near downtown and boats take to you to the nearby islands on a regular basis. Even though it is located in the northwest, climate is moderate with the average summer temperature in the mid-70s F and the average winter temperatures of mid 30s F. it does rain often though! Washington State does not tax social security and does not have income tax, which is attractive to retirees.

## The heartland:

*Boise, ID*

Boise, Idaho, has a population of around 200,000, with approximately 1/3 of them being over 50 years of age. The city is the home to Boise State University, which offer multiple programs for individuals over the age 50 including life-long learning classes, field trips and much more. The city also has an art theater, philharmonic orchestra and ballet dancing. If you like rugged terrain, this city offers plenty of opportunity for hiking. The state of Idaho does not tax social security, but is not on the list as a tax-friendly state and has an income tax rate of close to 7%.

*Lincoln, NE*

Lincoln, Nebraska has a population of around 250,000 people (28% over the age of 50 years). This is a city which is known for its parks. In fact there is at least one park within half an hour from your residence no matter which part of the city you live in. The University of Nebraska in Lincoln offers varieties of courses to seniors ranging from music to Spanish and even spoken Chinese language. The state of Nebraska does tax social security income and has a state income tax close to 7%.

**The sunshine state:**

*St. Petersburg, Clearwater beach, FL*

This area has a population in the vicinity of 250,000 people of which at least 36% are over 50 years of age. Activities that you can do in this area include theaters, which feature broadways shows, museums including the famous Dali museum for arts and other ones which features works of Famous artists such as Monet. There are abundant beaches and restaurants with varieties of cuisines that you and your family can enjoy and the city is located within one hour from Disney World. The nearby Colleges and Universities offer courses for seniors, where you may be allowed to audit or even teach students if you have the proper qualifications. Florida is considered a pension-friendly state, does not tax social security and has no income tax.

Other cities to consider for retirement include:

Ames, IA
Ashland, OR
Asheville, NC
Athens, GA
Beaufort, SC
Brunswick, ME
Davis, CA
Duluth, MN
Fayetteville, AR
Fort Collins, CO
Huntsville, AL
Northampton, MA
St. Luis Obispo, CA
Williamsburg, VA

## Retiring in a foreign country

Retiring in a country other than the US was a foreign concept to most physicians until recently. This concept is gaining popularity partly due to the changes in the world economy and partly due the advent and expansion of the use of the internet worldwide.

The economy of the world in changing with improved standards of living around the world. The internet is also providing the much needed connectivity to families and friends so that people can be in touch with family members and friends on a daily basis using programs such the Skype or other video conferencing technologies. The availability of the internet is also making it possible for people to access important issues in life such as bank accounts and retirement accounts, 24 hours a day, seven days a week.

While saving money has always been important to retirees, the recession and the financial crises of 2008 led to a significant drop in the total value of retirement accounts for many people who were either in retirement or were anticipating retiring. This combined with rising taxes and health-care costs in the US have made it a necessity for many people to seek alternative parts of the world as a retirement refuge. If you find the right place for you, you may be able to live comfortably on half the budget that you may need to maintain the same standard of living in the US. Some of the countries where this is possible include Ecuador, Belize, Panama and Costa Rica. Countries located in central American and south America. In some parts of these countries, the quality of life is good, the pollution is less and the quality of health care is acceptable.

There are conferences held annually on this topic. One such an example is "International Living". It has seen a significant jump in attendance for their annual seminar on retiring outside the U.S., where they bring in experts to answer questions on everything from financial planning and real estate to foreign currencies, expat taxes and legal issues. A few years ago, they used to get about 150 to 175 people. That more than doubled to 400 last year and this year, they're looking for a venue that can hold 500.

One of the important issues for people who are contemplating retirement in a foreign country is the availability of and the quality of health care. It is surprising to hear from many people who have already lived in some of these countries for many years in retirement that the medical care in some of these countries is available, affordable, and often just as good as the health care in other countries including the US. One of the downside to receiving health care outside the US, is that Medicare DOES NOT cover the care rendered outside the US. Some retirees have gotten around this by flying back to the US on "Medicare runs". The American Medical Association (AMA) also offers to physicians a type of insurance that is for catastrophic medical coverage. Part of the coverage is to fly you back to the US if you get ill abroad. You inquire more about this type of insurance by calling the AMA insurance agency.

Americans usually hear about other countries when there the media reports on ban news, but rarely hear about other countries in other contexts. It is very interesting however, to hear from some Americans who live abroad on how safe some places are including cities in countries such as Mexico. Take for instance the city of Merida, 4 hours west of Cancun, Mexico. According to testimonies from retired Americans who have live there for years, you hardly hear of any crimes in that city and the cost of living is very reasonable.

Some of the cities in central and Latin America may even be economically more stable with it comes to issues such as Real Estate. For instance home prizes did not drop as much as in the US during the economic and housing collapse of 2008. Prizes are more reasonable too. Few years ago (as of 2010) a developer built condos for rent and sale in the city of Cotachi in Ecuador, a nice city close to the Andes mountains for expectorates and retires. You could rent a condo for under $ 200.00 per month or buy one for under $ 60,000.00. You could have a nice meal at a good restaurant in one of these cities for under $ 5.00. Because the cost living is considerably less, inflation is less of a problem. If your condo rent is $ 1500.00 and the rent goes up by 10% a year over 5 years, you could end up paying $ 2000.00 per month 5 years from now, however, in one of these countries, if your monthly rent is $ 200.00 and the rent increases by 10% a year over 5 years, your monthly rent may still be under $350.00, which is still manageable. The same thing would apply to cost of food.

Planning to retire in Europe on the other hand may not be as attractive as central and Latin America because of the depreciation of the US against the Euro. However, if you search for places that are under the radar and you are willing to experience a different life style, you may still be able to find places that are affordable to spend your retirement in (continue reading..).

It's important to remember that living in a foreign country is very different than living in the US or visiting as a tourist. When you go to one of these countries as a tourist, you are likely to have a different experience compared to living in that country for an extended period of time. You have to embrace the experiences of living in another country and the changes that come with it, both the pros and the cons. For example, you may not be able to find your favorite brand of cheese, drink, liquor that you enjoy, your favorite restaurant that you have gotten accustomed. The best way to find out about retiring in a foreign country is to go to that country for several months. Rent a place. See what it's like to get around. Go to the "supermarket" and deal paying for your own utilities. See how easy it is to hook up an internet or a phone line. Explore if the language barrier or the new culture are going to be a problem for you. And just see if this is what you want your life to be like. You may also consider talking to other Americans who have been living in the area for many years. The bottom line is that you need to do your homework and plan for such an adventure over a period of few years instead of jumping in the ocean without adequate knowledge of what it is like to live in a foreign country.

In random order, here are some places to retire outside the US as reported by the AARP magazine, which it considers them "under the radar".

*Central Velley, Cost Rica:*
Costa Rica is Located between Nicaragua (to the north) and Panama (to the south) in Central America. Estimates indicate that there are approximately 50,000 Americans live in this Central American country. One of the main advantages of Costa Rica is the better quality of its health care, which sets it apart from some of the other countries. Because the country DOES NOT have a military, a significant portion of the country's Gross Domestic Product (GDP) is spent on health care. The central Valley area is more laid back considering that it

is further away from the major tourist cities, but it is still within a reasonable distance from major cities considering that Cost Rica is a relatively small country. Real Estate is not as cheap as it was several years ago, but it is still affordable for a retiring physician.

*Languedoc-Roussillon, France:*
This region is located on the Mediterranean Sea with hilltop village that overlook the sea. It is close to major cities for a weekend trip to any one of them, including Paris. The climate is very mild most of the year and the region is rich with medieval culture and castles. The area is a real melting pot with people from the US, the United Kingdom, the Netherlands and Germany. It is true that it would be very expensive in a large city in France such as Paris, but in this city the standard of living is affordable. France is considered to have one of the best health care systems in the world and that is important during retirement.

*La Marche, Italy:*
This charming city is located in the east cost of Italy on the Adriatic sea. It has a combination of mountains and beaches. Because Italy is such a narrow country, this city is still close to major cities such Milan, Florence, and Venice. You can rent a place for around $ 750.00 a month, but the rent goes higher and may reach $ 1500.00 a month as you get closer to the beach. The city has many fantastic restaurants, vineyards, and beautiful beaches. *La marche,* has one of the best fish dishes in Italy.

*Buenos Aires, Argentina:*
Buenos Aires is the capital of Argentina, a country in South America with a population of about 36 million, half of whom live in the province of Buenos Aires, where the capital is located. 95% of the population are white and of Italian or Spanish descend. Spanish is the official language of Argentina. The country went through an economic crisis in early 2000, but since then the economy has improved and as a

result the country has become more affordable for retirees and others who would like to live in a city that has a rich culture with plenty of museums, beautiful cathedrals and opera houses. Buenos Aires is also known to be the home the tango. The city is very scenic and is not very far from the beaches in the neighboring country, Uruguay. You can rent an apartment for under $ 800.00 per month or buy a condo or an apartment condo in a community known for its expatriates for under $ 300,000.00.

*Corozal, Belize:*
Belize is a relatively small country located in Central America with a population a little bit over 300,000.00 people. This is the most sparsely populated country in Central America. Most of the population lives in Belize city, the major business city and the country's port city. Corozal, is a city in Belize with a population of close to 10,000.00 people. One of the most convenient features of Belize is that English is the official language and most people speak English, which makes communication easy and no language barriers here. It is very easy to get residency status and the country offers significant benefits to retirees. The country has lots of white-sand beaches with opportunities for outdoor swimming, boating, biking at a relatively low cost. Real Estate is also very affordable. You could purchase a water view condo for a very reasonable prize.

*Granada, Nicaragua:*
Located in Central America, Nicaragua is a lot like its neighboring country Costa Rica with beautiful beaches, rainforest, and volcanoes. It is very affordable to live here and the AARP reports that there close to 10,000 Americans living in Nicaragua.

*Cascais, Portugal:*
Portugal is a country in Europe located northwest of Spain and the only country it is attached to. The rest of the country is bordered by

the Atlantic Ocean. The official language is Portuguese. Cascais, is a nice laid-back city only 15 miles from the capital, Lisbon. The country is part of the European union and therefore, deal with the Euro, but it is a very affordable place to live and people are very friendly. Cascais is a coastal town located on the Atlantic Ocean and therefore it has plenty of beaches and golf courses. You could buy a nice small house for under $ 250,000.00.

Other places to consider for retirement outside the US, include:

Portaviarda, Mexico
Boquete, Panama
Costa del Sol, Spain
Panama city, Panama (Donald Trump is building condos there)
Chiang Mai, Thailand
Sibu, Malaysa

## Disclaimer

The information contained in this book is considered general information related to the field of medicine as a profession and the financial and emotional ramifications of becoming a physician.

The information contained in this book is NOT intended to constitute legal or medical advice. The information contained in this book was compiled from sources deemed accurate at the time of writing of this book, with the passage of time neither the authors, nor the publishers guarantee its accuracy, or the accuracy of information in other sites accessible through links herein. The authors and the publishers makes no representations or warranties, either express or implied, as to the accuracy of any information in this book and neither the author not the publisher assume responsibility for any errors or omissions contained therein. No one shall be entitled to claim detrimental reliance on any views or information, whether provided by or accessed through this book or to claim any duty on our part to update the information in this book to protect the interests of those reading the book. In no event shall the authors or the publishers be liable to a reader of this book who has made decisions (financial or otherwise) or has taken actions based on reliance on information contained in this book. The reader should consult appropriate experts in their respective fields before making any decision with regard to a career or a financial or other decision.

# Selected References

1. Your Doctor's Education" in JAMA, Sept. 6, 2000.
2. Carris J. Analyze This. The Hospitalist. 2010; 14(5): 1, 14-15
3. Physicians owned practices fade. Wall Street Journal, Nov 8th, 2010.
4. Chang WW. Split Personality. The hospitalist 2010;14(11):1,4-6.
5. Journal of the American Medical Association, September 2010 issue.
6. www.bankrate.com accessed December 23, 2010.
7. Pewresearch.org accessed November 2009
8. www.ama-assn.org accessed November 2009, January 2010, and July 2010
9. www.kff.org accessed October 2010
10. New Algorith guesses SSNs using date and place of birth. Ars Technica. July 2009.
11. Fisher R, Ury W. Getting to yes.
12. cms.gov/OfficeofLegislation/. Accessed March 31, 2011
13. Rochlin JM, Simon HK. Does fellowship pay? What is the long-term financial impact of a subspecialty training in pediatrics. Pediatrics 2011;127(2):254-260
14. www.taxpolicy.org accessed June 11 and July 13, 2011
15. Historical table 13 at "Corporation income tax returns: Balance sheet, income statement, and tax items for income years. Expanded version. Tax years 1990-2008. http://www.irs.gov/taxstats/article/0,,id=175846,00.html. Accessed august 12, 2011.
16. CNBC.com; accessed multiple times.
17. The Moment of Truth. Report of the National Commission on Fiscal Responsibility and Reform. Section 3.3.5 reduce excess payments to hospitals and medical education. December 2010. Available at: http://www.fiscalcommission.gov

18. The budget control act of 2011. Public Law 112-25 of the 112th United States Congress, Title 4. The joint Select Committee on Deficit Reduction. Available at: http://www.gpo.gov

19. Graduate medical education financing: Focusing on educational priorities. Medicare Payment Advisory Commission Report on Congress: Aligning Incentives. Chapter 4. June, 2010. Washington, DC. Available at: http://www.medpac.gov.

20. Iglehart, J. The Uncertain Future of Medicare and Graduate Medical Education. NEJM 2011. 365(14), 1340–1345.

21. www.pewresearch.org accessed multiple times in 2008-2013

22. www.aarp.org accessed multiple times in 2012

23. www.ama.org

24. John K. Iglehart. N Engl J of Med 2011; 365:1340

25. www.ssa.gov accessed multiple times between 2011-14

26. Fitzgerald JEF, Caesar B, (2012). "The European working time directive: A practical review for surgical trainees". *International Journal of Surgery* **10** (8): 399–403.

27. Robinson, S. (August 14, 2004). "Antitrust Lawsuit Over Medical Residency System Is Dismissed". *New York Times*.

28. Wilkey, Robert N. (April 2011). "The Non-Negotiable Employment Contract: Diagnosing the Employment Rights of Medical Residents". *Creighton Law Review* 44: 705.

29. Bates DW, Czeisler CA (2004). "Effect of reducing interns' work hours on serious medical errors in intensive care units". *N Engl J Med* **351** (18): 1838-44

30. Drazen JM (2004). "Awake and informed". *N Engl J Med* **351**(18): 1884.

31. New ACGME Standards for Resident Duty Become Effective July 2011 Article written by Laurie Barclay, October 14, 2010

32. Gupta, Sanjay (June 15, 2001). "AMA expected to take up resident work hours". *CNN*. Retrieved 28 August 2012.

33. Public Citizen. Retrieved 28 August 2012

34. Wilkey, Robert N (2003). "Federal Whistleblower Protection: A Means to Enforcing Maximum Hour Legislation for Medical Residents". *William Mitchell Law Review* 30 (1)

35. Lowe, MD, Merlin C (August 26, 2009). "Have Resident Work Hour Restrictions Compromised Training - a Pediatrician's Perspective". *Doctor's Lounge.* Retrieved 28 August 2012

36. Gottlieb, S. (1997). *USA Today* 126: 20–20

37. Croasdale, Myrle (Jan 30, 2006). "Innovative funding opens new residency slots". *American Medical News.* Retrieved 29 August 2012

38. Reinhardt (2002). *Health Affairs* 21 (5): 28–32

39. Nicholson and Song; Song, D (2001). "The incentive effects of the Medicare indirect medical education policy". *Journal of Health Economics* 20 (6): 909–933

40. West, C. P.; Shanafelt, T. D.; Kolars, J. C. "Quality of Life, Burnout, Educational Debt, and Medical Knowledge Among Internal Medicine Residents". *JAM 2011;*306 (9):

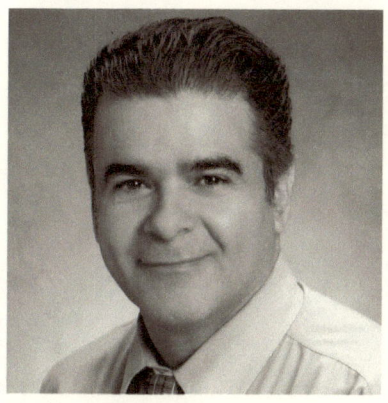

Rashed Hasan, MD, FAAP, is board certified in pediatrics and pediatric critical care. He has practiced in the United States for more than twenty years, and he has served on the academic faculty at Michigan State University, Harvard Medical School, and the University of Toledo. He is currently a professor of clinical pediatrics at the University of Toledo.

www.ingramcontent.com/pod-product-compliance
Lightning Source LLC
Chambersburg PA
CBHW031814170526
45157CB00001B/47